Terminal Illness

A Guide to Nursing Care

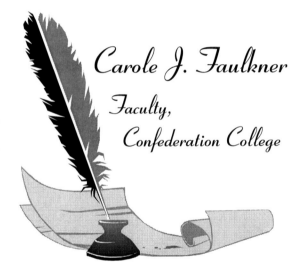

Terminal Illness

A Guide to Nursing Care

Charles Kemp, MSN, RN

Instructor, School of Nursing

Baylor University

Dallas, Texas

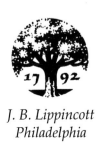

J. B. Lippincott
Philadelphia

Acquisitions Editor: Margaret Belcher
Sponsoring Editor: Kimberly Oaks
Production Manager: Janet Greenwood
Production Editor: Mary Kinsella
Production: Berliner, Inc.
Cover Design: Larry Pezzato
Printer/Binder: RR Donnelley & Sons Company, Crawfordsville

Photographs reproduced with permission of Deborah Hunter.

Kemp, Charles, 1944–
    Terminal illness: a guide to nursing care / Charles Kemp.
        p.   cm.
    Includes bibliographical references and index.
    ISBN 0-397-55123-1
    1. Terminal care.   2. Nursing.   I. Title.
    [DNLM. 1. Terminal Care.   2. Nursing Care.   WY 152 K32t 1995]
    RT87.T45K45   1995
    610.73′61—dc20
    DNLM/DLC
    for Library of Congress   94-16166
                                                          CIP

6 5 4 3 2 1

Any procedure or practice described in this book should be applied by the health care practitioner under appropriate supervision in accordance with professional standards of care used with regard to the unique circumstances that apply in each practice situation. Care has been taken to confirm the accuracy of information presented and to describe generally accepted practices. However, the authors, editors, and publisher cannot accept any responsibility for errors or omissions, or for any consequences from application of the information in this book, and they make no warranty, express or implied, with respect to the contents of the book.

Every effort has been made to ensure drug selections and dosages are in accordance with current recommendations and practice. Because of ongoing research, changes in government regulations, and the constant flow of information on drug therapy, reactions, and interactions, the reader is cautioned to check the package insert for each drug for the indications, dosages, warnings, and precautions, particularly if the drug is new or infrequently used.

To My Family
Leslie and David Kemp

Acknowledgments

This book would not exist without help and support from many people. I thank my teachers, Stephen Levine, Al Shapero, Dan Foster, Dorothy Pettigrew, John Reed, Elisabeth Kubler-Ross, and Steve Gaskin; the ones who helped me through the night, Robin Williamson, Mike Heron, Ron Hunter, Jerry Garcia, and the rest of the guys; the brave men of C Company, 1st Battalion, 26th Marine Regiment; General Chesty Puller; my companions on the journey, Tim Baker, Jim Jackson, Bill Finch, Chuck Maxey, David Overton, Becky Wilkerson, Ron Cowart, Paul Thai, Mom Than, Syl Benenson, Lynn Dorsey, Marion Anema, Jennifer Donovan, Ron Bowie, Lance Rasbridge, Thao Dam, Lek Keovilay, and Doug Puryear; Mark, Sabra, and Ed; my companions in hospice, Jimmie Boyd, Laura Neal-McCollum, Kathy Little, Bob Weisberg, Linda Wassenich, Gay Mallon-Frank, Joyce Overton, Debora Hunter, and all the rest (we really did it); Jan Viola and Jean Mitchell; my friends and colleagues at Baylor, especially Phyllis Karns, Mary Nowotny, Barbara Worth, Martha Sanford, Melanie McEwen, Eunice Warren, Beth Rodgers, Leslie Hussey, Alice Pappas, Linda Garner, Leonard Brown, and Ross Prater; my students; the book's editor, Michel DeMatteis, who helped make this a better book; Nancy Berliner, the good people at J.B. Lippincott, especially Margaret Belcher; and Jeff Wiseman (Jeff—Call Home!).

If I could sing only one song . . .

The Photographs

The photographs in this book were taken by Debora Hunter, Associate Professor of Art at Southern Methodist University. After being with her father as he died, Debora developed an interest in hospice care. Through her volunteer work with hospice patients, she worked to promote understanding of the human process of dying. These pictures are part of an extended documentary project entitled "Waiting: Portraits of the Terminally Ill." We are all deeply grateful for Debora's gift.

Preface

Great advances were made in the first several decades of contemporary care of patients with terminal illness. Brompton's cocktail, the stages of dying, and the hospice concept once were revolutionary. Now, Brompton's is obsolete, stages passé, and hospice programs are everywhere. Yet, the state of care of patients with terminal illness still has a long way to go: Despite advances in terminal and palliative care, pain and symptoms of terminal illness remain poorly managed in too many patients. In part because of inadequately managed symptoms, and for other reasons, many patients never have an opportunity to live as well as they might during their terminal illness. Denied peace and dignity, some are unable to work toward the reconciliations that so many seek.

Terminal Illness: A Guide to Nursing Care is a third-generation book in contemporary terminal care (following *On Death and Dying* and *Nursing Care of the Terminally Ill*) and is addressed directly to the practitioner and serious student of terminal care. As a practical tool, it concerns itself with patient and family needs and with how to facilitate meeting those needs. This book is based on experience, research, and field-tested theory. It is patient- and family-centered, and is oriented toward prevention.

In 17 years of work and/or teaching in hospice care, I have found that essentially all nurses and others interested in this field want to learn what to say and do when working with a person who is dying. Few have any abiding interest in learning theories and hypotheses of terminal illness, except as they apply to practice and application (antonyms of theory). Other books may present information *about* the care; this book is a tool for *doing* the care.

Conceptual Framework

There are three major organizing concepts to *Terminal Illness: A Guide to Nursing Care*.

First, effective care of persons who are terminally ill includes competent action in all areas of human needs: physiological, psychosocial, and spiritual. The book presents fundamental concepts, issues, problems, and interventions in each of these areas.

Second, while there is always individual variation, some terminal illness, such as cancer, are relatively predictable in their natural history. Knowing the natural history and attendant problems allows practitioners to anticipate what physiological problems may occur, and to act first to prevent them; or failing prevention, to recognize and treat problems early on and thus minimize their effects.

Third, superior care proceeds concurrently along two parallel tracks:

- competent action in all areas of human needs; and
- "watching," or being present, in spirit as well as in body, with the person who is dying (and/or their family).

Thus, in the first track, caring means aggressive action on the part of the nurse to manage problems and facilitate the patient and family's ability to manage problems. In what may appear paradoxical, caring in the second track means accepting suffering and frailty and, despite being unable to manage all problems or relieve all suffering, staying or "watching" with the patient and family. It is here, where it *seems* as though there is nothing more that can be done, that terminal care reaches for its highest and deepest goals. It is here, facing and enduring the presence of overwhelming suffering and fear, that we approach the fulfillment of an ancient and essential human function: the priestly function of accompanying another through suffering, and to the awesome finality of death.

Organization

The book is divided into five parts. Problems and interventions are detailed in all the chapters.

Part I, *Psychosocial Care and Issues,* presents terminal illness from the perspective of patient and family, and covers psychological and social issues, spiritual issues, major faiths, grief and bereavement care, and sociocultural issues. Chapters directed particularly to the nurse are on ethical issues and on stress and the health care provider.

Part II, *Pain Management,* is divided into three chapters. The first chapter discusses principles of pain management, the second covers classification and assessment of pain, and the final chapter is a comprehensive and detailed discussion of exactly how to manage the various pain syndromes.

Part III, *Physical Care: Problems and Interventions,* addresses the major problems, other than pain, of terminal illness. Problems are divided into chapters as follows: neurological, respiratory and cardiac, skin, oral, gastrointestinal, genitourinary, dehydration and fatigue, oncology emergencies and paraneoplastic syndromes, and imminent death.

Part IV, *Metastatic Spread: Implications for Patient Care,* presents a summary of the natural history and attendant problems of the 18 most common tumor sites that each cause more than 5,000 deaths annually in the United States. This section allows the practitioner to anticipate, and thus prevent or minimize, at least some of the problems and complications of advanced disease. It is divided into chapters on cancers of major organs, the female reproductive system, gastrointestinal, urinary tract, and blood/lymph and skin.

Part V, *Management of Other Terminal Illness*, covers diseases other than cancer that lend themselves to palliative care. These include AIDS (and opportunistic infections), degenerative neurological disorders, Alzheimer's and related disorders, and cardiovascular and chronic obstructive pulmonary diseases.

Contents

Terminal Illness

A Guide to Nursing Care

I PSYCHOSOCIAL CARE

DIMENSIONS AND ISSUES

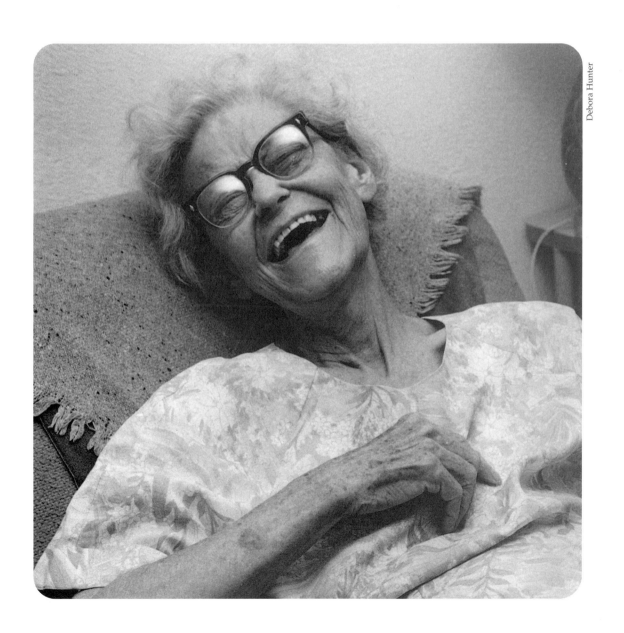

Introduction

The improvement of psychosocial care of patients with terminal illness has been a major advance in modern health care. From the 1940s–1960s, the era that marked a gradual decline in the incidence of dying as a family and community affair and before the advent of hospice care, the patient and family were too often made irrelevant to the purposes of modern curative medicine. As a consequence of exalting cure at all costs, immense suffering frequently resulted—often with no attendant extension of life span.

There is, however, some essential individual and social human quality that moves us toward attaining dignity and meaning in life. In terminal care, this quality was manifested in the 1960s, primarily through the efforts of the hospice movement; through the work of Edwin Shneidman, Avery Weisman, Elisabeth Kübler-Ross, and other well-known clinicians; and through the work of many unnamed and unknown nurses, physicians, and others. Along with symptom management, quality of life in terminal illness situations and dying with dignity became priorities of care.

This section addresses an array of psychosocial issues typical of the situations of people who are dying and of their families. Along with lengthy chapters on individual and family psychosocial needs and problems, there are also chapters on spiritual care, the major faiths, sociocultural issues, and grief and bereavement care. The section ends with chapters on ethical issues and on the stress associated with the situation of health care providers.

Although specific direction is provided on various situations and problems, there is no general information given on counseling: a complete discussion of counseling, or helping behaviors, is beyond the scope of this book. However, several broad points on psychosocial care are helpful to keep in mind when working with people who are dying:

- The first step in addressing psychosocial needs and problems of people who are dying is to manage distressing physical symptoms. Few people caught up in suffering from severe physical problems can muster the emotional strength to deal with psychosocial problems.
- The essence of helping, caring, or effective intervention in the nurse-patient relationship "is the engagement, the identification of the nurse with the patient" (Morse et al., 1992, p. 819). This "connected" engagement helps the nurse focus on the patient's response to illness, whether physical or emotional, and thus increases the likelihood of providing

the needed care. Staying completely focused on a person who is suffering and dying is terribly difficult. "The hardest state to be in is one in which you keep your heart open to the suffering . . .and simultaneously keep your discriminative wisdom. . . . It takes a good while to get the balance." (Ram Dass, 1978, p. 1).
- Trust is an essential component in all communications. The patient must trust the nurse to (1) always tell the truth, and (2) be competent. Trusting and being honest with oneself and the patient are central in the process of engagement.

The nurse's fundamental beliefs about humankind and caring have a profound influence on the quality of care provided and the response of the patient to the practitioner and the situation. While basic beliefs are infinite in number and variation, several are notable in having a positive effect on all concerned.

- Human beings have intrinsic worth. It is not necessary to believe that all humans are "good" or noble. There is reason to believe that many are not! However, if the practitioner operates from the perspective that people have at least the potential for worth (which may not always be apparent), then the relationship is more likely to be productive.
- The purpose of terminal care is to relieve suffering. This may seem obvious, but it bears explication that the practitioner intentionally and specifically seeks to relieve the physical, emotional, and spiritual suffering that often accompanies the process of dying. To understand the concept of relieving suffering is to achieve profound insight into the meaning and purpose of terminal care. Understanding this concept fosters the commitment to caring and to the patient that is the core of effective terminal care. It also brings hope to people who might otherwise feel a great sense of hopelessness.
- Relieving suffering requires a high level of competence and is an active, even aggressive endeavor. Effective terminal care is not a matter of passively letting people die or simply administering large amounts of analgesics. It requires finely honed assessment skills, in-depth knowledge of disease processes, and tenacity in patient advocacy.
- Terminal care is not always a successful endeavor. No matter what is done, most patients will suffer to some extent, and some will suffer terribly. Suffering may be physical, mental, and/or spiritual. It is imperative that the practitioner be able to stay gracefully in the presence of people who are suffering.
- It is worthwhile to help uncover, or help actualize, the worth, beauty— or whatever one calls—the positive potential of people. The time of dying is the last chance many people have to finally become who they really are, rather than who they pretend to be. Dying can be a time of reconciliation with God, self, and others. For many, achieving this reconciliation is not easy. It requires facing the absolute truth about the way life was lived in relation to what might have been. The practitioner

who sees intrinsic value in this process is the one most likely to play a meaningful part in reconciliation. Practitioners must also accept that some patients will never achieve reconciliation.

- There is always hope. An effective practitioner always has and always gives hope. The hope is not necessarily that the patient will not die (although many patients hold that hope to the very end), but rather that suffering will lessen, reconciliation be achieved, a goal met, meaning found, or any number of other highly likely possibilities. It should be added here that the hope of not dying should not be taken from one who clings to that particular hope.

- Patient, family, and practitioner share dynamic responsibility for what happens in the process of dying. The practitioner gives the patient and family the benefit of her or his knowledge and expertise so that patient and family are able to make informed decisions about what is happening and what will happen. By "dynamic responsibility," I mean the practitioner must be an expert willing to take control when necessary and give up control when possible. A practitioner who must always be in control will have difficulty providing terminal care. At the same time, a consistently effective practitioner will have a powerful sense of responsibility in giving the best possible care. If this sounds somewhat paradoxical, so be it; we are dealing with paradoxical beings at their most extreme moments of life.

- Working cooperatively with others is necessary. A host of providers can and should be involved in the care of a human being in the final days of life. These include the obvious (family, nurses, doctors, chaplains, volunteers, aides, and so on) and the perhaps not so obvious (neighbors, relatives, family minister, work colleagues, and others in the social sphere of the patient). This leads to a key point in providing care: many people, professionals and others, have no experience in providing effective care, and thus derive great benefit from help in knowing what to do. The expert practitioner, acting as a consultant or case manager plays an essential role in getting people organized. In terminal situations, people who are organized and who know what to do and when to do it, are generally able to find purpose and meaning in what they do. People who are disorganized, who do not know what to do or when to do it, generally feel a sense of inadequacy and frustration. Working cooperatively with others also includes getting help for oneself as a person.

- Living or working with uncertainty is acceptable. For the practitioner, the human need for understanding, order, and predictability must be set aside in terminal situations; even as the practitioner provides or creates as much understanding, order, and predictability for others as is possible in the situation.

While there are other beliefs or attitudes that positively influence the quality of care provided and the response of the patient to the practitioner and the situation, the above are basic to providing quality care.

References

Ram Dass. (1978, December). Introduction. *Hanuman Foundation Dying Project Newsletter*, 1.(Available from the Hanuman Foundation.)

Morse, J.M., Bottorff, J., Anderson, G., O'Brien, B., and Solberg, S. (1992). Beyond empathy: Expanding expressions of caring. *Journal of Advanced Nursing. 17*, 809–821.

Psychosocial Needs, Problems, and Interventions: The Individual

This falsity around him and within him did more than anything else to poison his last days.

(LEON TOLSTOY, THE DEATH OF IVAN ILYCH)

The process of dying creates unfamiliar psychosocial problems and brings old ones into focus. The complexity of these problems—new and old, large and small, individual and family—is overwhelming at times. This section presents common problems, processes, and interventions in terminal illness—all of which do not necessarily apply to every person and circumstance. They are offered here as a means of understanding and helping in complex situations.

Profile of the Dying

Caring for people who are dying is based, as much as possible, on appreciation and understanding of the experience of living with terminal illness. While each person goes through terminal illness in a different way, there are often many similarities in the experience and/or responses to it.

An important point of departure in viewing the experience of and response to terminal illness is the recognition that each person is different. A fundamental rule in effective care is to approach each person without preconceptions. At the same time, it is important to be aware of and responsive to cultural differences, gender and sexual orientation issues, problems common to various diagnoses—in short, any related circumstances or means through which sense can be made of confusing situations. So, while approaching each individual without preconceptions, the nurse is prepared for predictable patient/family responses.

One way to begin appreciating the person who is dying and his or her experience is to work toward understanding the "whole" person. Every person comes to their time of dying with unique life experiences; with strengths and weaknesses, with some psychosocial and spiritual issues resolved and some unresolved. Seeing and accepting all that a person brings to their

Charles Kemp: TERMINAL ILLNESS: A GUIDE TO NURSING CARE. © 1995 J. B. Lippincott.

last days honors the wholeness of the person. If each patient is seen and appreciated—both in their fullness and in their incompleteness—then the care given is based on the reality of that patient, and is thus more likely to succeed.

Appreciating the person also means appreciating who he or she is in the present moment. For many of us, facing death is the greatest challenge of our lives. Some of us meet that challenge with great courage and dignity; others meet it with less courage or less dignity. Nearly all of us meet it in the best way we can.

THE PROCESS OF TERMINAL ILLNESS

To understand and appreciate the person who is dying also implies understanding and appreciating their experience with illness. Some practitioners hold narrow views of particular patients; for example, as hospice patients, surgical patients, or chemotherapy patients. Such a view is incomplete. Having a terminal illness is often only the last stage in a long process beginning with struggle, temporary victories/remissions, setbacks, hope, and despair, and continuing with more struggle, changes in direction, more hope, more despair, and so on.

Typically, the process begins with an ominous symptom. That symptom, or symptoms—a persistent cough, bleeding, lump, or pain—brings fear and often denial. Eventually, the symptom cannot be ignored and help is sought. In the process of assessment, testing, and waiting for results there is hope, fear, anxiety, and denial. Receiving the diagnosis and discussing treatment and prognosis are overwhelming and confusing situations. Waves of hope and fear wash over the person, and many people sense that our common illusion of living indefinitely is shattered by reality. At a time like this, few people are capable of processing all they are hearing, and afterwards they will often ask: "What exactly is wrong with me, and what does it mean to me?" (Follow-up at this point in the process—including clarifying what the patient understands and providing correct information about what was misunderstood—is a classic nursing intervention.)

Among the components of various treatments for terminal illnesses are many that, unfortunately, bring with them a host of side effects and other problems. The physical side effects and difficulties caused by some cancer treatments, for example, are generally well documented. One relatively unrecognized problem, however, is that of negative expectations in relation to pain—the most feared aspect of cancer other than death. How do so many people with cancer come to believe that their pain will be uncontrollable?

One explanation may be that postoperative pain (a common aspect of diagnosis and treatment for a variety of tumor types) is often under-treated, and when under-treatment is preceded by the usual preoperative promise—"We'll control your pain after surgery"—then a negative expectation, or response, to similar words later in the disease process is created.

Side effects and other treatment problems also give the patient and their family intimations of suffering and mortality. Persons unfamiliar with cancer, AIDS, and other catastrophic illnesses often are surprised at how sick patients can become. The prospect of advanced disease becomes overwhelming.

Treatment often results in remission of disease or diminished disease-related problems. Hope rises, but the specter of mortality and more intense suffering lurks in the background. When symptoms recur, hope falls. With the vast array of both legitimate and spurious treatments available, the patient and family may find themselves on a veritable rollercoaster ride of responses. At some point, however, people tire, hope wanes, and the prospect of suffering and mortality becomes reality. Everyone involved is emotionally and physically exhausted: tired of hoping and failing; tired of sickness; tired of worry; tired of feeling tired. It is a deep weariness that surpasses all previous experience.

Terminal Illness as a Developmental Stage

Having advanced disease is an important developmental stage in the life of a person and in the lives of that person's family. Within the disease's overall developmental stage, there are a series of smaller stages, sometimes referred to as "the process of cancer." This process is adaptable to other diseases discussed in this book.

Colin Murray Parkes, one of the pioneers in the care of people with terminal illness, wrote that cancer is a process that forces everyone involved gradually to give up assumptions about life. There is a series of setbacks, each causing a negative reaction, followed (hopefully) by acceptance of the loss. These setbacks are characterized as "crisis points," or "partial deaths," the responses to which have positive or negative effects on subsequent crises (Parkes, 1978, p. 52; Shneidman, 1978, p. 153). Sullivan gave profound insight into the opportunities presented by these crisis points when he wrote, "It is at the developmental thresholds that the chance for notable favorable change" is the greatest (1953a, p. 247).

Thus, every crisis point, or stage, in the process of cancer is a developmental threshold and an obvious intervention point, offering an opportunity for responses that are growth-producing or not. Even positive changes—remission, for example—are stressful and provide opportunities for positive or negative responses.

Terminal illness is a developmental stage in the life of the family/social system as well as in the life of the person who is dying. In some cases, except for the patient's physical needs, the family is the focus of care. (Please see chapter 2.)

Erikson's developmental stages and psychosocial crises, shown in Table 1.1, help in understanding patients and families (Holland, 1993). Although ages and psychosocial crises suggest general directions in the care of patients and families, it is Erikson's last stage that is broadly applicable to terminal situations, *regardless of the patient's age or developmental stage.* In many respects, terminal illness is a struggle to maintain or achieve integrity rather than despair.

These stages can help guide counseling. For example, a major issue for an adolescent who is terminally ill may be feelings of alienation from the all-important peer group. Or the young adult may feel a terrible isolation and grief over intimacy never achieved. Alienation from the group or problems of intimacy can thus be used as starting points in counseling.

TABLE 1.1
DEVELOPMENTAL STAGES/PSYCHOSOCIAL CRISES

Stage and typical age	Psychosocial crisis
Infant (birth–2 years)	Trust vs. mistrust
Toddler (2–4)	Autonomy vs. shame and doubt
Early school age (5–7)	Initiative vs. guilt
Mid-school age (8–12)	Industry vs. inferiority
Early adolescence (13–17)	Group identity vs. alienation
Late adolescence (18–22)	Individual identity vs. role diffusion
Young adult (23–30)	Intimacy vs. isolation
Middle adult (31–50)	Generativity vs. stagnation
Later adult (50–death)	Integrity vs. despair

In looking at a person's life, the nurse may see past, unresolved psychosocial crises emerge as major conflicts in dying. Conversely, earlier crises resolved in an effective manner can serve as points of strength around which the patient may rally. A fundamental technique in crisis intervention is to help the person in crisis to use past coping skills to adapt to the current situation. This technique is frequently applicable in terminal care. Helping a person recall how he or she handled receiving the original diagnosis (if it was well-handled), for example, may bring to mind strengths and coping skills that were forgotten in the current crisis.

Psychosocial and Related/Interrelated Problems

LOSS AND GRIEF

Much is lost in the process of dying, including some or even most of the following:

- physical health;
- the belief in remaining healthy indefinitely—of living indefinitely;
- confidence in the certainty, order, predictability, and security of life;
- family;
- roles, identity;
- job, employment;
- being productive, feeling competent;
- independence;
- control (of bowels, of life—everything);
- people thought to be friends;
- things, e.g., possessions;
- the future;
- superficial relationship with God;
- hope;
- meaning.

Not everyone experiences all these losses, but everyone experiences at least some of them. Valued, comfortable aspects of life, beliefs, illu-

sions, and much more all inevitably fall away. Nothing can be done to prevent some of these losses. What can be done is to modify, or change the responses to them.

The natural response to loss is grief. A number of contemporary theoretical constructs of the stages of grief have been proposed since Lindemann's pioneering work (1944). To the extent that they delineate and normalize certain expressions or experiences of grief and mourning, they are helpful. In terms of predicting behavior, they are less helpful. Most can be summarized as having two themes: (1) phases of avoidance, confrontation, and reestablishment; and (2) recognition of the difficulties and necessity of engaging in "grief work" to resolve the loss (Cooley, 1992).

The power of grief should not be underestimated. Not only does grief have profound effects on individuals and families, it also has profound effects on the human race as a whole. "Grief appears prominently in all great systems of thought (religious and philosophical), although it does not always go by that name" (Carse, 1980, p. 8).

Grief and mourning may include responses such as denial, shock, anger, guilt, sadness, or depression. (Depression is different from sadness in that it is an "abnormal extension of overelaboration of sadness and grief" [Stuart & Sundeen, 1991, p. 1008].) A significant problem in grief is that different people (e.g., family members) move through it at different speeds. Loss and grief are further discussed in the section on families, and in greater detail in the chapter on grief. Depression is discussed as a separate category in this chapter.

Basic interventions/responses to persons experiencing the overwhelming losses in dying include the following:

- Acknowledge the losses and their magnitude. Saying simply (words to the effect), "You're really losing a lot," can bring relief to the person who is grieving for the losses that dying and death bring. It tells the person that you understand not what the person feels, but *that* the person feels. In other words, connection is made.

- Help the patient explore losses and their meaning. Whether losses are physical beauty, a loving relationship, meaning in life, or whatever, the opportunity to talk about and understand them promotes growth in the process of dying. It is not necessary for all these losses to be accepted, resolved, and forgotten. Some are resolved and forgotten; others remain painful; and still others serve as a means of growth and change. Losses such as a (perhaps comfortable) superficial relationship with God or dependence on physical beauty can result in significant personal growth.
- Help the patient resolve conflicts and complete unfinished relationships. As noted under the list of losses, dying means losing the future, i.e., the common illusion of living indefinitely.
- Help the patient explore what is left. The person who is able to grieve about loss of beauty, relationships, and old meanings in life may find that physical beauty passes and the loss is not great; loving relationships thought to be gone live on in the heart; and meaning in life may change and deepen as growth occurs.

LONELINESS AND ISOLATION

Charles Bukowski once wrote: "If you want to find out who your friends are, get yourself a jail sentence" (1969, p. 208). Substitute the words "terminal illness" for "jail sentence" and this thought conveys the idea that dying can be hard, lonely work. Often, friends fall away, or are not available in the most difficult times. Many people go through the dying process emotionally, spiritually, or physically alone.

And no matter who or what is there, in flesh or faith, everyone, sometime during the process of dying, in one way or another, conceives of themselves as utterly alone. This age-old, uni-versal conception of isolation in the face of death is reflected, for example, in the depiction of the death of Christ by the authors of the New Testament, in psalms and in Christ's cry as he died:

My God, my God, why hast thou forsaken me?

(PSALM 22:1; MARK 15:34)

Aloneness or despair, however, are not the full measure of what is inherent in dying—they are only a part of it. The process of living and dying, as a whole, determines the quality of life in dying. This is not something the nurse tells the patient; it is what the nurse lives and imparts to the patient.

The loneliness inherent in the process of living and dying is obviously affected by the presence of others. The *quality* of the presence is what is important, and not everyone who is present must be alive. A loving memory may often bring more comfort than a living person, and sometimes people seem to need permission to call on memory for comfort. A nurse might say, for example, "Tell me what you valued most about your wife? What would she say to you if she were here now. What would you say to her?"

Two superficially contradictory forms of valued presence in the process of dying are:

- the presence of one who works consistently and skillfully to manage symptoms and problems;
- the presence of one who "can be silent with us in a moment of despair or confusion, who can stay with us in an hour of grief and bereavement, who can tolerate not knowing, not curing, not healing, and face with us the reality of our helplessness . . . " (Nouwen, 1974, p. 34).

One of these presences does everything; one does nothing. In reality, both are doing what the patient needs. As noted earlier, there is still loneliness, but the suffering is not so great.

One curiosity in the cases of a significant

number of dying people is the change that often occurs in the dynamics of their inner circle of close friends and family: new people appear; others who seemed distant or weak gain new strength; or faith may deepen and sustain those who never considered themselves particularly religious before.

FEELINGS OF USELESSNESS

Feelings of uselessness arise from the physical and emotional/social limitations that come with terminal illness. These feelings of uselessness are probably greatest in cultures or social systems that value people primarily for what they accomplish and achieve. In Western cultures, this "being-by-doing" ethic is so powerful that even elderly people, sick unto death, are troubled by being unable to "do." The drive to "do" may also function as a means of avoiding dealing with "being."

Feelings of uselessness can be approached in several ways:

- When possible, help the person be—not feel, but be useful. This is accomplished by getting the patient involved in his or her own care, by helping them participate in decisions, and, in general, by including the patient as much as possible in normal life activities.
- One of the most helpful things to do for a person who is dying is to help that person help others, rather than remaining simply the object of others' care and protection. Terminal illness often brings great insights into the meaning of life. Reciprocal sharing of feelings and knowledge can turn passive patients into vital partners in possession of an important gift they can leave behind. Nurses (and their present and future patients) benefit from asking patients what they can share with them about being in their situation.
- Explore losses and, whenever possible, help the patient achieve resolution or acceptance.

ANGER

Anger is a response to anxiety or threat, and may be expressed directly or indirectly. Although often ascribed to the patient's response to their illness, anger in terminal illness may arise in reaction to other issues. This displacement of anger to illness is actually less threatening than when the anger is directed to its underlying target of self or others.

Regardless of how it is expressed, anger is an important theme in many lives. Expressed directly, excessive anger may result in a chronically hostile life of rage and conflict. Excessive anger that is repressed (unconscious mechanism) or suppressed (conscious effort to forget or not express) may result in a life characterized by depression, superficiality, or passive aggressive behavior. A pattern of internalizing anger may also predispose some to certain physical diseases (Carson et al., 1988). The stress of terminal illness often brings anger sharply into focus. Old, unresolved anger emerges and becomes a central issue in the process of dying.

Common targets for anger include individual family members, the entire family, health care personnel, the disease, institutions, self, fate, and/or God. Some anger is reasonable, justifiable, and should be expressed. Enmeshment in anger, however, is destructive. If expressing anger is a lifestyle, or if there is a pattern of repressing or suppressing anger, change is difficult. Among the ways anger may be expressed are rage, quarreling, sarcasm, exasperation (fault-finding), withdrawal, depression, and bitterness (Beck et al., 1988).

Chronically angry people drive others away with anger and blaming. Anger then has a cyclic nature, in which anger promotes isolation, isolation promotes anxiety, and anxiety promotes more anger.

A process for understanding and addressing anger as a problem includes these steps:

- Understand one's own response to anger. Being with a person who is angry can be extremely difficult. It is difficult not to have a negative emotional response to the angry person, especially when the anger is directed at oneself (the practitioner). Not so apparent, perhaps, is that the angry person probably also has a negative response to him or herself.

- Accept that anger or irritability is present in many people who are dying and, in fact, is considered a natural part of the process of dying by some, e.g., Kubler-Ross (1969).
- Help the person verbally express the anger and name the object of the anger.
- When anger is reasonable, or justifiable, and the object or precipitating factor can be changed, then facilitate the change.
- Help identify the precursors to angry feelings; the situations, words, behaviors, and feelings that trigger anger.
- Help identify the underlying feeling; e.g., betrayal, frustration, anxiety, etc. This can be done by discussing with the patient what was occurring and what he or she was feeling just before getting angry. This is best done when the person is not angry.
- Help identify alternatives to anger as ways of expressing feelings of frustration, anxiety, etc. The patient or family member can discuss or practice with the nurse more productive ways of expressing the feelings.
- Help identify consequences of angry behavior.
- Because anxiety underlies much anger; and because anxiety and poor self-concept are related, assisting the patient or family member to examine and improve self-concept may also be helpful. (See also sections on uselessness and anxiety.)

ANXIETY AND FEAR

Anxiety is "apprehension or uneasiness that results from the anticipation of danger, usually of intrapsychic origin and therefore unconscious." Fear on the other hand, is "apprehen-sion resulting from a consciously recognized, usually external, threat or danger" (Nicholi, 1978, p. 34). Along with sadness and/or irritability, fear and anxiety are "normal for patients with advanced cancer" (Miller & Walsh, 1991, p. 27) and certainly for other patients with life-threatening illnesses. Although anxiety and fear are often indistinguishable in the patient's experience and expression, we need to consider them here, at least theoretically, as separate concepts.

Anxiety is the "most common form of psychological distress" in patients with cancer (Holland, 1993, p. 1023). It may be experienced as diffuse dread and attributed to fear of of the disease, of dying, of non-being, or of being dead. However, anxiety arises primarily from tension associated with not having fundamental interpersonal needs met. In some cases, anxiety may also be a result of disease process, e.g., abnormal metabolic states, hormone-secreting tumors, paraneoplastic syndromes, or pain; or of disease-related factors, including medication side effects, medication withdrawal, or painful procedures (Holland, 1993). The great problem of anxiety in general, and the terrible anxiety felt by many who are dying is that its etiology is generally outside the awareness of the individual (Sullivan, 1953b). In general, anxiety must be addressed in the context of the illness as well as interpersonally. Interventions to address the problem of anxiety include:

- Manage symptoms and other problems.
- Decrease the unknowns in the disease process and in the care given. The patient and family should be given as much information as they are able to absorb about their situations. There is no better judge of how much a particular person can tolerate than that person themselves. Over-protection often is a misdirected kindness. Understanding helps promote a sense of control or order.
- Involve both the patient and family in the patient's care. Teaching skills to help build

a sense of purpose and competence can, to a great extent, replace anxiety.

- Help the patient talk about his or her anxious feelings (without insisting that it be called anxiety). This intervention alone is helpful for many because expressing and discussing the feeling brings it more into awareness, making it less mysterious and threatening.
- As anxiety is recognized, assist the patient to identify associated feelings or threats. Associated feelings point to the threat underlying the anxiety. Fear of abandonment is a very common threat. Some threats may be realistic; some are not. Both should be acknowledged as valid for that patient at that time.
- Understanding the feelings or threat underlying the anxiety allows the nurse and patient to explore together the meaning of the threat or feeling. A person who is anxious about the prospect of abandonment may have a legitimate concern in the here and now or may be dealing with a life-long conflict.
- While not usually prescribed as a counseling technique, frequent and realistic reassurance is often helpful for a patient who is dying. The reassurance is not that the patient will not die, but that he or she can go through the process—one step at a time, and not alone.
- For some patients, it is necessary to set limits on talking about anxiety. Scrutiny of interactions in which anxiety is endlessly discussed may show that the nurse is not helping the patient move beyond talking about the anxiety.
- Anti-anxiety medications should be considered. Benzodiazepines, especially the short-acting agents, such as alprazolam (Xanax) are most commonly used. Other medications (Holland, 1993; Wilson, 1989) include:
  1. Chlorpromazine (Thorazine), 12.5–25 mg PO every 6–8 hours is "the most effective sedative in the dying" according to Wilson (1989, p. 31).
  2. Amitriptyline (Elavil), 25–50 mg PO at night helps with sleep and depression, as well as anxiety. Tricyclic antidepressants are also helpful in managing pain, especially neuropathic pain (Panerai et al., 1991).
  3. Lorazepam (Ativan), 1–3 mg every 8–12 hours to start, increasing up to 10 mg/24 hours. A larger dose can be given at night.

Note that doses for amitriptyline and chlorpromazine are smaller than those given for psychiatric disorders.

Anxiety is a complex problem that is too often confused with fear and too often attributed to external and identifiable events. Some anxiety is normal in any patient who is dying. Fear, on the other hand, results from a consciously recognized, usually external, threat or danger. The following is a list of common fears related to death, and the potential responses to them.

- Fear of death itself, perhaps as annihilation, or as "not being"—e.g., "not me!" Many people, regardless of their religious faith, at some time in the process of dying can experience this fear. The fear of death itself is one of the great existential challenges of life, something everyone must face, and there are no quick or easy answers to "why," or to "how" this is accomplished.

  We should be especially wary of assuming that a patient's religious faith can supply the answer to these questions, or to the crisis of death itself. Even individuals of strong faith can feel abandoned by their God at some point during the process of dying. To respond arbitrarily to such a crisis with prayer or with words from holy scriptures may be to deny the dying person the fullness of their own doubt and experience. The nurse remains with the person who is dying in the time of their darkness as well as in the light. Sometimes only going through the darkness with a person can help them find the light.

- Fear of punishment for sins: death, from the point of view of many religions, brings with it a judgment from God, according to which there will be either punishment or reward. In psychological terms, death forces people to come to terms with a final self-judgment: What have they made of their lives? Rationalists may deny, or term "superstitious," the belief in a judgement by God after death, while some religious fundamentalists may deny the individual's right to judge themselves. Again, the tendency to look for quick and easy answers to the doubts and confusion posed by this final reckoning of an individual with his or her life should be avoided. Exploring mistakes and regrets can be productive when feelings of guilt and fear of punishment are present in the individual. Patients (or family members) can be asked what they would like to be different if life could be lived over again. This is one of the most potent questions to ask in the process of dying. While some people may feel they have, in fact, committed great sins, many may judge themselves harshly (and expect that God will judge them in the same way) for seemingly trivial transgressions. Guilt imposed by parents or by others is another common, but often unrecognized factor. Terrible and lifelong guilt often occurs when people have been abused as children. The process of helping a patient deal with fear of judgment and guilt includes helping the person:
  1. express guilty feelings;
  2. identify the source of guilt;
  3. accept responsibility for that for which he or she is responsible, and reject responsibility for that for which he or she is not responsible;

  4. accept the forgiveness of others and understand blame from others;
  5. identify and accept positive aspects of self;
  6. forgive her or himself—many people have great difficulty forgiving themselves. Those who are able to fully accept their own mistakes and failings, and fully accept forgiveness, can experience a powerful healing. Involving a chaplain or minister in these efforts is a part of nursing care in these situations, but making a referral *is not providing care*, and we are in the business of caring.

- Fear of dying as a mysterious and/or horrible process: Fear of dying may be related to ideas about the manner in which the person expects to die. Fantasized events are almost invariably worse than the reality. Determining what expectations the person has about her or his death and judiciously furnishing factual information on the manner in which people actually *do* die generally relieves this fear.

- Fear of the symptoms of terminal illness—unrelieved pain is the most feared symptom (Miller & Walsh, 1991). Fear of suffocation also frightens many. Fear of unrelieved symptoms often is based on unfortunate experiences in the earlier stages of illness, or on experience with other people's dying. While assurances that symptoms will be controlled helps, prompt attention to symptom relief is the most effective intervention.

DEPRESSION

The sadness common in terminal illness is often described as depression. Sadness is a normal response to many situations, and although including some aspects of depression, it is distinguished from depression by generally responding to supportive interventions (Wilson, 1989) and by a lesser degree of impairment in cognitive functioning (Robinson & Fleming, 1989). Depression, on the other hand is a pathological state that does not respond to supportive interventions (Wilson, 1989). Hopelessness is common in depression. Please also see the discussion of suicide following this section.

American Psychiatric Association diagnostic criteria (APA, 1987) for a "major depressive episode" include at least five of the following being present nearly every day during the same two-week period:

1. depressed mood—the "essential feature";
2. markedly decreased interest or pleasure in daily activities—often seen as apathy;
3. significant weight loss or gain;
4. sleep changes, especially insomnia;
5. psychomotor agitation or retardation;
6. fatigue;
7. feelings of worthlessness or excessive guilt;
8. diminished cognitive ability;
9. recurrent thoughts of death and/or suicide (pp. 218–222).

The APA notes that "even when associated with the full depressive syndrome," uncomplicated bereavement is "not considered a mental disorder" (APA, 1987, p. 222). Risk factors for depression in terminal illness include, but are not limited to, personal or family history of depressive episode(s), alcoholism, and unresolved grief (Wilson, 1989).

Clearly, the determination of depression is a major challenge in the context of the complex psychological and physical matrix of terminal disease. Among the factors confounding diagnosis are: similar symptomatology (fatigue, weight loss, thoughts of death); the presence of acute, and often chronic, grief; and the frequent presence of pain or other symptoms. In practical terms, an accurate diagnosis is not necessary, and many patients who do not meet the criteria for a major depressive episode are treated with anti-depressants.

Tricyclic antidepressants are the mainstay in the pharmacological treatment of depression or depression-like distress in terminal illness (Wilson, 1989; Massie et al., 1991). The efficacy of tricyclic antidepressants in treating depression is well known. Less known perhaps is that they are effective in treating insomnia (Kaye, 1990) and in treating the neuropathic pain that may occur in AIDS, multiple sclerosis, cancer, and other diseases (Please refer to chapters 10–12 on pain.) Further indication for using this class of medication is the mutually reinforcing relationship of pain, physical deterioration, and depression common in patients with advanced disease (Coyle et al., 1990).

Amitriptyline (Elavil) is a commonly used tricyclic antidepressant. Lower starting doses, e.g., 10–25 mg at bedtime, are given to older or debilitated patients (Kanner, 1987). Psychostimulants, such as dextroamphetamine in the morning, may be effective (Massie et al., 1991) but are not commonly used.

Independent interventions with patients with depression or depression-like distress include:

- Evaluate for external causes, including uncontrolled symptoms, medications, and syndromes known to cause depression. Medications that can cause depression include methyldopa, reserpine, barbiturates, diazepam, propanolol, prednisone, dexamethasone, as well as some chemotherapeutic agents (Massie, et al., 1991). Some metabolic, nutritional, endocrine, and neurologic disorders can cause depressive symptoms, notably abnormalities in potassium, sodium, or calcium; and hyperthyroidism and adrenal insufficiency (Massie et al., 1991).
- Maintain or improve physical status. The patient may be apathetic about medications, hygiene, diet, and other aspects of physical care, and thus require direct intervention.
- Be aware of one's own response to unrelieved depression. Working with a person

who is depressed can be depressing and frustrating—especially when, as is frequently the case, the depression is refractory to supportive care and other interventions.

- Throughout the course of care, help the patient set achievable (usually small) goals. These may be related to self-care, expression of feelings, or anything else relevant to the patient's concerns. While not curative in themselves, achieving these goals gives objective proof of success and can build self-esteem in a person who generally sees him or herself as unsuccessful.

- Help the patient directly express and accept feelings of sadness, worthlessness, guilt, and other feelings common with depression. A major challenge in such expression is the tendency for some patients to ruminate endlessly about sadness, poor self-image, guilt, and hopelessness. When expression of feelings become repetitive or consistently result in greater depression, the nurse should help the patient:
  1. identify attitudes or other factors that contribute to the feeling(s);
  2. identify origins of those attitudes or factors;
  3. identify realistic and unrealistic aspects of such attitudes or factors;
  4. explore the possibility that irrational beliefs or attitudes can be reexamined and perhaps rejected.

- Anger often underlies depression. Expressing and accepting anger may be central to overcoming depression.

- Help the patient do something for another person. This helps decrease the self-absorption of depression.

The process of expressing, accepting, and exploring feelings, achieving success in small goals, and helping another person contributes to a sense of control over self and the situation. Ultimately, the patient may experience alternatives to her or his depressed mood.

SUICIDE

Although the exact rate of suicide among cancer patients is unknown (Saunders & Valente, 1988), the incidence is higher among patients with cancer than among the general population, and is likely to be under-reported (Holland, 1993). The rate of suicidal ideation among patients with advanced cancer exceeds 25% and is clearly linked with depression (Coyle et al., 1990). Thoughts of suicide occur in almost all patients with cancer (Holland, 1993). Among patients with AIDS, suicide risk is extremely high (Cohen, 1992) and likely exceeds that of patients with cancer (D. Overton, personal communication, June, 1993). In patients with multiple sclerosis, suicide may account for more than 25% of deaths (Sadovnick et al., 1991). Risk factors given for depression apply also to suicide: personal or family history of depressive episode(s), alcoholism, and unresolved grief. Having a terminal illness is itself a risk factor, as are inadequate social support, recent knowledge of terminal prognosis, and poorly managed symptoms. A history of suicide attempt(s) indicates very high risk (McClean, 1987). The risk is increased by the common presence of large amounts of narcotics, barbiturates, and other medications easily used for suicide.

Suicidal ideation may not be apparent in the context of terminal illness. With death a central issue and feelings of despair not uncommon, nurses may not take particular note of behaviors that might otherwise indicate suicide risk. Clues that alert the nurse to the possibility of suicide in persons who are not terminally ill are functional behaviors in terminal illness, e.g., giving away possessions, sudden desire to make a will, and talking about death. Nevertheless, clues often exist. Despair, for example, is not a state of mind to accept without concern in patients.

The primary indication of suicide risk is the patient talking indirectly or directly about suicide. Examples of *possible* hints about suicide include statements such as: "I wish it was over with. Anything would be better than this." "I wish there was a way to finish this." Persons with persistent despair/hopelessness or depression should also be evaluated for risk.

- Evaluation is direct and begins with asking, "Are you thinking about killing yourself?" Questions about suicide are difficult to ask, but there is no substitute for direct questions. If the answer is "yes," the degree of risk is determined by the interrelation of the following factors: feelings of hopelessness, specific plan, talk of method, time, and other details, and lethal, available method. A firearm is the most lethal, but other means are also lethal. Extremely high lethality (the patient feels hopeless; has lethal means; intends to use the means in a specific way at a specific time soon) is often an indication for hospitalization and, in some cases, a call for emergency personnel. Such a patient should not be left alone. A few very determined individuals commit suicide after giving only the slightest hint to those around them that they intend to take their lives.
- Remove the most lethal means of suicide. It is not possible, however, to remove all means from a home. It is important for the nurse to get help at this point. Suicide intervention should not be an individual effort.
- As with intervening in other manifestations of psychological distress, an engaged relationship is most effective. Interventions suggested under the headings above for "loneliness" and "depression" are appropriate for a person who is suicidal.
- Suicidal ideation in a person who is not historically suicidal may be relatively transitory. The risk of suicide decreases if such a person is supported through the crisis of despair that leads to the thoughts of suicide. Support for any person considering suicide includes an overall increase in care.
- A "no-suicide contract" is an effective intervention (Rawlins, 1988). In this *written* con-

tract, the patient agrees that she or he will not hurt or kill her or himself during a specific time period; that if such thoughts or feelings arise, she or he will contact the nurse or other involved person, and that if the nurse is difficult to contact, the patient will keep trying.

LOSS OF SEXUAL INTIMACY

Sex and intimacy are central issues in human behavior. They are sources of immense joy and immense pain to people of all ages and cultures. The varieties of their meaning and expression are infinite. It is impossible to predict what sex and intimacy might mean to a particular individual who is dying, or to his or her partner. But it is likely to mean *something* to them. The loss of sexual intimacy may generate feelings of loss, loneliness, uselessness, or all of these and more.

While terminal illness is not usually a time of great libido, sexual or physical intimacy may be sorely missed. Most practitioners, however, are ill-prepared to discuss sex (Auchincloss, 1991). Even when the need is obvious, such as in persons with gynecological cancer, few practitioners are willing to try (Jenkins, 1988). Patients with AIDS often present with major sexual problems, especially in earlier stages of the disease. The nurse's purpose is not to provide sex therapy, but rather to identify problems of the whole person, and to at least try to support the person in coping with the problems.

Many nurses (and other professionals) are reluctant to bring up sex in patient or family assessments. The best way for most practitioners is simply to ask in a direct manner. The nurse might ask, "What has this illness meant to your sex life or your special times together?" (Note that there is an assumption that the illness has had an effect.)

Common etiologies of sexual dysfunction in terminal illness include emotional problems, physical aspects of the disease itself, physical aspects of treatment, and medications.

- Psychological difficulties are the most frequent cause of sexual dysfunction (Sawczuk, 1989). The psychosocial factors that most often affect sexuality in the patient or sex partner (Lamb, 1991), include alteration in body image, decreased self-esteem, role changes, attitudes, beliefs and misconceptions, anxiety and/or depression, and lack of availability of a partner.
- Physical aspects of cancer related to sexual dysfunction include: genital tumors, fistulas, pain, dyspnea, nausea, and similar problems (Lamb, 1991). Hodgkin's disease and tumors adjacent to genitalia, or related nerve plexi or the spinal cord, often cause sexual problems (Anderson & Schmuch, 1991). Other diseases associated with sexual dysfunction are AIDS, multiple sclerosis, Parkinson's disease, epilepsy, diabetes mellitus, arteriosclerosis, chronic renal disease, hepatic disease, chronic lung disease, heart disease, and endocrine disorders (Sawczuk, 1989). (Please see chapter 27 for information specific to AIDS.)
- Physical aspects of treatment that are most troublesome are surgery for prostate cancer, pelvic exenteration, abdominal (especially colon) surgery, and mastectomy (Anderson & Schmuch, 1991). Whether from disease, treatment, or both, fatigue is a problem for many patients. Both radiation and chemotherapy also may create problems (Lamb, 1991).
- Medications that commonly cause sexual dysfunction include antihypertensives, antidepressants, antipsychotics, and opioids. Alcohol also causes sexual dysfunction (Sawczuk, 1989).

As noted earlier, most nurses (or physicians, social workers, psychologists, etc.) are not well-prepared to provide sex therapy. Realistically, it is highly unlikely that there is anyone available who is better able to deal with sex problems than is the nurse. Interventions include:

- Bringing the problem into the open: This alone is farther than many people ever go in dealing with changes in sexuality.
- When the problem is one that can be readily addressed (for example, patient or partner feeling that sexual desire is wrong "at a time like this"; poorly maintained colostomy or wound dressing; pain, etc.), take appropriate action. Action could include: giving information to correct misconceptions, teaching wound or colostomy care, or managing symptoms.
- Many problems are less readily addressed. Severe depression, for example, results in loss of virtually all pleasure (anhedonia), including pleasure from sex or intimacy. Whether the etiology of the sexual difficulty is resolved or not, it is generally helpful to teach the partner of the affected person about the etiology of the sexual problem.
- Some problems are insurmountable. Persons with invasive vulvar disease or penectomy are unable to have sex as before. In situations in which the etiology cannot be changed, it is still possible at times to help the patient and partner explore alternatives. One alternative is to change the focus from sexual dysfunction to intimacy. The process of changing the focus includes:
  1. Help the patient and partner openly admit and face the losses suffered and resultant grief.
  2. Explore with one or both persons the meaning of sex to them. Alternatives to intercourse—oral sex, etc.—may emerge in such discussions.
  3. Give permission or encourage the patient and/or partner to try alternative(s). Too often, people quit sleeping in the same bed or even in the same room because of the illness. At times, lying down together is all a couple can do. Yet the comfort each can give the other by

the simplest touch, or just close physical proximity, can be beyond measure.

MANIPULATION

When all aspects of life spiral out of control, small wonder that many patients resort to manipulation as a means of control. Not all manipulation is problematic. One of the challenges that manipulation provides for practitioners is that it often works effectively as a means of meeting dependency needs. The patient may then be reluctant to stop. In terminal situations, manipulation may take the form of frequent calls for attention. These calls may not be direct requests for help, but instead may manifest as a series of problems: running out of medication on the weekend; delayed reporting of problems; family conflict in which the patient refuses care or a family member refuses to give care; threats and stipulations ("If you don't do this, then I won't do that."); angry outbursts; splitting staff and/or family; over-dependence; and so on. The key to recognizing dysfunctional manipulation is seeing a pattern of direct and indirect demands that have negative consequences.

Once staff realize they are being manipulated, the response too often is to label such patients manipulative and respond with avoidance, rigidity, or passive-aggressive retaliation: "She's not going to manipulate me!" or,"We are, after all, only trying to help, and there are plenty of *other* people who want our help." These reactions may be more prevalent among hospice and other similar types of staff, and staff members may also have a few dependency needs of their own.

Patients with a history of chemical dependency, antisocial personality disorder, or borderline personality disorder present major challenges with respect to manipulation. A clinical nurse specialist or related consultant should be utilized.

In working with patients who over-use manipulation, it is important to involve all other staff on the case. Otherwise, the patient is likely to redirect the manipulative behavior to whomever will best respond as the patient desires. Interventions include:

- Remain aware of personal feelings engendered by the manipulative behavior. Resentment, anger, and pity are common. Do not deny these feelings, but do not share them with the patient. Rather, observe your own feelings, understand them, then set them aside. Sharing responses to or feelings about manipulation with the team is helpful. You are not alone!
- Carefully organize care, especially schedules. The patient and family should have full understanding of who will do what and when it will be done. A written plan should be given to the patient and family.
- Set and consistently follow limits on behavior. Be very careful of setting too many limits or requirements. In other words, choose your battles carefully, and be sure that no harm is done to the patient.
- Focus patients' attention on their own behavior rather than on the staff's. Some people are incredibly skilled at diverting attention from the initiating behavior to others' responses.
- Allow socially acceptable expressions of anger. Then help patients relate the anger to their underlying feelings—often, the feeling present will be one of being out of control, or inadequate.
- Help the patient explore the feelings leading to manipulation. Understanding those feelings helps lead to their acceptance. Once underlying feelings are exposed and accepted, they may no longer need to be acted out through manipulation.
- As the patient works toward accepting underlying feelings, the nurse plans and implements the care in such a way that there is maximum patient involvement in both planning and implementation.

DEPENDENCE

Dependence and manipulation are related, hence interventions are similar in some respects. Some aspects differ, and they will be discussed separately. There is a time for dependence and independence and a time when one or the other is dysfunctional. It is not uncommon for patients to be ambivalent about the extent to which they are dependent on others. Some patients may deny that they are dependent (even as they avoid independence). As with patients who are manipulative, a lifelong pattern of dependence is unlikely to change in the last stages of life. To intervene with patients who are overly-dependent:

- Stay aware of personal feelings engendered by the behavior. It is beneficial to the nurse to take note of the extent to which patients becomes dependent on him or her. A pattern of dependent patients offers insight into the nurse's behavior.
- Carefully organize the care. Activities that the patient can perform should be specified. These are determined by physical and psychological potential. Given enough time, hopefully there will be progression toward some degree of independence.
- Set and consistently follow expectations. For extremely dependent individuals, expectations should not be too high. If, for example, the patient is expected to perform certain hygiene measures and does not, what options exist other than performing them for him or her?
- Help the patient identify consequences of dependency, and explore what can be done to become more independent. But be careful of providing the solutions!
- Help the patient explore feelings associated with dependency. Some of the most passively dependent patients are filled with the greatest repressed or suppressed anger. Expressing anger will be anxiety-provoking for such people. Please see the discussion of anger.

- Throughout the course of care, help the patient gradually increase independence. Almost any increase addresses several of the human needs discussed in the following section.

Dying, Death, and the Human Needs Model

Human needs, the things fundamental to existence as humans, have been identified by various sources (Baylor University School of Nursing [BUSN], 1991). While differing in some detail, most human needs models are essentially similar to one another. Understanding basic human needs serves to increase understanding of the process of dying and of the stresses inherent in it.

The first psychosocial human need (or cluster of related needs) is *understanding, order, predictability.* Logically, of course, everyone should understand that in the sense of the human death rate (100%, with untold millions of replications) dying and death are orderly and predictable. But we are not all that logical.

For we will never die!

(SOLZHENITSYN, 1983, P. 104).

Besides the specter of imminent death, people are also confounded by the manner of dying. "Like this? No warning?" Or, "Like this, so slow and wasting away?" When death comes from a terminal illness, the nurse can help create a sense of understanding, order, and predictability in several ways:

- Demystify the disease and process of dying. Assessing patient and family ideas about what is happening, and will happen, in the process of dying often reveals many misconceptions. Increasing the understanding of the process helps the situation become more manageable.

- Help plan the care with patient and family involvement in planning, and with their involvement explicit in the plan. The patient and family thus know who will do what and when. The sense of order created by this planning can literally be a lifeline to the patient.

Adequacy, competency, and *security* is another grouping of needs. These needs are a special problem for persons who want to be in control of every situation. Dying may be seen as the ultimate loss of control, and death as the ultimate failure of competence. This is particularly problematic for persons whose identity is tied to performance. What can a person who is dying do, and how secure can he or she feel? Some find that there is nothing to do, and the insecurity is absolute. Others find there is everything to do and, as a result of competent doing, find perhaps the greatest security of their life! This is the last and often the greatest task in life: to die well. It is the sum of a life; a kind of comprehensive final exam, in which all knowledge and experience is applied. Those who face it squarely with whatever pain and incompleteness they may feel, find that they were, after all, well-prepared. Those who do not face it, or who try to overpower it, find the task more difficult. These needs can be addressed in several ways:

- Early in the process of dying, patients and families are helped to gain control of the situation and care. See the sections on psychosocial needs/problems of families and on teaching the family, in chapter 2. Symptoms are competently managed.
- It is a tradition, or ideology, for many people in the helping professions not to encourage patients, but rather to continually throw them back on their own devices or past means of coping. The literature focuses to an overwhelming extent on the nurse being *empathetic*; and sympathy and encouragement seem to be viewed almost as character defects

in a practitioner. But sometimes, it is very appropriate to be sympathetic, or to simply encourage the patient (Morse, Bottorff, Anderson, O'Brien, & Soldberg, 1992); to let them know that they can do this and do it well. Indeed, what a marvelous opportunity this is to give someone the gift of courage.

The need for adequacy, competency, and security is perhaps most deeply challenged in parents whose child is dying. Such an occurrence calls into question the parent's fundamental human role of parenting/protecting the child. As with other situations, it is necessary to shift the focus of care; in this case, from protecting the child from death to protecting the child from as much suffering as is possible.

A third group of needs is *self-esteem, worth*, and *identity*. The person whose identity or sense of worth comes only from "doing," or from other external sources, may also have greater difficulty with these needs. Some realize that all the time spent seeking esteem from external sources was largely wasted. Those whose physical attractiveness is a primary source of self-esteem can be devastated by the effects of disease. Self-esteem is exactly what it says it is: esteem of self by self. Paradoxically, its genesis is in relationships with others, primarily with parents (Satir, 1967). Terminal illness gives people a last opportunity to understand how they got their ideas about themselves. It is also a last opportunity to evaluate and acknowledge "achievements, ability, and personal value, as well as to recognize and accept limitations and less desirable characteristics of self" (BUSN, 1991, p. 413). To address issues of self-esteem, worth, and identity, the following interventions are helpful:

- Help the patient express feelings about him or herself. Expression of negative feelings may precede positive ones, and be cathartic and accompanied by intense emotion. There is often tremendous grief over years of feeling bad about self in general, or about

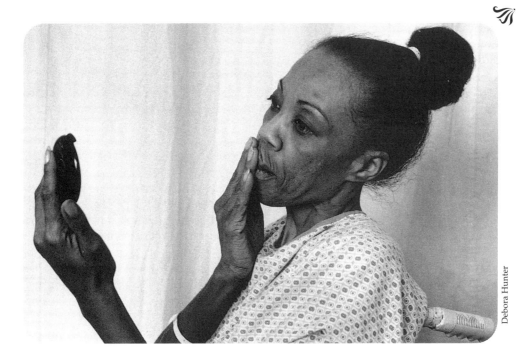

Debora Hunter

some particular aspect of self. Grief may also be expressed about the current situation, both in relation to dying and to changes in the body, in relationships, and in other issues.

- Once negative feelings are expressed, they can be examined and perhaps put into perspective. Some people carry with them emotional burdens, such as guilt and negative self-appraisal, for half a century or more. Saying words to the effect that, "you can let it go now" may be the permission they need to cease the judgment.
- Having expressed and examined the negatives, the positives may then be seen—with assistance. This is a great truth of human nature: positive aspects often cannot be seen or acknowledged until the negatives have been dealt with.
- Maintain hygiene and grooming to the end.

Personal growth and *fulfillment* together make up an important classification of human needs. Dying brings the message that all which has been put off until another day must now be done—"Now or Never." Will life be fulfilled or not? There are many means of growth. One person may write poetry or otherwise express that which has not been expressed; another may resolve conflicts, while yet another may come to accept self. Meeting previously noted needs may be preliminary to this, or working toward satisfying this need may be part of meeting those other needs. Interventions to help patients with this need include the following:

- Explore with the patient what is unfinished or unexpressed in his or her life. Some people may think there is no hope for growth, sometimes because of the illness, but more often because they simply have not grown or been fulfilled for many years.
- Encourage the patient to try to grow in whatever direction he or she needs. Even an attempt at growth is growth.

Love, belonging, and *approval* comprise the last group of human needs, as presented here. When all is in disorder; when competence is a dim memory; when growth is lost; when faith trembles and hope wanes, what is left that can help? Love.

So faith, hope, love abide, these three;
but the greatest of these is love...

1 CORINTHIANS 13:13

As expressed in this well-known quote from the Bible, love has a unique power in all our lives.

The patient who has, or has had, love is far more likely to grow and be fulfilled in the process of dying. Paradoxically, the more love and fulfillment in a person's life—the more a person has to lose by dying—the easier the dying. The less a person's life is characterized by love and fulfillment—the less a person has to lose by dying—the harder the dying.

What can be done for a person without love? Compassionate care—to remain by the side of the dying person and "watch with them"—is the best answer. Our human legacy decrees that all of us will be sorrowful and lonely at some point in (or throughout) the process of dying. And stripped of everything else, what the dying person needs the most is someone to simply be present, in body *and* in spirit, with them through this darkest "night of the soul." This is *primary spiritual care*; it is, in fact, the very bedrock of hospice or terminal care. When there is nothing left to do, there is still this love to give: to watch with the person facing death in despair.

There is often no thanks in such work. Some patients cannot say "thank you," even if they wanted to. But this "watching" can bring us full circle in our own spiritual journey, for what we do is for ourselves as much as for the patient. It is our gift to the patient; but the patient's gift to us is the opportunity to participate in the work of humanity.

Other Perspectives on Dying and Death

Works by several authors on concepts dealing with the care of the dying have contributed significantly to efforts to understand human perspectives on dying and death. With a better understanding of these perspectives, we can more easily deal with the awe, as well as with the trivialities, inherent in dying and death. What these concepts do is to break into manageable parts something (a human dying) that is too much to comprehend as a whole. Having some understanding of the parts, we are then better able to understand the whole.

No one concept, as expressed in these works, is better or worse, more or less useful, than another. However, some concepts may be more suitable for a particular nurse to use; or may be used to greater advantage in understanding a particular patient. These concepts can be seen as sets of different tools, for different workers, for different jobs. They help give direction to care.

Avery Weisman has spent more than two decades studying people who are dying. His book, *On Dying and Denying* (1972), is a significant contribution to the field of thanatology. Weisman developed the concept of "appropriate death," a death in which the following qualities characterize the person who is dying:

- Relatively pain-free, suffering reduced, emotional and social impoverishments kept to a minimum.
- Within limits of disability, operate on as high and effective a level as possible (even though only token forms of fulfillment can be offered).
- Recognize and resolve residual conflicts and satisfy whatever remaining wishes that are consistent with present situation and ego ideal.
- Be able to yield control to others in whom one has confidence, with the option of seek-

ing or relinquishing significant key people (Weisman, 1976).

These characteristics serve well as basic or generic goals in caring for people who are dying.

James Birren is lesser known in thanatology. His "tasks" of the person who is dying (1964) apply very well to patients and families, and also give direction to care:

- Manage reaction to pathophysiology. Implicit in this task is that the nurse manages the symptoms of the pathophysiology.
- Prepare for separation. We might ask from what, both good and bad, is a particular patient separating?
- Manage the prospect of transition to unknown state.
- Deal with the question of how life was lived in relation to what might have been. This is a potent question that includes at least two major issues: mistakes made and, simply, the way life worked out. We all understand making mistakes in life. There may also be issues beyond the control of the person who is dying. For example, nobody chose to be abused as a child, to have breast cancer at age 32, to be a refugee, or to watch a loved one go through Alzheimer's disease. Life is "unfair" for many. And, while a person may have surmounted his or her fate, pain often remains. This task is related to the concept of life review, but goes more directly to the issue of problems that may decrease quality of life. Patients can be helped to address this task if the nurse says words to the effect that, "In looking at your life, what do you wish had been different?" As noted elsewhere, a curiosity of humans is that it is common to be unable to see the positives in life until the negatives are faced. Unfortunately, some have great difficulty facing negatives and regrets without assistance. It must also be noted that facing negatives does not guarantee that positives will then emerge without assistance. The nurse

who builds a working relationship with patients and then helps them to face negative aspects of self may be rewarded by seeing significant growth in the patient.

Any discussion of dying and death should include Elisabeth Kubler-Ross' stages of dying. Her book, *On Death and Dying* (1969), literally blew wide open the secretive and misunderstood way in which people were dying (and continue to die) in the United States. Kubler-Ross' concept of stages, and some of her other ideas, received considerable criticism. We would do better to thank her for the work she has done—and the price she paid. The stages of dying identified by Kubler-Ross are denial, anger, bargaining, depression, and acceptance. These are most useful if examined as states of mind common to people who are dying rather than as sequential stages. It is also helpful to remember that Kubler-Ross considers these stages, or states of mind, as "helpful" guidelines, rather than as absolutes (p. 82). Her stages are as follows:

- *Denial* is a defense mechanism that can be healthy or unhealthy. In psychiatric terms, denial is unconscious. As popularly used in relation to people who are dying, denial may also be a conscious effort to not think about what is happening, or a mix of belief and disbelief. Whatever the case, experience shows that many people go back and forth between denial and acceptance throughout the process of dying.
- *Anger* replaces "not me" with "why me?" Anger about being terminally ill, or about the fact that one's spouse or child is terminally ill, is common. This anger is often an expression of feeling overwhelmed or frightened. Anger in the process of dying may also be part of a lifelong pattern of responding to stress with anger. Finally, although we operate in a world that constantly looks at and judges psychosocial processes and needs in terms of psy-

chopathology, it is well to remember that anger may sometimes be appropriate and justified. The fact is that health care staff and institutions sometimes treat people with insensitivity, and even, at times, with gratuitous cruelty.

- *Bargaining* is an old tradition; throughout literature, and even in the Scriptures, man has sought to bargain for life with both God and the Devil. However, no matter what the bargain offered, death comes. Bargains can sometimes be made to fulfill some wish; indeed, lack of fulfillment of a wish or need may slow death, even when it seems physiologically overdue and desired by all concerned. In a real sense, bargains may also be struck to achieve peace of mind.
- *Depression* comes when the preceding defenses have run their course and are no longer functional; when the person realizes, "Yes, I too will die." Operatively, we might best think of this "depression" as grief. The person experiences a deep sadness over the many losses already experienced and the prospect of separation from "life's web of connectedness" (Carse, 1980, p. 5).
- *Acceptance*, as Kubler-Ross sees it, is more than a state of mind in which the person says, "Okay, I accept that I will die." Acceptance is closer to Merton's "freedom and transcendence . . . that nobody can touch" (Merton, 1968, p. 342). It is enlightenment, or a sense of grace. The patient has accepted him or herself, is looking squarely at infinity, and does not fear.

Edwin Shneidman is a pioneer in the study of suicide. He has also contributed significantly to the understanding of people who are dying from terminal illness. *Death: Current Perspectives* (1976) is one example of his work. Another, more personal, contribution is *Voices of Death* (1980). This last is a lovely, healing book.

Shneidman says that "one dies as one has lived in the terrible moments of one's life" (1980, p. 112). Thus, responses to previous dif-

ficulties presage responses to terminal illness. These may include: "stoicism, rage, guilt, terror, cringing, fear, surrender, heroism, dependency, ennui, need for control, fight for autonomy and dignity, and denial" (p. 111).

Shneidman (1980) offers the following "principles, goals, and beliefs" in psychotherapeutic work with persons who are dying.

- Increased psychological comfort. Shneidman emphasizes the need for comfort in "a grim situation."
- Autonomy of the individual. This includes the individual having control of treatment, maintaining a sense of dignity, and being "as free as possible of unnecessary pain" (1980, p. 114).
- The importance of transference. Transference, positive, negative, or ambivalent, is operative in any therapeutic relationship. All can be helpful in the therapeutic process, and positive transference can provide great comfort.
- Limited goals. Few people die "right on psychological target" (1980, p. 120) with everything worked completely through. This is supremely important to understand. Expecting or desiring all or many patients to reach a state of complete acceptance dooms the nurse to disappointment in his or her abilities, and also, perhaps in the very real, although vastly differing, abilities of patients.

Final Note

Humans are remarkable in their strength and adaptability. The adversity of dying enables some to resolve relationships past and present, and thus bring their lives to completion.

"Entering healing beyond ideas of life and death, we become who we have always been, that which preceded birth and survives death.."

(LEVINE, 1987, P. 290)

References

American Psychiatric Association. (1987). Diagnostic and statistical manual of mental disorders (3rd ed., revised). Author: Washington, D.C.

Anderson, B.L., & Schmuch, G. (1991). Sexuality and cancer. In A.I. Holleb, D.J. Fink, & G.P. Murphy (Eds.), *Clinical Oncology*. (pp. 606–616). Atlanta: American Cancer Society.

Auchincloss, S. (1991). Sexual dysfunction after cancer treatment. *Journal of Psychosocial Oncology. 9*(1), 23–42.

Baylor University School of Nursing. (1991). Self study report. Dallas, Texas: Author.

Beck, C.K., Rawlins, R.P., & Williams, S.R. (1988). *Mental Health-Psychiatric Nursing*. (2nd ed.). St. Louis: C.V. Mosby.

Birren, J.E. (1964). *Relations of development and aging*. Salem, New Hampshire: Ayer Press.

Bukowski, C. (1969). *Notes of a Dirty Old Man*. San Francisco: City Lights Books.

Cooley, M.E. (1992). Bereavement care: a role for nurses. *Cancer Nursing. 15*(2), 125–129.

Carse, J.P. (1980). *Death and existence: a conceptual history of human mortality*. New York: John Wiley & Sons.

Carson, R.C., Butcher, J.N., & Coleman, J.C. (1988). *Abnormal psychology and modern life*. Boston: Scott, Foresman and Company.

Cohen, M.A.A. (1992). Biopsychosocial aspects of the AIDS epidemic. In G.P. Wormser (Ed.), *AIDS and other manifestations of HIV infection* (2nd ed.) (pp. 349–371). New York: Raven Press.

Coyle, N., Adelhardt, J., Foley, K.M., & Portenoy, R.K. (1990). Character of terminal illness in the advanced cancer patient: Pain and other symptoms in the last four weeks of life. *Journal of Pain and Symptom Management. 5*(2), 83–93.

Holland, J.C. (1993). Principles of psycho-oncology. In J.F. Holland, E. Frei, R.C. Bast, D.W. Kufe, D.L. Morton, & R.W. Weischselbaum (Eds.), *Cancer medicine* (3rd ed.) (pp. 1017–1032). Philadelphia: Lea & Feiberger.

Jenkins, B. (1988). Patient's reports of sexual changes after treatment for gynecological cancer. *Oncology Nursing Forum. 15*(3), 349–354.

Kanner, R.M. (1987). Pharmacological management of pain and symptom control in cancer. *Journal of Pain and Symptom Management. 2*(2), S19–S22.

Kaye, P. (1990). *Symptom control in hospice and palliative care*. Essex, Connecticut: Hospice Education Institute.

Kubler-Ross, E. (1969). *On death and dying*. New York: MacMillan.

Lamb, M.A. (1991). Alterations in sexuality and sexual functioning. In S.B. Baird, R. McCorkle, & M. Grant (Eds.), *Cancer nursing: A comprehensive textbook* (pp 831–849). Philadelphia: W.B Saunders.

Levine, S. (1987). *Healing into life and death*. Garden City, New York: Anchor Press.

Lindemann, E. (1944). Symptomatology and management of acute grief. *American Journal of Psychiatry, 101*, 141–148.

Massie, M.J., Heiligenstein, E., Lederberg, M.S., & Holland, J.C. (1991). Psychiatric complications in cancer patients. In A.I. Holleb, D.J. Fink, & G.P. Murphy (Eds.), *Clinical oncology*. (pp. 576–586). Atlanta: American Cancer Society.

McClean, L.J. (1987). Patterns of self-destructive behavior. In J. Haber, P.P. Hoskins, A.M. Leach, & B.F. Sideleau (Eds.), *Comprehensive psychiatric nursing*. (pp. 700–718). New York: McGraw-Hill.

Merton, T. (1968). *The Asian journal of Thomas Merton*. New York: New Directions Books.

Miller, R.D., & Walsh, T.D. (1991). Psychosocial aspects of palliative care in advanced cancer. *Journal of Pain and Symptom Management. 6*(1), 24–29.

Morse, J.M., Bottorff, J., Anderson, G., O'Brien, B., & Soldberg, G. (1992). Beyond empathy: Expanding expressions of caring. *Journal of Advanced Nursing, 17*(6), 809-821.

Nicholi, A.M. (1978). History and mental status. In A.M. Nicholi (Ed.), *The Harvard guide to modern psychiatry* (pp. 25–40). Cambridge, Massachusetts: The Belknap Press of Harvard University.

Nouwen, H.J.M. (1974). *Out of solitude*. Notre Dame: Ave Maria Press.

Panerai, A.E., Bianchi, M., Sacerdote, P., Ripamonti, C., Ventafridda, V., & DeConno, F. (1991). Antidepressants in cancer pain. *Journal of Palliative Care. 7*(4), 42–44.

Parkes, C.M. (1978). Psychological aspects. In C.M. Saunders (Ed.), *The management of terminal disease* (pp. 44–64). London: Edward Arnold.

Rawlins, R.P. (1988). Hope-despair. In C.K. Beck, R.P. Rawlins, & S.R. Williams (Eds.), *Mental Health-Psychiatric Nursing* (pp. 263–292). St. Louis: C.V. Mosby.

Robinson, P.J. & Fleming, S. (1989). Differentiating grief and depression. *Hospice Journal. 5*(1), 77–88.

Sadovnick, A.D., Eisen, K., Ebers, G.L., & Paty, D.W. (1991). Causes of death in patients attending multiple sclerosis clinics. *Neurology. 21*(5), 1193–1196.

Satir, V. (1967). *Conjoint family therapy*. Palo Alto: Science and Behavior Books.

Saunders, J.M., & Valente, S.M. (1988). Cancer and suicide. *Oncology nursing forum. 15*(5), 575–581.

Sawczuk, I. (1989). Impotence. In T.D. Walsh (Ed.), *Symptom control*. (pp. 265–270). Oxford: Blackwell Scientific Publications.

Shneidman, E.S., (Ed.). (1976). *Death: Current perspectives*. Palo Alto: Mayfield Publishing.

Shneidman, E.S. (1978). *Deaths of man*. New York: Quadrangle/The New York Times Book Co.

Shneidman, E. (1980). *Voices of death*. New York: Harper and Row.

Solzhenitsyn, A. (1983). We will never die. In D.J. Enright (Ed.) *The Oxford book of death.* Oxford: Oxford University Press.

Stuart, G.W., & Sundeen, S.J. (1991). *Principles and practice of psychiatric nursing.* St. Louis: Mosby Year Book.

Sullivan, H.S. (1953a). *The interpersonal theory of psychiatry.* New York: Norton.

Sullivan, H.S. (1953b). *Conceptions of modern psychiatry.* New York: Norton.

Weisman, A.D., (1972). *On dying and denying.* New York: Behavior Publications.

Weisman, A.D. (1976). Appropriate and appropriated death. In E.S. Shneidman (Ed.), *Death: Current perspectives.* (pp. 503–506). Palo Alto: Mayfield Publishing.

Wilson, P. (1989). Depression. In T.D. Walsh (Ed.), *Symptom control.* (pp. 89–97). Oxford: Blackwell Scientific Publications.

Psychosocial Needs, Problems, and Interventions: The Family

Initially, I was like a rock while other members of the family broke down in tears. Eventually my wife reacted by accusing me of not caring about her. It was a huge relief to her when she first saw me weep.

(PEDERSEN, 1991, P. 390).

The first step in addressing psychosocial needs and problems of the patient and family is to manage the patient's physical symptoms. At times, psychosocial problems are part of the etiology of physical problems, hence addressing psychosocial issues is also part of managing physical problems.

Review of Family Concepts

Several concepts of family dynamics are helpful in understanding families in terminal situations:

- *Family Systems Theory* Taken together, the members of a family make up the family system. A change in one part of the system changes the rest of the system. There are often subsystems of two or more persons within the family system. Family systems range from rigid (closed) to flexible (adaptive) to diffuse (chaotic or no system). The ability to adapt to change is essential to maintaining optimal function in the family system. The changes inherent in a terminal illness may be the greatest changes a family ever faces.
- *Communications* Accurate and direct communications within the context of (a generally) positive emotional climate are essential to effective functioning. Metacommunications, verbal or nonverbal, indicate the meaning of what is communicated. "Humans cannot *not* metacommunicate" (Satir, 1967, p. 76). One of the most damaging mistakes in terminal care is telling secrets to one family member and excluding the others—e.g., telling the family that the patient is dying but not telling the patient.
- *Rules, Roles, and Themes* Every family has overt and covert rules, roles, and themes that may or may not be recognized by any/all family members or by others outside the family. Rules affect the various roles and boundaries of each family member. Roles should be age-appropriate and boundaries clear. Rules may range from

Charles Kemp: TERMINAL ILLNESS: A GUIDE TO NURSING CARE. © 1995 J. B. Lippincott.

positive to negative in content and function. Universal, or rigid rules, roles, and themes—such as the role of the person who is *always* bad or *always* good, or the theme that a particular family *never* has conflict or *always* has conflict—are often problematic because they do not allow for the fullness of human expression.

When a family member is dying, all of the above concepts of family dynamics are affected to some extent. The system must change to adapt to the situation. At the moment of a family member's impending death, more than ever before, when the truth is hardest to bear, it must be told. Rules and roles must change in some respects, but not in others. For example, children (including adult "children") may need to feed and clean a parent and yet remain the "child" of the parent.

The Process of Terminal Illness: Appreciation and Understanding

Caring for families of people who are dying is based, like the care for the patient, on appreciation and understanding of the experience of going through a terminal illness with a loved one. While each person goes through this process differently, there often are similarities in the experience and/or response to it.

Although there is disagreement about the definition of family, there is one constant: each family is different. Families may consist of relatives living together or apart; of heterosexual or homosexual couples; of unrelated people who depend on one another; and even of people who are living and people who are dead (the memory of a loved one is a powerful presence in some families).

Just as it was suggested that the practitioner work to understand the fullness of the person who is dying, so should he or she work to understand and appreciate the fullness of the

family of the person who is dying. The family and the patient have a mutual history. Probably they have helped, hurt, sustained, and disappointed one another. They have done things together and apart. There are things they never got to do, that they would do over again if they could, and that they wish they had not done. If we can see and appreciate the family and individuals within it in the fullness and incompleteness that each family and person brings to dying, then we can make an enormous step in the care given.

Many families find that facing death is the greatest challenge of their life together. Death brings irrevocable change to the family. The effects of terminal illness on the family as a whole and on individuals within the family, are profound. Common responses include anxiety, depression, anger, and guilt (Clark, 1990). Different families and different individuals within the family meet the challenge (or do not) in different ways.

Like the person who is dying, families go through the up-and-down experiences of illness and treatment. Hope springs up and is dashed. There are bad times and, hopefully, good times. Ultimately, there is the realization that a loved one will die. The crisis points discussed under psychosocial needs and problems of the individual apply also to the family. The family that goes through these crisis points with the patient is most likely to help the patient through the process of dying; *and*, in turn, be helped by the patient (Holland, 1993). The developmental stage for the family in a terminal illness case is usually integrity vs. despair; or mutual aid vs. uselessness (Cullen, 1987).

At times, the family is the focus of care. The basic concept in caring for a family when a loved one is dying is much like the basic premise of family therapy and the "identified patient." When the family gets better, the patient also gets better (Satir, 1967). The family is often the focus of care when the patient is a child.

Psychosocial and Related Family Problems

LOSS AND GRIEF

(Please also see Chapter 6.) Everyone loses something in the process of dying. Family and survivor losses are similar to the patient's. Family losses may include:

- Physical health: as a result of the physical and emotional demands of providing care, some caregivers take as much as a year to recover their strength. Some never recover.
- The idea of living forever; of health forever: the dying and death of a loved one generally destroys this illusion, if it exists.
- Confidence in the certainty, order, predictability, and security of life in general, as a family and as individuals: in this and in other losses, control is a central issue.
- Family structure: at a minimum, the family structure changes. Depending on who dies and the relationship, a permanent void may result from the death.
- Roles, identity: some loss of role and identity of survivors is a given with any death of a loved one.
  A person who takes his or her identity from the person who is dying, or who has a symbiotic relationship with that person, obviously losses far more that one who has his or her own identity separate from the other. One of the more striking forms of symbiosis, or enmeshment, is *douleur à deux,* a disorder characterized by "shared suffering, mutual dependency, fluctuating sick role, and decreased socialization" (Kassirer et al., 1988, pp. 46–47). For the frail, elderly, and isolated survivor, the death of a spouse or other loved one may literally be the death of self.
- Feelings of competence, usefulness: if beating death is the goal, then loss and defeat are certain. If doing the best job possible to relieve suffering is the goal, then . . . even then, everyone involved may sometimes feel beaten down, but at least not useless.
- Independence: this loss is sometimes unrecognized by practitioners, and sometimes unexpressed by a particular family member. Independence, or a semblance of it, is lost when the person who dies was the survivor's primary link to the outside world. This is a problem especially for elderly, isolated persons.
- People thought to be friends: much is learned about who is a friend and can be depended on, and who cannot.
- Financial security: terminal illness is an irredeemable financial disaster for some families. When this is the case, there may be great resentment toward the patient by the family, and the patient may also resent him or herself.
- Superficial relationship with God or faith: on the surface, losing a superficial relationship with God or faith might seem like a positive event. But such a relationship may be a very comfortable relationship; it may also serve as a precursor to, or foundation for, a deeper relationship with faith.
- Hope: the (common illusory) hope that life will go on unchanged forever is lost. Other hopes, such as that life may go on a little longer, or that strength will be found, can replace the hope of living forever.
- Other more relative, or particular, losses, defined and experienced in each unique family.

Not every family or survivor experiences all these losses, but some experience many or most of them. Valued comfortable aspects of life, beliefs, illusions, and more fall inevitably away. In many cases, nothing can be done to prevent these losses. The fundamental issues are response to the loss and what, if anything, will replace the loss.

Grief is the normal reaction to loss and "any interference with it (is) useless or even harmful"

(Freud, 1917, p. 239). Grief is the long, sad, road to recovery. "The deep capacity to weep for the loss of a loved one and to continue to treasure the memory of that loss is one of our noblest human traits" (Shneidman, 1980, p. 179).

Families and patients often grieve for different losses, present and anticipated, at different speeds during the process of dying. Although anticipatory grieving cannot be completed until after the actual loss (Parkes, 1987), sometimes the grief work seems done, while the patient lives on. When this occurs, there may be emotional distancing between family and patient, with the patient treated unconsciously as if she or he is no longer completely within the family.

An obvious difference in family and patient grief is that the patient's grief dies with him or her, while the family's lives on, and may intensify. Like any other human behavior or experience, grief and mourning may be carried to extremes in behavior or length. What constitutes "extremes" is subject to debate. Grief is discussed in depth in Chapter 6.

LONELINESS AND ISOLATION

It is not only the person who is dying who finds him/herself lonely and isolated. Isolation for the family occurs when friends and other family members do not respond with their physical or emotional presence; when the enormous demands of care result in some family members—who are usually carrying on with their normal work schedule—being completely deprived of free time; and when others have no understanding of the magnitude of the pain or process of caring for a loved one who is dying. Thus, isolation can be the physical, psychological, or spiritual absence of others. One of the most isolating situations is when others seek to comfort through inappropriate cheer, or through "transform(ing) bad into good or pain into privilege" (Kushner, 1981, p. 23).

In addition to the isolation experienced by many who give care to a loved one, there may also be an anticipatory isolation that is related to anticipatory grief: When the job is done, only emptiness is the reward.

Key factors contributing to isolation are that many people do not know how to ask for, or how to accept help, and many do not know how to offer or give help. Too often, needs for help are expressed amorphously: "I wish someone would just help me in some way." Attempts to help may then be met with the message that the help attempted is the wrong help, or that it is not being done correctly. Offers to help are frequently expressed in a summary manner: "Let me know if there is anything I can do to help." While these kinds of offers are perhaps sincere, the usual outcome is that no help is requested, and no help is given.

When a family's life is characterized by isolation, there is little the practitioner can do to change the situation other than to decrease isolation through her or his own presence, or through enlisting the help of volunteer or other types of programs. When the family is, to some extent, engaged with others, whether other family and/or the community, isolation can be decreased in several ways:

- Teach how to ask for very specific help at specific times, e.g., grocery shopping twice a week, fixing a meal every Saturday, taking out the trash four times each week, organizing medical bills, etc.
- Teach that except for the one or two most dependable people, "on-call" requests should be avoided. As previously noted, two forms of presence (of others) are especially valuable. They are (1) the person(s) who competently perform certain tasks and (2) the person(s) able to be with one who is suffering. Most people can do one or the other.
- Teach that asking for help is not only "okay," but that it will probably need to be done a number of times. If, for example, the family's church and/or clergy is unhelpful,

rather than just swallow the hurt, the family can learn to confront the church in a positive and effective manner.

In the same manner in which friends sometimes are "discovered," rising to meet the needs of a person who is dying, so may friends be discovered who can help meet the needs of a dying person's family.

USELESSNESS

Family members' feelings of uselessness often emerge from the physical and emotional/social limitations that are a part of terminal illness. No matter how hard the family works, no matter how much they care, no matter how much money is spent, despite the prayers, despite everything—the object of the efforts continues dying. It is helpful, however, to remember that the patient's survival is not the only object of the effort. The well-being of the family is also at stake. They are also trying to help themselves by maintaining the family system. Control is, of course, a central issue. Feelings of uselessness can be approached in several ways (please see also the discussion below on Helplessness):

- Help family members be—not feel, but *be*— useful. In general, the family should be involved in as many aspects of care as possible. This includes children. A young child's contribution may consist only of bringing the patient a glass of water. Any contribution helps children (as well as adults), both during the dying family member's illness itself and later on, when the family confronts the death. The section below on Teaching the Family gives greater detail on family involvement.
- Help the family understand—and feel as though they are making an investment in— the goals of palliative care.
- Explore feelings about the situation in general, and about regrets in particular.

HELPLESSNESS (OF PATIENT AND FAMILY)

Helplessness is related to, and in some ways similar to feelings of uselessness. There is, however, a dimension of helplessness that is best examined alone: terminal illnesses seem, or in some respects really do have an inexorable quality, rolling mercilessly along to their inevitable end as patient, family and everyone else concerned stand helplessly by. Behaviors and attitudes that served patient and family well during the phase of illness when cure was possible are no longer as functional when cure is not possible.

An underlying dynamic in helplessness is feeling incompetent. Caring for a person who is dying is no small feat, under any circumstances. In modern Western culture, the difficulties inherent in caring for a person who is dying are compounded by smaller families, urban isolation, work schedules, complex technologies of patient care, and inexperience in providing care. Feeling helpless and incompetent means that some people never try to help. They are then left with the unescapable knowledge that, whatever the reasons, they did not help. Feelings of helplessness can be addressed in several ways:

- Move the focus of care consciously from cure to care. The goal of care then shifts from the patient not dying to the patient living as well as possible.
- Involve the patient and family in care. Even when the family is financially able to pay for total patient care, competently providing at least some care is beneficial both during the process and afterward.

ANXIETY AND FEAR

The discussion on anxiety and fear covered in Chapter 1, under Individual Psychosocial Needs, also applies to the family.

It is not only the body that dies, but "irreversible damage (is done) to the web of connectedness between persons," and it is within that connectedness that we experience life, or meaning in life (Carse, 1980, p. 4). As is true in other psychosocial issues, the frail elderly and/or isolated family members are at tremendous risk. For many, beyond the (in itself terrible) horizon of a life partner dying, and the attendant grief, may lie the prospect of continuing life alone in a nursing home, and/or suffering physical and mental deterioration.

ANGER/CONFLICT

The discussion of anger covered in Chapter 1 under Individual Psychosocial Needs also applies to the family.

It would be hopeful to think that when a loved one is dying, the family sets aside differences and rallies around the dying person. Of course, this does happen in many cases; in others it does not. Grief, anxiety, fatigue, and other dynamics place enormous stress on the family. Old, unresolved conflicts, hurts, and resentments surface and, in some families, the dying process becomes a battlefield. There are times when the atmosphere in a patient's room resembles that of a psychological war zone. In most families, at some point in the illness, it seems that some sort of conflict is bound to emerge.

When the family has a history of conflict, and current interactions are characterized by dysfunctional conflict, it may be wise to recall the principle of limited goals (Shneidman, 1980). In some situations, the goal may be practitioner-oriented, and limited to not responding negatively to conflict so as to be able to maintain contact with the patient.

In most families, anger and conflict *can* be resolved. The process for understanding and addressing family anger and conflict is similar to that used in individual situations:

• Understand one's own response to anger. This is especially important when the prac-

titioner comes from a family in which conflict was a theme, *or* where conflict was repressed.
• Accept that anger and conflict are normal responses to the stress of terminal illness and of providing care.
• Help family members verbally express the anger rather than act it out in a destructive or indirect manner.
• Help identify the precursors to angry feelings, and the underlying feeling, e.g., betrayal, frustration, anxiety, etc. Helping family members identify underlying feelings is promoted by discussing what was occurring and what individuals were feeling before the conflict began. This is best done when the conflict is not active.
• Help identify alternatives in expressing feelings of frustration, anxiety, etc. The patient or family member can discuss (or role play with the professional) more productive ways of expressing the feelings.
• Help identify consequences of angry behavior.
• Because anxiety underlies much anger, and because anxiety and poor self-concept are related, assisting the patient or family member to address self-concept may also be helpful.

DEPRESSION

(Please also see Chapter 6 and the definitions and discussion of depression in chapter 1.)

Sadness and other aspects of depression are common in families in which someone is dying; but clinical depression is less usual. The absence of sadness may be more problematic than sadness. Extreme or incapacitating sadness or depression also indicates problems perhaps beyond the immediate one of the dying family member. In reality, who and what is dying is not just a person, but also dreams unfulfilled, hope lost—the essence of life itself.

As with the individual person who is dying, clear identification of depression in a family member may be extremely difficult. Interventions discussed in Chapter 1, for the dying individual, hold true for that individual's family members as well. While depression is not classically seen as a family problem (in the same way as, for example, eating disorders are), having a family member with depression is certainly a family issue. The possibility of family members attempting suicide should also be considered, especially after the patient dies.

LOSS OF SEXUAL INTIMACY

The dimensions of sexuality that are more specific to the spouse, or partner, of the dying person than to the patient are most often related to the issues of (1) sexual feelings that, due to illness or other reasons, the patient does not share; and (2) confronting the loss of sexual activity after the patient dies. It may be inappropriate to address these issues with the patient and spouse, or partner, together. Indeed, these are issues that are seldom brought up in *any* context. They are most likely to develop into problems in need of understanding and guidance when the patient and spouse, or partner, are young; when the patient's illness is lengthy, e.g., myasthenia gravis; or when the illness is one whose effects include decreased libido, e.g., multiple sclerosis.

Interventions to help a spouse or partner deal with sexual feelings or impulses might include listening *without making judgements*, and assisting with finding sources to help guide spouses or partners when they are in doubt. Sexual desire is a very private matter for most people; in addition, a consequence of that privacy is that there is scant opportunity to develop objective perspectives. Thus, most people who struggle with issues of sexuality are left alone with their thoughts, feelings, desires, and impulses. There are few opportunties to speak of them to others, and even fewer chances of finding good advice when actions are in doubt. Apart from making our-

selves available to listen objectively to others' sexual problems, the practitioner can help locate pertinent information among the range of self-help and other books available on the subject of sexuality.

In any case, people who struggle with sexual feelings nearly always respond positively to the opportunity to talk about their struggles (the practitioner is usually advised to avoid discussion of too specific desires). Cognitive interventions are helpful in most instances. These include:

- Helping the person to recognize the consequences of behavior. One of the curiosities of sexual desire is that logic often seems to be absent in the contemplation of actions. Simply talking through potential consequences may be immensely helpful.
- Helping the person to identify situations that result in strong desires (stimulus-response cycle) and in other precursors to action, and to develop strategies to avoid such situations, if possible.
- Teaching techniques that interrupt the stimulus-response cycle. Avoidance, interruption, and diversion are proven methods for finding and maintaining the balance and self-control necessary to acting according to beliefs and principles.

On the whole, however, it would be wise to remain aware of the fact that the the stress of frustrated sexual feelings and impulses during the time of illness, and after the death of a spouse or partner, is a little-explored area in which there is much pain and great ignorance.

CAREGIVER FATIGUE

The fatigue experienced both by those who are dying and by those who are watching a loved one die is all-encompassing. It is physical, emotional, and often spiritual; it is also more than the sum of these.

Working in hospice and in other similar settings, where human life is constantly ebbing away, means experiencing people in their true guises, as they really are: often contradictory, contrary, manipulative, worrying, working, loving, steadfast, and oftentimes, in the final analysis, capable of moving beyond themselves in outpourings of love and hard work. Many are lifted up; some are not.

As with other aspects of terminal care, fatigue in the caregiver often has a cyclical nature. First, there is physical labor, coupled with sleep loss. Because of grief, anxiety, and other psychological issues, the labor seems harder to do and sleep more difficult to accomplish and less restful. Isolation, both in terms of the decreased presence of others and the unfulfilled expectations of help from others, adds to the stress. To put it in another way, for many, this is the hardest work they have ever tried to accomplish, with the least confidence and support they have ever experienced; and they are often doing it when they are old and when they have fewer physical, and, in some cases, emotional resources. Another facter is that the number of hours spent providing care may have less of an impact on fatigue than does the degree to which care-giving impinges on the caregiver's schedule (Jensen & Given, 1991).

Fatigue negatively affects the physical health of caregivers. Besides contributing to general debilitation and to risk for stress-related illness, fatigue is also one of the major reasons why caregivers neglect their own health, frequently ignoring diet restrictions and medication compliance. Increased use of alcohol, tobacco, and/or mood-altering drugs may occur, along with misuse of prescription drugs.

Like grief, fatigue may be considered a given in caring for a terminally ill loved one. While fatigue obviously is a problem for many, it may also be viewed as a sort of coping mechanism; as a confirmation of the experience. Caring for a loved one who is dying is a duty prescribed by the most ancient traditions and customs of humankind. The word "role," as in "your role as the caregiver," does not adequately describe the situation: carrying out the duty of caring for a dying loved one is part of being fully human. Those who fulfill this duty come away from it exhausted but fully aware that, on the very deepest levels of human existence, they did the right thing. Tired? Of course. The nature of duty is that it is seldom easy, and that it usually involves much sacrifice; if it were easy and free of cost, we would call it something else.

Caregiver fatigue can be addressed, and to some extent prevented as follows:

- Try to understand the extent of the fatigue. Directly acknowledge the fatigue and sacrifices made in providing care. Many people will deny that they are overly tired or that they are sacrificing to provide care. This does not mean they do not benefit from the acknowledgement. Both during the ordeal and when it is over, words of understanding and acknowledgement are remembered.
- The caregiver's health status should be regularly assessed and action taken based on the assessment. The caregiver's health status is directly related to the quality of care given to the patient and to the patient's well-being.
- Hospice and other, similar services provide immense help to families and patients. Scheduling services to fit with the caregiver's schedule is extremely important. Helping families organize themselves, their friends, or their church can have a profound impact on the situation. This is discussed in the following section.

Teaching the Family

In the United States and in other technological societies, most people do not know what to do when a family member is dying. Scattered families, the technological nature of dying, and

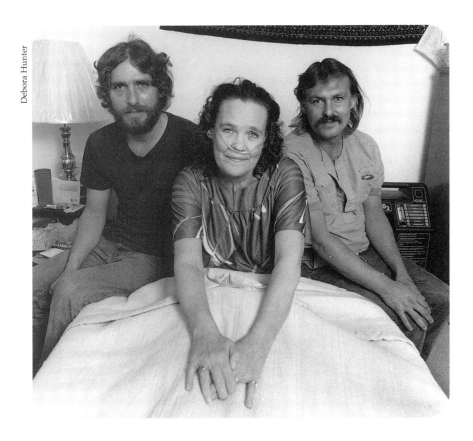

Debora Hunter

other factors are well-documented as playing a part in this phenomenon (e.g., Kastenbaum & Aisenberg, 1976; Feifel, 1976; McNulty, 1978).

In the absence of extended families or of experience in caring for persons who are dying, a central question is, what do families and others need to be taught to adequately provide care for a family member who is dying? Some of the answers are obvious: methods of catheter care, medication administration, pump usages, etc., must be taught to family members. But caring for a loved one goes far beyond technical care. Families and others need to understand the organization of physical care, the process of dying, and what to do emotionally and spiritually, as well as how to carry out procedures.

When people know what to expect, the process of dying is not a terrible mystery. When people feel competent to care for a family member, they are far more likely to participate in the care. When people understand and participate, the situation is still extremely difficult, but it tends to go better.

GOALS IN TEACHING THE FAMILY

The first step in teaching is to determine family/patient goals and how these and practitioner goals can fit together. The best way to determine goals is to consult with the people involved. Discussing goals of care gives the practitioner the opportunity to further assess the family, and the family the opportunity to begin assessing themselves. A standard of openness is set when the family is involved directly and early in the process of providing care. And, not surprisingly, the question of goals often results in family members learning (to their great surprise) that they expect and want different things.

Some families or family members are unable to discuss goals of care. These families or individuals tend to have great difficulty going through the process of terminal illnesses.

TEACHING/LEARNING NEEDS

Teaching and learning needs vary according to patient problems, family strengths, and other factors. The paragraphs below discuss typical areas of need.

- While not usually considered a teaching/learning need, probably the most important thing to teach family members is who you, as the practitioner, are, what you will do to help, and how to locate you in an emergency. It is immensely helpful for the family and the patient to learn what will happen in the course of care and how to get help in difficult times. Giving this information begins the process of addressing the overwhelming sense of isolation and helplessness experienced by many families.
- Medications should be understood, including what, how much, and when to give; adverse effects; when to discontinue and/or to ask for help; how to keep track of medications (see Part II—Pain Management); and when to obtain refills. (For example, Saturday night is a bad time to run out of Dilaudid!)
- Technology, even the simplest kind, is often mysterious and intimidating to families and patients. If power equipment is used, e.g., pumps, the family needs to know how to turn it on and off, how to regulate flow, how to handle minor malfunctions, and who to call if problems cannot be corrected. If equipment is basic, e.g., catheter, NG tube, etc., caregivers should know how to

recognize and resolve problems, and who to call if problems cannot be resolved. For any sort of technology, caregivers should know how to prevent problems.

- How to provide physical care, again including basics, is often completely new information to many people. Physical care can be divided into three areas: understanding and dealing with existing problems, preventing problems, and general comfort.
- Disease progression is a sensitive and complex matter and the practitioner must find a way to resolve conflicting demands—like anticipating to family members the likelihood of specific problems occurring and teaching about those problems, and, at the same time, ensuring that family and patient are not burdened with unnecessary information. Areas to consider teaching about include: (1) early recognition of and action to take for oncology emergencies and other problems (based on tumor type and metastases, or for persons with AIDS, signs of opportunistic infections, medication side effects, etc.); and (2) what to expect and do as the disease progresses. What to do when the patient dies is almost always an issue.

Clearly, the preceding five areas of teaching and learning are not inclusive, are not in the correct order for every patient/family, and cannot all be taught in one encounter.

In some families, more than one person provides care. *Clear division of responsibilities* is extremely important in preventing conflict and gaps in care. One person may be in charge of the catheter and the medications; another person may pay bills and call around for sitters. The procedure for dealing with more than one caregiver is discussed in the following section.

ORGANIZATION

Whether there is one caregiver or five, the care must be organized. Failure to organize care increases fatigue and conflict and often results in a breakdown of care. Organizing care does not just happen; nor is it something that many families can do on their own. The practitioner assists in organizing care as follows:

- Explain to the caregiver(s) and the patient that organization is necessary to meet their goals. It is necessary because (1) the work of care is very heavy and is usually more than one person can do; and (2) dying and grief are lonely matters, and other people can help, especially if they are part of the process.
- Have the family make lists of (1) what help they need now and will need later; and (2) everyone who has offered to help or who might help. Different people have different skills and should be utilized accordingly. Some will be most helpful with shopping and errands, others with cooking and cleaning, others with reading or companionship, others with organizing bills and so on. There are many ongoing jobs that must be done, even in the midst of dying. Every family presents with a unique constellation of social support. Probably the best way to pull together a support system is for the family to go through their address book, name-by-name, and then to consult their church directories, civic clubs, places of employment, and any other such listings. The list of names resulting from such a search may be smaller than anticipated. The list will grow smaller as contact is made and help requested.
- Help the caregiver fit tasks and helpers together. It is nearly always a mistake to ask friends for help "in general." Be specific and people will be more helpful. Where there is not a fit between tasks and helpers, a social work and/or volunteer service agency may be able to come to the rescue.

A common problem when working on involving others is that one or several family members may want to do everything. Sometimes, when people have enough time and energy, this is possible. Other times, the desire to do everything may function as a way of dealing with guilt or conflict. Attempting to do everything when such a feat is impossible may also function as a means of justifying a failure of the care effort, and thus hospital or nursing-home placement.

It may be obvious to an outsider that the person who wants to do it all cannot handle the workload. But often, the person who wants to do it all will be unable to see that he or she is virtually ensuring failure of the care effort. When this is the case, the practitioner can help the caregiver explore her or his perceptions of self as caregiver, and of others who might help. It is essential to set very clear expectations for helpers in order that they do the best job possible, and in order to encourage caregivers who are possessive to accept their help.

TEACHING EMOTIONAL CARE (AND HOW TO MEET NEEDS)

In part, teaching emotional care means teaching concepts discussed under psychosocial needs and problems. Family and patient benefit from learning about and helping one another. Some families and patients require no teaching about needs or emotional care; some teach the practitioner; and others need the help.

Teaching emotional care may also include teaching innovative ways of meeting needs. The people involved have basically the same needs they did before. This may seem like a simple concept, but the practice of it is more involved. A major problem in meeting these needs is that people are limited by thinking of meeting them exactly as they were met before the illness. If, for example, the need of belonging was met in some part through church activities, the common perception is that the only way to meet the need through church is to go to church for the whole service. Why not make a one-time increase in analgesic and go just long enough for communion and a hymn? Why not make a video or audio recording of the church service? Why not have a small Sunday school class in the patient's home? Why not? Because people are in the habit of doing things in a particular way and nobody thought of doing it in any other way; and because people think in terms of how they met the need in the past, rather than how the need might be met now.

CHILDREN

The fundamental purposes of any family or parent with children are to protect the children and provide means of growth. Thus, when someone in a family is dying, there is often an almost primitive urge to shield the children from the situation (Gibbons, 1992). And, in fact, some shielding is appropriate. Just as young children do not benefit from knowing all the details of adult sexuality, so do they not benefit from knowing all the details of dying. However, as difficult as it may be, children must be told the truth about dying and death.

There are numerous articles on children and death; many use the works of Piaget, Erickson, or other developmental psychologists as a basis for understanding how children view dying and death (Backer, Hannon, & Russell, 1994). In some ways, this treatment of the issue tends to relegate dying and death to a lifeless, isolated area in which it becomes merely another concept to grasp or understand. Other factors besides developmental issues play important and sometimes dominant roles in how children view, and react to, dying and death.

A child's psychosocial life experiences or circumstances, for example, are very important in how that child views, and reacts to, dying and death (Backer, Hannon, & Russell, 1994). A child who has grown up in a neighborhood in which drugs and violence are a part of life may have more experience with death than do many adults who live in other circumstances.

Refugee children may have seen mass death. Such children may be numbed or dissociated from pain and death; they may also have very strong reactions.

The extent, or lack of, family social networks and support also plays a part in a child's view of, and responses to, dying and death (Silverman & Worden, 1992). Social support comes from both family and friends.

Gender is yet another factor that can affect the expression of feelings to dying and death—if not to the experience itself. Children, as well as their parents (especially older parents), may often reflect gender stereotypes. Girls can tend to express and confide more, while boys may tend to be less expressive (Silverman & Worden, 1992).

Overall, there are three variables that deeply affect a child's view of and response to dying and death: who dies, how the death occurs, and who survives. The death of a close family member is obviously more troubling than that of a neighbor, and the nature of the child's relationship with the surviving parent, or other family members, also plays a part.

How the death occurs is the variable in which family and caregivers can exert some influence, because it not only encompasses the degree to which the death was a surprise or expected, and the degree of suffering and related issues (appearance, smell, etc.), but also the extent and nature of the child's involvement in the dying process (Gibbons, 1992). Attempting to separate or protect a child from the process may only make the process more frightening and mysterious. Later, there may be reports from the "protected" child that she or he did not know exactly what was happening; only that something "big and bad" was happening. When the process is a hidden mystery, some children may feel somehow responsible for the events. On the other hand, just as it is generally a mistake to attempt to hide the situation from children, so is it also generally a mistake to force inappropriate situations on them. There is no formula for calculating how much is "too much," or "too little." A good, general rule is to make decisions based on sensitivity to a child's response. It is also important to keep in mind that children do not deal with life (and death) in the same way that adults do. In grief, many children, for example, "do not wish to talk about feelings or events as much as they want to reminisce" (Silverman & Worden, 1992, p. 103).

Erikson's developmental stages and psychosocial crises (see chapter 1) give practitioners great insight into where to *begin* working with children in families in which someone is dying. Assessments and interventions directed to the child can, at least initially, be structured around these developmental stages. Work with the parents should include: teaching or reminding them that the child's natural development goes on, to some extent, regardless of other events; and helping the parents understand how to deal with development-related issues. For example, primary issues for a six-year-old center around initiative vs. guilt. Left to her or his own devices, a six-year-old child is likely to figure out something to do (on her or his own initiative) to help the person who is dying. Support of this initiative, no matter how impractical the idea is, tips the balance toward reinforcing initiative. Rejecting the idea, especially in an irritable or ridiculing manner, tips the balance toward guilt. Note that Erickson's childhood stages usually center around action on the part of the child and, further, that they all imply parental support for the action.

In the case of young adolescents, responses to someone in the family who is dying can be complicated by issues of peer-group identity, which may result in the adolescent feeling pressure to choose between family and peers, and may appear more problematic. Many girls and boys in early adolescence are capable of providing superb care for family members, and sometimes group identity issues can be deferred to some extent; or they can be handled effectively with the help of school teachers and staff. Some adolescents may attempt to play the role of savior for a parent who is dying, or for the bereaved parent who is left behind. This can sometimes be an attempt to avoid dealing with their own pain; it can also sometimes be an expression of maturity. In either case, the young person will need help with her or his own feelings, both during and after the experience.

Piaget's work in cognitive-affective development also provides insight into how children view and experience dying and death (Backer, Hannon, & Russell, 1994). In general, children tend to progress from the egocentric and magical thinking of the preoperational period (2–7 years), to an increasing intellectual realization of the finality of death in the concrete operations period (7–11 years), and onward to an understanding of the implications of dying and death in the formal operations period (Phillips, 1975).

It is clear that many factors affect how children and adults view and experience dying and death. Using developmental concepts helps in understanding children, but is not a substitute for understanding individuals. It is important, both before and after the death, that the child maintain connection with a parent, sibling, or other loved one who died. Before the death, connection is maintained through helping with care. After the death, connection is maintained through participation in mourning rituals, openly grieving, treasured keepsakes, and reminiscing.

References

Backer, B.A., Hannon, N., & Russell, N.A. (1994). *Death and dying: Understanding and care* (2nd ed.). Albany, NY: Delmar.

Carse, J.P. (1980). *Death and existence.* New York: John Wiley and Sons.

Clark, J.C. (1990). Psychosocial dimensions: The family. In S.L. Groenwald, M.H. Frogge, M. Goodman, & C.H. Yarbro (Eds.), *Cancer nursing: Principles and practice* (3rd ed.) (pp. 365–372). Boston: Jones and Bartlett.

Cullen, S.I. (1987). Family dynamics. In J. Norris, M. Kunes-Connell, S. Stockard, P.M. Ehrhart, & G.N. Newton (Eds.), *Mental health-psychiatric nursing: A continuum of care.* (pp. 199–222). New York: Delmar.

Feifel, H. (1976). Attitudes toward death: a psycholog-
ical perspective. In E.S. Shneidman (Ed.), *Death:
Current perspectives* (pp. 423–429). Palo Alto, CA:
Mayfield.

Freud, S. (1917). Mourning and melancholia. In J. Stra-
chey (Ed.), *The standard edition of the complete psychological works of Sigmund Freud (Vol. 14)*. London:
Hogarth Press.

Gibbons, M.B. (1992). A child dies, a child survives: The
impact of sibling loss. *Journal of Pediatric Health Care,
6*(2), 65–72.

Holland, J.C. (1993). Principles of psycho-oncology. In
J.F. Holland, E. Frei, R.C. Bast, D.W. Kufe, D.L. Morton, & R.W. Weischselbaum (Eds.), *Cancer medicine*
(3rd ed.) (pp. 1017–1032). Philadelphia: Lea &
Feiberger.

Jensen, S. & Given, B.A. (1991). Fatigue affecting family caregivers of cancer patients. *Cancer nursing,
14*(4), 181–187.

Kassirer, M., Cahill, J., Leskowitz, E., Osterberg, D. &
D'Amelio, R. (1988). Douleur à Deux. *Journal of pain
and symptom management, 3*(1), 46–49.

Kastenbaum, R. & Aisenberg, R. (1976). *The psychology
of death*. New York: Springer Publishing.

Kushner, H.S. (1981). *When bad things happen to good people*. New York: Avon.

McNulty, B.J. (1978). Out-patient and domiciliary man-
agement from a hospice. In C.M. Saunders (Ed.),
The management of terminal disease (pp. 154–165).
London: Edward Arnold.

Parkes, C.M. (1987). *Bereavement: Studies of grief in adult
life* (2nd ed.). Madison, CN: International Univer-
sities Press.

Pedersen, K. (1991). Dying with dignity. In M. Abiven
(Facilitator), Round table: Dying with dignity (pp.
389–391). *World Health Forum, 12*(4), 375–399.

Phillips, J.L. (1975). *The origins of intellect: Piaget's theory*.
San Francisco: W.H. Freeman Company.

Satir, V. (1967). *Conjoint family therapy*. Palo Alto, CA:
Science and Behavior Books.

Shneidman, E. (1980). *Voices of death*. New York: Harper and Row.

Silverman, P.R., & Worden, J.W. (1992). Children's reactions in the early months after the death of a parent.
American Journal of Orthopsychiatry, 62 (1), 93–104.

3

Spiritual Care: Needs, Problems, and Interventions

When death is near, many people turn instinctively to faith, to God. Spiritually and philosophically, death—the enemy, the end—becomes "an invitation to new life" (Carse, 1980, p. 9). But an invitation is not a map. The invitation may be only the explication of the need for a new life, without the understanding that a new life is possible, or how it can be found. Spiritual care can provide help in exploring that possibility, and achieving it.

Many nurses feel ill-prepared to provide spiritual care and thus avoid addressing spiritual issues, even when the need is great (Stepnick & Perry, 1992). Reasons for avoiding providing spiritual care include the following:

- Some nurses lack the spiritual preparation to provide spiritual care: personal doubts and uncertainties may result in their feeling inadequate to help patients in these matters. Other nurses have no doubts or uncertainties about spiritual matters, and may thus think of providing spiritual care only in terms of their own personal beliefs. It is difficult to offer effective spiritual care in either of these two extreme cases. In the first, elements of faith or knowledge are missing; in

the second, elements of humanity or humility are missing. In both, the spiritual preparation to minister to others, especially to those of a faith different from one's own, is lacking.

- Most nurses lack basic educational preparation related to spiritual care. These subjects may be only cursorily defined in some undergraduate or graduate programs, and there is little in the nursing literature about them (McGuire & Sheidler, 1990). What does appear is often limited to descriptions of various religious beliefs related to death or illness.

These two factors, and other barriers, stand in the way of nurses and others providing beneficial spiritual care. In this chapter, we will examine what methods exist—despite the difficulties presented by personal uncertainties, ignorance, or prejudice—to allow practitioners to offer spiritual care to patients, families, and others. The issue of personal spiritual preparation is a good starting point.

Charles Kemp: TERMINAL ILLNESS: A GUIDE TO NURSING CARE. © 1995 J. B. Lippincott.

Providing Spiritual Care: Spiritual Preparation

It is neither necessary, nor perhaps desirable, to be a person of absolute convictions; in short, to have all the answers to spiritual questions related to life and death. Spiritual care is not a matter of providing the *right* answers or explanations; even less is it a matter for argument. The essence of spiritual care is being present in the face of suffering, helplessness, fear, and despair. "Being present," i.e., right there, consistently, day after day, with a person who is dying, is *primary spiritual care.* Being present, or "watching" meets a fundamental spiritual need, represented by the simple words below from the Bible, recounting the turmoil of Jesus Christ before his own crucifixion.

"My soul is very sorrowful, even to death; remain here, and watch with me ."

(MATTHEW 26:38)

This presence, or watching, requires the will to face one's own and others' suffering, helplessness, fear, and despair. It does not require conquering, understanding, coming to terms with, or even accepting these difficult psychological states of being (Friedlander, 1976). At least initially, simply being present and watching with another requires only the will to consistently be there; to come back again and again. Zerwekh (1991, p. 879) writes, "If the nurse can remain present beside a dying person, that compassionate presence converts the experience into a triumph of love and human community."

Of course, it does not always feel like a triumph. More often it feels like unbearably hard work. It is perhaps a part of our particular Western socialization to define triumph as exultation or happiness; for example, the joy one feels after winning a game, or obtaining a desirable grade. Real triumph, the kind that can be felt by people who endure terrible tri-

als—like psychologically surviving incest, living through combat, or persevering in the face of continual defeat—is not a "happy" business. It runs deeper than that. Those who achieve this kind of triumph turn their attentions inward, listening to truth, secure in the knowledge that they have, by choice, faced what few willingly face, and that they have not been conquered by suffering, fear, helplessness, and despair—although those who have triumphed are very familiar with those states.

The first part of spiritual preparation, then, simply consists of "doing the job," achieving the perseverance necessary to remain present and to "watch" with the dying person. The second part consists of exploring one's own spiritual resources, in searching for and discovering a spiritual foundation for self and work; that is, a source of meaning beyond self and work, which may also include participation in teaching, in prayer or meditation, in ritual, or in any other formal or informal mode of spiritual exploration and fulfillment. It is not that one finds all the answers—and certainly never "perfection." One interpretation of this search is the idea that people can be helped to grow beyond themselves and their egos, to experience life on more than just the material level, by actively participating in religious rituals where "universal values" are served by tradition (Frankl, 1969, p. 64).

Of course, many people who draw on faith for support are not necessarily religious (O'Conner, Wicker, & Germino, 1990). We probably all know people of faith who operate effectively in the world and who do not participate in religious activities. Nevertheless, in *this* work, in caring for the dying, in helping people and their loved ones face the hour of death, practitioners operate in the midst of enormous suffering, continually confronted not only with others' but also with their own mortality. Both we, as practitioners, and our patients will benefit if we are possessed of the strongest possible spiritual foundation.

Providing Spiritual Care: Spiritual Needs, Problems, and Practices

Spiritual needs (Baylor University School of Nursing [BUSN], 1991; Conrad, 1985; Levine, 1984) include the need for the following:

- Meaning
- Hope
- Relatedness to God
- Forgiveness (or acceptance)
- Transcendence

These needs, examined separately below, often overlap with one another (Conrad, 1985) as well as with many other needs and issues.

An individual or family inability to meet or fulfill these needs may be expressed in many ways. Miller and Walsh (1991, p. 27) examined "psychosocial aspects of palliative care" and determined that "emotional distress" in patients with advanced cancer most commonly includes anxiety, sadness/depression, fear, irritation, loneliness, and anger. Any or all these could be related to the above spiritual needs. Fulfilling spiritual needs aids in alleviating these expressions of distress.

MEANING

One of the common tasks, or stages, in theoretical constructs of the human experience is that of life review, or some similar activity. Inherent in this activity is the search for meaning—in the individual's life, as it has been lived. Meaning includes the reason for an event or events; the purpose of life; and the belief in a primary force in life (BUSN, 1991). For some people, meaning may be found in a review of external achievements. More frequently, the search is a moral or spiritual search, often dwelling on mistakes and inadequacies. But there is more to this question of meaning than a simple search

through the past. Meaning may also include the meaning of dying, of human existence, suffering, and of the remaining days of life (Conrad, 1985; O'Conner, Wicker, & Germino, 1990). The absence of meaning in one's life—meaninglessness—is expressed in many ways, often through hopelessness and despair.

MEANING: INTERVENTIONS

Questions of meaning, faith, hope, and similar issues are usually best addressed directly. The search for meaning in life as it has been lived is facilitated by asking the patient questions such as, "If you had your life to live over again, what would you like to be different and what the same?" This can be an enormously productive question in terms of the issue at hand, of communications in general, and of the nurse-patient relationship.

There are, however, two "dangers" in such questions: First, the question may bring up suppressed material and thus result in pain for the patient. This is not uncommon, and family members may resent the nurse bringing up such matters. But it is important to understand that the pain is already there—conveniently hidden, perhaps, but there. Second, the patient may begin to dwell obsessively on a past circumstance or transgression. In this case, as discussed in chapter 1, the patient is usually obsessing on some aspect of the problem as a means of not completely coming to grips with it. In this case, it is necessary to (1) listen to the problem, and (2) help the patient further explore the problem, and its associated feelings, in depth.

The meaning of dying and suffering are difficult to understand in terms of psychological explanation. They can be addressed by questions such as, "What does it mean to you that this (dying and suffering) is happening?" This is a very serious question, and often gets serious answers.

Often paramount to the question of suffering is the question, "Why me; why am I suffering?" This is a tough question, especially for the nurse who feels obliged to provide an answer. Providing an answer may even prove to be a sort of trap that functions to stifle exploration of the suffering and its meaning. For some patients—those who belong to formal religious groups, or who have grown up with a formal religious background—helping them to find and reread passages from the sacred books of their own faiths may provide the best kind of "answer"; and every faith is rich in examples of compassionate reaction to human suffering.

Another way of confronting these questions is to consider with the patient the fact that the meaning of human existence is addressed directly by many people exclusively from the point of view of their *own* existence. When their own existence, then, is shattered and characterized by emptiness, all of human life seems empty and broken. Many people have the idea that they are the only ones who feel empty, inadequate, or broken. Exploration of how and why a person feels this way, coupled with a gentle reminder that others also feel this way, may be helpful.

Contemplating the questions mentioned above may lead to other questions: about forgiveness, acceptance, punishment, and even transcendence. They may lead also to patients questioning the meaning of the remaining days of their lives, and the prospect of what might be done to make the most of that time. Meaning for the future is especially a problem for those patients in whom meaning in the past was habitually extracted from external achievement. However, there is almost always room for internal achievement, or personal growth, and most people remain very alive to the universal human hunger for personal and interpersonal growth. In the context of dying, the opportunities for that growth are numerous, and the chances for their success are very high (Sullivan, 1953).

Psychosocial means of helping patients grow or work through problems and relationships are presented in chapters 1 and 2. In this section, the focus is on meeting the need for meaning in whatever amount of life remains to the patient. Many people are amazed at the idea that there is hope for meaning in the weeks or months of remaining life. Simply presenting the possibility of meaning is a valuable intervention.

Of course, meaning must be found by the person who seeks it, and cannot be given arbitrarily by another (Frankl, 1969). But help in the search may be given in several ways. Some patients need help in sorting through what is realistic and what is unrealistic, given their circumstances. Few can write a book, for example, but many can write a poem. Few can achieve perfect interpersonal relations with all others, but many can improve a relationship. Few can achieve spiritual perfection, but many can pray.

Nurses and other caregivers also help give meaning to life by the act of consistently dispensing their loving care, whether or not meaning and hope can be achieved by the patient. It is in fact here, in the "eclipse" of meaning and hope, that strong faith has proved to many to be the most essential factor (Fackenheim, 1976, p. 511). The person who is dying may or may not notice that meaning can exist where strong faith abides; still, it is there. "What our patients need is unconditional faith in unconditional meaning" (Frankl, 1969, p. 156).

HOPE

Hope is an important factor in dealing with stress, in maintaining quality of life, and, in some cases, in continuing life (Conrad, 1985). Dimensions of hope (Nowotny, 1989), or attributes of a hopeful person, include:

- confidence in the outcome;
- ability to relate to others;
- possibility of a future;
- spiritual beliefs;
- active involvement; and
- strength that comes from within.

While hope is seen by some as being in conflict with the realities of terminal illness (Corless, 1992), a person who is dying may hope for many things: to live another day; for relief from suffering; for a good death; for a healed relationship; to see a loved one; or even to not die. No matter how sick a person is, more often than not, on some level, there is always the hope to not die. In terms of psychology, this is perfectly reasonable, but in terms of disease progression, very unlikely.

HOPE: INTERVENTIONS

The dimensions of hope identified above give guidance in helping patients and families find hope within terminal illness. Building or strengthening dimensions that are lacking, and reinforcing those that are stronger, facilitates the growth of hope. Nowotny (1992) offers suggestions for each dimension:

- Confidence in the outcome: This is a challenge. Realistically, the outcome is that the person will die. Recall, however, that how one goes about dying—psychologically, socially, and spiritually—is not predetermined. In terminal illness, many patients ask three important questions—though not necessarily out loud. First, there is the question of cure, then there is the question of symptoms and problems, and finally, there is the question of whether the process can be gotten through, i.e., "Can I do this well?" (D. Foster, personal communication, 1991). Thus, the nurse helps build hope by focusing on this question of how the patient goes through the process. The nurse's self-confidence, confidence in the patient, and ability to identify and support patient and family strengths all influence the patient's confidence in the outcome. Christians, Jews, Muslims, Buddhists, Hindus, and others all have a definitive belief in outcome, i.e., in what happens after

death. These beliefs can bring enormous confidence in, or acceptance of the outcome (after death).

- Ability to relate to others: interpersonal relations are fundamental to mental health; the absence of relationships creates hopelessness, and activities that support relationships help build hope. Relationships need not be with persons in physical proximity. People already dead can even be central in some people's lives. Relationships that encourage spiritual growth can also be sought in both formal and informal religious settings and organizations.

- Possibility of a future: religions offer the only possibilities about the future (after death) that allow their believers substantial hope for redemption and an after-life. But what believer has not at some point thought, "What if . . . there is only nothing—or there is only hell?" The more devout the doubter, the more difficult it is for them to express their doubts, and the greater the conflict. The response to such doubts can be two-fold: first, stay with and support the patient, whether they are doubting or not; second, help the person who doubts to refer back to their religion, by providing reading materials, facilitating visits by their clergy, etc. Apart from questions about the "greater" future, there are also questions about the day-to-day future. With cancer or AIDS, the cliché, "one day at a time" is no longer a cliché, but a mighty truth. The present and short-term future is so momentous that the long-term future can often be left to itself as the day-to-day struggle goes forward.

- Spiritual beliefs: spiritual well-being clearly has a positive effect on persons with life-threatening illness (Carson & Green, 1992; Kaczorowski, 1989). Over the course of a life, many people fall away from the faith of their early years; some never had a faith. There is the possibility that many people who long for faith are not aware of what they long for. The time of dying is a good time to have another look at faith. If a visit to a place of worship is not physically possible, a visit from clergy could be very helpful. The songs and rituals of a patient's faith may be even more comforting than counseling. Patients who had few spiritual resources in their early years may wish to be seen by a chaplain. Religious rituals that can take place at a bedside (for example, for Christians, communion) should be offered. Audio tapes of devotional music (available at many specialized religious bookstores) may work wonders.

- Active involvement: this principle is covered primarily in chapters 1 and 2, and, at least superficially, usually has less to do with spiritual aspects of hope than it does with psychosocial aspects. The underlying principle of active involvement is autonomy. In the context of spiritual care, this means that the patient is free to choose, and to be in charge of, her or his own spiritual direction, and the practitioner facilitates this by providing an atmosphere, or milieu, of acceptance.

- Strength that comes from within: it is essential to use the patient's own strengths in exploring the often grim psychological and spiritual landscape of terminal illness. Anything other than recognition and validation of the patient's own feelings, strengths, and weaknesses means that full exploration—hence full understanding—is unlikely. Practitioners should be willing to leave the patient alone with the unanswered questions that the patient must face. This may be difficult, but necessary: Each person needs to discover and personally experience their own doubts and fears. "In religious matters it is a well-known fact that we cannot understand a thing until we have experienced it inwardly" (Jung, 1953, p. 338).

RELATEDNESS TO GOD

Many secularists, and even some authors writing from a spiritual perspective, view relationships with other people as a fulfillment of spiritual needs (Karns, 1991). Although relationships with others are essential and even, in some cases, exalting, nevertheless, with some slight exceptions, in the case of caring for those who are dying, the focus is on relatedness with God, or with whatever represents God—the concept of the eternal, universal, all-knowing, etc.

While the concept of God differs everywhere, God is infinitely available to all people, and to people of all faiths. The God of Judaism, Christianity, and Islam is clearly explicated. Hindus also believe in "One God, who can be understood and worshiped in many different forms" (Green, 1989, p. 50). Buddhists can believe in a divine "force" or "being," as expressed by the Buddha. Jung has written that the presence or acknowledgment of God among virtually all peoples of all religions is evidence of God as a universal archetype, i.e., an "imprint" of God on the psyche (Jung, 1953, p. 339).

While God is conceived of in many ways, the essential characteristic universally present for all is that God is infinitely more than human. This is central to the comfort to be derived from relatedness to God.

RELATEDNESS TO GOD: INTERVENTIONS

While God, in the many manifestations of religious belief, ancient and present, is always conceived of as greater than ourselves, there has also always been a corresponding conception that humans can act as instruments, or representatives, of God. Through one's own "spiritual" work, no matter if one is consciously "religious" or not, and despite whatever personal failings may exist, there is always the possibility of allowing our conception of God to work through us, or, as one Christian writer put it, of allowing "the Holy Spirit to touch another person through you" (Karns, 1991, p. 13). Working with love, care, respect, and diligence is the right way to practice with people who are dying, no matter what one's religious or non-religious persuasion. Working in this manner, with a "spiritual foundation," allows the concept of God that each person carries within them to touch another, something Karns called "the highest form of spiritual care" (1991, p. 12).

It goes without saying that this idea of working with a spiritual foundation is not the same thing as being religion's marketing department. In providing spiritual care, the message is the care itself, and not any effort to convince a patient to believe as someone else does.

FORGIVENESS OR ACCEPTANCE

A moral, or spiritual review of life on the part of someone who is dying generally uncovers the kind of defenses that help so many of us to get through painful situations in life. Suddenly, all the events, circumstances, and actions of a lifetime, including mistakes of commission and omission, are revealed to us. Guilt may become a central factor. Some see this process primarily as one related to sin, repentance, forgiveness, and punishment (Conrad, 1985), although for all of us, mistakes or sins—as defined by all major spiritual and moral belief systems—are a part of our lives.

It is important to remember, and to remind the patient, that some guilt experienced by people is related to events or circumstances completely beyond the control of the sufferer; for example, in the case of a parent whose child has died, or of adults who have psychologically survived the ordeals of childhood incest, or of growing up with alcoholic parents. In all of these examples, the adults are likely to experience terrible guilt due to a distorted sense of

their own sins or responsibilities in connection with the painful circumstances of their lives.

FORGIVENESS OR ACCEPTANCE: INTERVENTIONS

The concepts of forgiveness (common to the Judeo-Christian ethic) and acceptance (an explicit element of Hindu and Buddhist beliefs) are central to almost all faiths or religions, even though their interpretations may differ. For example, when working with Hindus and Buddhists in terminal situations, it may be more beneficial to think in terms of acceptance rather than forgiveness (see chapter 4 for a detailed review of the beliefs and practices of five major religions).

Whatever our own beliefs, or the beliefs of our patients, it is important to remember that we cannot confer forgiveness, and that teaching acceptance is a major challenge. What we *can* do is manifest forgiveness and acceptance through providing consistently loving care, and thereby hold out to the patient the possibility that forgiveness and acceptance can be found. No matter what our religious or non-religious persuasion, it is our duty to practice this form of charity. Moreover, by manifesting these qualities, we are, again, allowing the concept of God that we all carry within us to work through us and to touch others.

The idea of this form of intervention, which appears to be passive rather than active in nature, is a difficult one for many nurses, who are accustomed to operating as problem-solvers. A practitioner impatient to get at the "problem" often impedes the expression of spiritual needs like these. The patient's need of forgiveness and acceptance is a profound issue, very different in nature from other kinds of practical problems faced by nurses in their everyday work, and it cannot be resolved through the usual psychological and/or pharmacological channels. It can only be approached though our quality of care—through the example of our own charity.

TRANSCENDENCE

Transcendence is a quality of faith or spirituality that allows one to move beyond, to "transcend" what is given or presented in experience—in this case, the suffering and despair so often inherent in dying. Whether one believes in transcendence as God-given or as a personal achievement, it is the quality that can bring us victory over, and carry us beyond, suffering and death. Transcendence redefines limited views of life (including suffering and death) and relationships (including with self, others, and with God). (O'Conner, Wicker, & Germino, 1990.) Transcendence is the means by which one finds meaning "retroactively . . . even in a wasted life" (Frankl, 1969, pp. 76–77).

TRANSCENDENCE: INTERVENTIONS

Like the need for forgiveness, the need for transcendence is a profound issue that cannot be approached as a problem in need of "solving," and interventions here also are limited to what can be accomplished through a quality of care that is persevering and patient. It is important to keep in mind, however, that transcendence can happen when a person loves as much as is possible—especially when they do not feel like loving, and when their loving does not seem to "work." Then, sometimes, personal limitations may be overcome, and a new, or greater reality revealed.

Reflections on Providing Spiritual Care

Providing effective care in the spiritual process of dying includes the following responsibilities, eloquently expressed by Zerwekh (1991):

- listening;
- diagnosing distress of the human spirit; and

- affirming the ultimate importance of spiritual concerns at the end of life.

These responsibilities may be met through the practice of "watching" with a person in the final time of life. The "simple and costly demand" of watching is to remain in the presence of pain, suffering, and failure (Saunders, 1978, p. 8). Watching is an active, spiritual practice that includes awareness of the pain in life and death, the hope for healing (forgiveness), awareness of the concept of God, hope for the possibility of transcendence, and acceptance of whatever happens.

The personal qualities that are helpful in providing spiritual care include the following:

- REALISM: Death is the end of a life on earth—definite and final. It is no comfort to hear words of false hope or comfort that hide the truth.
- HOPEFULNESS: This encompasses the hope for a better life in the present and in the future.
- TRUTHFULNESS: It is neither helpful nor philosophically possible to provide "good" answers to every question about suffering and death. The need is greater than that of merely knowing "what" is happening and "why." What *is* necessary is our loving presence.
- CONVICTION, OR FAITH: In the "valley of the shadow of death," faith can prove to be the most exalted quality.
- RESOURCEFULNESS: To be able to use effectively whatever resources are available. Since each patient presents with unique life experiences and needs, a primary resource to always consider is each patient's individual beliefs and strengths. Other resources include rituals they believe in, and the presence, or acknowledgment, of key people in their lives.
- ADVOCACY: Spiritual needs may sometimes be neglected in the many events surrounding

dying. Hymns and communion, for example, are often forgotten by all concerned. Where possible and advisable (where the patient's faith is known to the practitioner and where the desire has been expressed or understood), practitioners should attempt to fulfill patients' spiritual needs.(see chapter 4 for a detailed review of the beliefs and practices of five major religions.)

- SENSITIVITY: Openness to and acceptance of the patient's uniqueness is essential to understanding the person and to providing care. Keep in mind that dying is not routine for the person going through it.

- OPENNESS AND EXPECTATION: Be prepared. Ask yourself, "What is the potential in this situation?" "How can it be experienced most fully, for the patient and for myself?" Consider how the inherent experience can become a "gift," both from ourselves to the patient and from the patient/situation to ourselves. Through the act of being present, or watching, even in the midst of suffering and failure of the spirit, the nurse becomes a potent symbol of the God who is within us, and with the patient.

References

Baylor University School of Nursing. (1991). *Report of self-study*. Dallas, Texas: Author.

Carse, J.P. (1980). *Death and existence*. New York: John Wiley and Sons.

Carson, V.B., & Green, H. (1992). Spiritual well-being: A predictor of hardiness in patients with acquired immunodeficiency syndrome. *Journal of Professional Nursing*. 8(4), 209–220.

Conrad, N.L. (1985). Spiritual support for the dying. *Nursing Clinics of North America*. 20(2), 415–425.

Corless, I.B. (1992). Hospice and hope: An incompatible duo. *The American Journal of Hospice and Palliative Care*. 9(3), 10–12.

Fackenheim, E.L. (1976). On faith in the secular world.
In A.H. Friedlander (Ed.), *Out of the whirlwind* (pp. 493–514). New York: Schocken Books.

Frankl, V. (1969). *The will to meaning*. New York: New American Library.

Friedlander, A.H. (1976). Introduction to the questions after the storm. In A.H. Friedlander (Ed.), *Out of the whirlwind* (pp. 462–464). New York: Schocken Books.

Green, J. (1989). Death with dignity: Hinduism. *Nursing Times*. 85(6), 50–51.

Jung, C.G. (1953). Psychology and alchemy. In J. Jacobi, R.F.C. Hull (Eds.), *C.G. Jung: Psychological reflections* (pp. 338–339). Princeton, New Jersey: Princeton University Press.

Kaczorowski, J.M. (1989). Spiritual well-being and anxiety in adults diagnosed with cancer. *Hospice Journal*. 5(3/4), 105–116.

Karns, P.S. (1991). Building a foundation for spiritual care. *Journal of Christian Nursing*. 8(3), 10–13.

The Koran. Translated by N.J. Dawood (1990). New York: Penguin Books.

Levine, S. (1984). *Meetings at the edge*. New York: Anchor Books.

McGuire, D.B., & Sheidler, V.R. (1990). Pain. In S.L. Groenwald, M.H. Frogge, M. Goodman, & C.H. Yarbro (Eds.), *Cancer nursing: Principles and practice* (3rd ed.) (pp. 385–441). Boston: Jones and Bartlett Publishers.

Miller, R.D., & Walsh, T.D. (1991). Psychosocial aspects of palliative care in advanced cancer. *Journal of Pain and Symptom Management*. 6(1), 24–29.

Nowotny, M.L. (1989). Assessment of hope in patients with cancer: Development of an instrument. *Oncology Nursing Forum*. 16(1), 57–61.

Nowotny, M.L. (1992). Strategies to facilitate hope relating to dying using the Nowotny hope scale subscales. Unpublished manuscript.

O'Conner, A.P., Wicker, C.A., & Germino, B.B. (1990). Understanding the cancer patient's search for meaning. *Cancer Nursing*. 13(3), 167–175.

Saunders, C.M. (1978). Appropriate treatment, appropriate death. In C.M. Saunders (Ed.), *The management of terminal disease*. London: Edward Arnold.

Stepnick, A., & Perry, T. (1992). Preventing spiritual distress in the dying client. *Journal of Psychosocial Nursing*. 30(1), 17–24.

Sullivan, H.S. (1953). *The interpersonal theory of psychiatry*. New York: Norton.

Zerwekh, J. (1991). Supportive care of the dying patient. In S.B. Baird, R. McCorkle, & M. Grant (Eds.), *Cancer nursing* (pp. 875–884). Philadelphia: W.B. Saunders.

Spiritual Care: Faiths

In connection with the material discussed in Chap. 3 under spiritual care, and to enhance the practitioner's store of useful information on these issues, this chapter will focus on major religions. The following sections summarize the basic beliefs or tenets, and outline the beliefs concerning dying and death, in five different faiths: Judaism, Christianity, Islam, Hinduism, and Buddhism. The material is presented with a caveat: it is impossible to fully understand and communicate another person's faith. There are many denominational or sectarian variations in every major religion, many of them fiercely disputed, and there are infinite individual variations. Nevertheless, the following information will provide a foundation for an initial understanding of the religious backgrounds of the many different individuals with whom we work.

Judaism

Jews are descended from the Patriarch Abraham and were known initially as Hebrews, or Israelites. About 1300 BC, Moses, "the Lawgiver" was, according to Jewish belief, told by God to lead the Israelites, "my people," out of Egypt, where they lived under oppressors:

Come, I will send you to Pharaoh that you may bring forth my people, the sons of Israel, out of Egypt...

EXODUS 3:10

Judaism was born in oppression, and persecution has been a constant theme throughout its history (Carse, 1980). The Holocaust was a defining event for Jews, and its relation to the spiritual, psychological, and social lives of Jews is not yet completely developed, nor is its present development fully understood. Suffice it to say, the Holocaust may have the potential to play a conscious or unconscious role in the spiritual and psychological responses to dying, suffering, and death among those of the Jewish faith.

TENETS OF THE FAITH

Central to Judaism are: belief in one God, the Ten Commandments, and the glorification of God through the practice of belief, as evidenced through individual comportment, personal work, family life, moral behavior, etc. (Ponn, 1991). Ritual, sacred literature, the Law, sacred institutions, and "the people, Israel" are among the key "strands" of Judaism (Steinberg, 1975, p. 3–4).

Charles Kemp: TERMINAL ILLNESS: A GUIDE TO NURSING CARE. © 1995 J. B. Lippincott.

The sacred literature of Judaism (Bradley, 1963) includes:

- The *Torah*, which is found in every synagogue: At least one copy is written in the original Hebrew, on parchment, and includes the first books of the Old Testament; Genesis, Exodus, Leviticus, Numbers, and Deuteronomy. The word "Torah" may also be taken to mean "all teachings of Judaism."
- The *Mishnah*, which is an interpretation of the Law by generations of Jewish scholars. The Mishnah provides direction for daily life.
- The *Talmud*, which gives further insight into the Law and is significantly longer than the Mishnah.

Scholarship has always been a hallmark of Judaism, whose scholars pursue philosophical efforts to understand and explicate the nature of God, man, evil, and similar profound issues.

BRANCHES OF JUDAISM

As with other religions, there are differences among and within the various branches of Judaism. The three main branches in the United States are *Reform, Conservative* and *Orthodox*. Reform Judaism is a modern interpretation of the religion and is an effort to adapt to Western society (Bradley, 1963). Ritual and Talmudic practices play a lesser role, while fundamental beliefs remain. Conservative Judaism hews closer to ritual and reinterprets the Law for the times and society, but does not seek assimilation. Orthodox Judaism holds strictly to Talmudic teachings and rules. Either through intent, or as a result of religious behavior, Orthodox Jews tend to mix less than their brethren with the non-Jewish population.

The Sabbath, the Jewish holy day corresponding to Christian Sunday, begins before nightfall on Friday and ends when the first three stars appear on Saturday evening. For some conservative Jews, and for all Orthodox Jews, writing, traveling, switching on non-essential electric appliances (lights are nonessential; suction machines are essential), elective surgical procedures, and other activities are forbidden during this time period each week. Dietary law for this segment of the Jewish population explicates what foods or combinations of foods may and may not be eaten. Kosher foods are those that are slaughtered, manufactured, or prepared under specific circumstances and conditions.

A rabbi is the ideal provider of spiritual care; however, it is appropriate for a person of another faith to read from the Torah section of the Old Testament, or from Psalms. Tradition directs the family to support and encourage the patient, including staying at the bedside (Gordon, 1975). There is disagreement about whether or not full knowledge should be shared with the patient. Both positions are supported in scripture (Heller, 1975). It is paramount to provide information and spiritual care in a manner that supports morale (Scherman, 1984).

Deathbed confession and repentance, and blessing and ethical instructions to the family or others present, are traditional. The following is the "minimum confession:"

I acknowledge (give thanks) before You, Hashem, my God and the God of my forefathers, that my recovery and death are in Your hand. May it be Your will that You heal me with total recovery, but, if I die, may my death be an atonement for all the errors, iniquities, and willful sins that I have erred, sinned, and transgressed before You. May You grant my share in the Garden of Eden, and privilege me for the World to Come that is concealed for the righteous...

(SCHERMAN, 1984, P. 795).

Meaning has long been a major philosophical question among Jews, and Victor Frankl, who brought the question of meaning into focus for many non-Jews, developed his philosophy in a Nazi concentration camp. Hope for Jews includes the hope for "the people, Israel," for justice, for the Messiah to come, for reunification or reconciliation with God, and for the resurrection to come (Gordon, 1975; Heller, 1975; Ponn, 1991). As among people of other faiths, there are infinite variations of what is hoped for. Relatedness is clearly with God, who "chose" the Jews as his people. Forgiveness is asked in the deathbed confessional, and transcendence is found in the outcome of the lifelong struggle between good and evil.

IMMEDIATE AFTERCARE

The deceased person's eyes should be closed immediately after death, preferably by one of the person's children. The body should be straightened and covered. Some families will request that the body not be moved on the Sabbath. Autopsy is opposed but permitted, but no part of the body should be removed. Organ transplants are acceptable only after consultation with a rabbi. Burial should be within 24 hours of death, except that burial should not be on the Sabbath. Autopsy and related activities should be concluded quickly.

FUNERAL AND BURIAL PRACTICES

Most synagogues or communities have a burial society with whom certain funeral homes cooperate. This volunteer group prepares the bodies of members of the congregation according to Jewish law. "Death is death" in Jewish belief, and thus some of the trappings of Western funerals, such as cosmetics on the body, viewing the body, satin-lined coffins, and artificial turf around the grave, are unacceptable (Gordon, 1975, p. 47). The *Kaddish*, a formal ritual of prayer that praises God and extends through a number of days after the death, is said at the cemetery and elsewhere.

May He give reign to His Kingship in your lifetimes and in your days, and in the lifetimes of the entire family of Israel, swiftly and soon. Now respond Amen.

FROM THE MOURNER'S KADDISH.

Some hospice principles, to a remarkable extent, mirror Jewish mourning customs. There is a prescribed period of mourning, during which grief is expressed openly and in keeping with ritual. The first period of mourning is called *shivah*, and is divided into three days of deep grief, followed by seven days of mourning. During this time, personal adornment and vanities, including shaving, are forbidden, as are trivial discussions about matters other than the issue at hand. There are then thirty days of readjustment, followed by eleven months of remembrance and gradual healing. After a year, there is a ceremony during which the name of the person who died is inscribed in a room in the synagogue.

Christianity

Christianity began approximately 2,000 years ago with, according to Christian beliefs, the birth, teachings and miracles, crucifixion, and finally the resurrection of Jesus Christ (revealed in Christian scripture as the Son of God), all recounted in the New Testament, which, together with the Old Testament, constitute the Bible. Each of the events in Christ's life is enormously significant to Christians and may be generally summarized in the following beliefs:

- The birth of Christ occurred according to Old Testament prophecy:

  Therefore the Lord himself will give you a sign. Behold, a young woman (a virgin) shall conceive and bear a son, and shall call his name Eman'u-el...

  ISAIAH 7:14

Debora Hunter

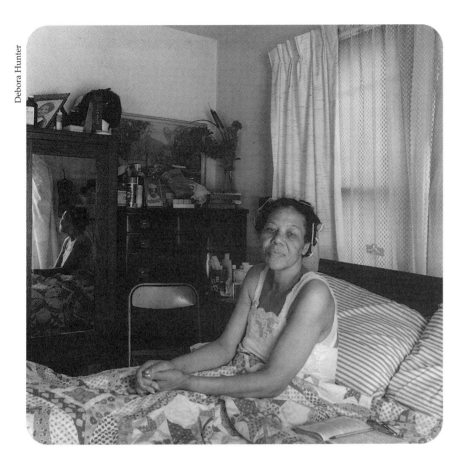

- The meaning of Christ's teachings, as recounted in the Bible, are sometimes hidden in "parables," but some also are direct and unmistakable:

  I am the resurrection and the life; he who believes in me, though he die, yet shall he live, and whoever lives and believes in me shall never die…

  JOHN 11:25–26

- A belief in the occurrence of miracles, like those wrought by Christ in the Bible, regarded by some as central to the faith, and by others primarily as illustrations of God's power.

- The crucifixion of Jesus Christ, which is described in the New Testament both as a religious-political torture and execution, and as the fulfillment of divine prophecy. The cross, on which Christ was crucified, is Christianity's powerful, primary symbol, representing both suffering and death and the hope of life everlasting, through the sacrifice of the Son of God.

- The resurrection of Christ, the greatest of the Christian miracles, which confirms Christian belief in life everlasting. After three days in his tomb, Christ rose from the dead, appeared and spoke to the disciples, was taken up into heaven, and sat down at the right hand of God (Mark 16:9–19).

The ultimate meaning of the death of Jesus Christ (God's sacrifice of His son) for Christianity is that salvation is available, through grace, for all those who believe in Christ. Christianity posits the universal presence of sin and offers a way, through belief in Christ's death and resurrection, of transcendence through God's forgiveness.

The Bible is considered by Christians to be the revelation of God. There are divisions within Christianity about whether the words of the Bible are meant to be understood in a literal fashion, or interpreted. There are two major groupings and numerous denominations within Christianity, and further divisions within these, some involved in serious dispute with one another about who truly represents "real Christians." The two major groupings are Protestants and Catholics (whose adherents believe in the "infallibility" of their highest spiritual leader, the Pope, who resides in the Vatican.)

The two important "sacraments" (or religious rituals) for Protestants are baptism and holy communion. Holy communion, or the "Lord's supper," should be made available to consenting Christians who are dying. Participating in this rite can have a healing effect on those who feel isolated or estranged. The Catholic sacraments most relevant in dying are the anointing of the sick and the holy Eucharist, the Catholic communion. These two rituals, along with confession to a priest, should be made available to consenting Catholics. Prayer and reading from the Bible are appropriate forms of spiritual care for all Christians. Passages that are most comforting include:

- Psalm 23: *The Lord is my shepherd*, preceded, perhaps, for a patient who is deep in a spiritual crisis of anger or estrangement, by one of the lament Psalms, e.g., Psalm 22: *My God, my God, why hast thou forsaken me?* The lament Psalms include 13, 38, 51, and many others.

- John 11:25–26: *I am the resurrection and the life . . .*
- John 14:1–4: "Let not your hearts be troubled . . ."
- I Corinthians 15:54–56: "O death, where is thy victory?"
- Matthew 6:9–13: "Our Father who art in heaven . . ."

The above passages, and many others, can be offered to consenting Christians as a simple recitation of sacred words—as an opportunity for opening themselves to the common connectedness and deep feeling inherent in ancient writings. Audio tapes of sacred music can also be very effective in providing spiritual support and connection with the "great community of faith."

A basic spiritual need for Christians includes the idea of persistent meaning in life—mainly a Western concept, and controversial at best, since the meaning of many lives may be small, or even negative. Christian faith, however, promises its believers that, through grace, meaning can be found for any life.

Hope in Christianity exists explicitly for personal salvation and for God's forgiveness, through faith.

Relatedness is to a personal God and Savior. It is essential to remember that any person of faith—any patient or any professional—can be deeply troubled by the inevitable moments when God, hope, grace, transcendence—all seem hidden, and the relatedness seems absent. In this case, Christian belief urges faithful perseverance, or "constant witness" (doing what you don't want to do when you don't want to do it) as a way of living the "unfelt faith," and as an alternative to despair.

Forgiveness of sin through acceptance of Christ is central to Christianity. It is through their belief in forgiveness and grace that Christians, according to the tenets of their faith, can transcend self, sin, and suffering.

Islam

Islam is based on the Word of God as revealed to the Prophet Muhammed in about 610 AD, and the adherents of this faith are known as Muhammedans, or Muslims. Islam repudiated the religious practices of Arabs at the time Muhammad received this revelation. It also repudiates the Christian belief in a Son of God. The scripture of Islam is the Koran, or Al Qur'an, which is believed to be infallible and unequivocal.

Islam has several main divisions, including those between fundamentalists and secularists; significant "denominations" of Sunni and Shi`a Muslims; and various schools, or sects, within the larger divisions.

The basic belief of all Muslims is in One God, *Allah:*

God! There is no god but Him, the Living, the Ever-existent one…

KORAN. THE IMRANS 3:1

This belief in One God, in Allah, is central to all Muslim belief (Rahman, 1966). Muslims also believe in angels, in Satan, in the *jinn* (spirits), in the Day of Reckoning and Heaven and Hell, and in the Prophets (e.g., Abraham, Moses, Jesus, and Muhammad—the Messenger of God). Both Judaism and Christianity are recognized by Islam, but not accepted, since Islam (like some other religions) rejects those faiths that do not acknowledge their most sacred beliefs—in this case, God's word as revealed to Muhammad.

TENETS OF ISLAM

Also central to Islam are the "five pillars of faith." These are (1) faith in the one God, (2) prayer five times each day, (3) alms-giving, (4) fasting (on holy days, from sunrise through sundown), principally during Ramadan, the yearly Muslim religious celebration, which lasts for one month during springtime, and (5) making a pilgrimage, known as the *hajj*, to the Islamic holy city of Mecca (the birthplace of Muhammad, in Saudi Arabia) whenever possible in one's lifetime (Cavendish, 1980). Friday is the most important day of worship for Muslims. Women and men are segregated during almost all religious and social events.

Marital and family relationships, individual behavior, prayer, and many other aspects of daily life are definitively prescribed by Islam, backed up by the teachings in Al Qur'an, which, unlike the Bible, is quite straightforward in its approach and written by the same hand, leaving little room for interpretation or discussion about whether or not it is the direct Word of God.

Cleanliness is a major issue for Muslims, who believe in washing their mouths, hands, and feet at least five times each day, before the five required daily prayer times. Showering is preferred over bathing and modesty is extremely important. Health care and personal hygiene care provided by persons of a different gender may be distressing to Muslims.

Dietary restrictions include pork and any meat not slaughtered according to custom. During Ramadan, Muslims fast from sun-up to sun-down each day of the month. Some interpret fasting to include all medicines, while others allow medicines during the day.

Family members and friends remain with the sick person 24 hours a day, and a close relative may even sit in bed with the patient. Most patients prefer to lie down facing Mecca. Consenting Muslim patients should be provided with the opportunity to confess their sins on their deathbeds, and other interventions would include making the Al Qur'an and/or readings from it available to consenting patients. Prayers are offered by family members or friends during the dying process and afterwards.

Spiritual needs of Muslims can be met, or addressed, as follows. Individualistic meaning in life, at least in the Western sense, is not a major issue in Islam. Hope is available in abundance for true believers in Allah, and in the words of the Al Qur'an. Relatedness to God is both clear and prescriptive and, according to Bradley (1963), the Muslim faith has more power in this sense than any other religion—in Islam, there is no doubt about who God is and who man is. Forgiveness is available, but exclusively for believers.

He accepts the repentance of His servants, and pardons their sins. He has knowledge of all your actions.

(KORAN, COUNSEL 42:25)

"When will the Day of Judgment be?' they ask. On that day they shall be scourged in the Fire, and a voice will say to them: 'Taste this, the punishment which you have sought to hasten!'"

(KORAN, THE WINDS 51:3)

Islam, like Christianity, also posits the resurrection of the body, final judgment, and assignment to heaven or hell. Transcendence is readily available for all Muslims who are undoubting, true believers.

AFTERCARE, FUNERAL AND BURIAL PRACTICES

Non-Muslims should not touch the body. Among some Muslims, the family is responsible for washing and preparing the body, and with others, a designated person from the community performs this function. Autopsies are permitted, but resisted. Organ donation is not allowed. The funeral should take place within 24 hours of death, and bodies are buried, preferably in a Muslim cemetary.

Hinduism

Hinduism is an ancient religion intimately intertwined with the development of life and culture in its birthplace, India. The practice of Hinduism as an organized, historical system began about 5,000 years ago. The sacred literature of Hinduism includes the earlier *Vedas* and the more recent (beginning in about 800–300 BC) *Upanishads*. There are numerous other examples of Hindu literature, notably, the *Bhagavad-Gita*, an epic of war and devotion.

TENETS OF HINDUISM

Hinduism has no creed or founder. It is a devotional theism (or belief in superhuman powers), taking a number of forms, with a philosophical background and a social system based on the concept of function, or *karma* (cause and effect in all action or inaction) and on "caste" observances. Hinduism depends on what a person is and does, on social conduct, rather than on any one belief. Most Hindus also believe in transmigration of the soul, or reincarnation (*samsara*) and look forward to an ultimate salvation (*nirvana*) in the form of release from the cycle of rebirth and death.

The popular practice of Hinduism incorporates numerous gods (diversity of belief is regarded as natural and inevitable), with one god singled out (usually according to sect) for most of the devotion. Practices include prayer and worship of images of gods in temples or private chapels, the making of pilgrimages, a belief in asceticism and the efficacy of yoga, and honoring and seeking the teachings of highly respected *guru*, or holy men.

The rigidity of the caste system, based on the idea that people are born to be what they are and that they cannot be anything else, and of other similarly confining Vedic beliefs regarding hope for a better life, helped promote the development of various sects (of which there are a large number, the most important being the Vaishnava, Saiva, and Shakta), some of which offer increased hope of salvation through devotion (Bradley, 1963).

Give me your whole heart,
Love and adore me,
Worship me always,
Bow to me only,
And you shall find me:
This is my promise
Who love you dearly.

(BHAGAVAD-GITA (A), P. 129)

The goal of Hinduism, i.e., salvation, is release of the *atman* or soul, from the endless cycles of suffering inherent in life. Many Hindus also adhere to dietary law (usually a strict vegetarian diet).

Hindu patients exhibit a strong preference for dying at home (Green, 1989b), which can result in decisions that, from a medical perspective, may seem incompatible with the patient's best interest. Some, who have the financial resources, will go back to India, to the sacred city, Varanasi, to die. Prayer, recitations, and hymns from Hindu scripture are appropriate in the process of dying. The presence of a Hindu priest is comforting. Health care staff should expect the priest to interact with them, with the patient, or with the family in a different way than would clergy from Western religions. Rituals surrounding dying and death include prayer and chanting, use of string and lustral water, and touching the patient with various objects (Green, 1989b).

Hinduism can be disconcerting for Westerners because it is so outside the experience of most non-Hindus. Hindus do not believe in proselytizing, and there has been little attempt to spread Hinduism among other peoples. Nor has there been much enthusiasm among Hindus to assimilate; inter-marriage is extremely rare. The spiritual needs around which this chapter is partially structured might be addressed by a Hindu as follows:

- The meaning of life is devotion to God.
- Acceptance of fate is central to Hinduism. One also hopes for a better life and, ultimately, for release from rebirth.

- Everything is related. Relatedness to God (as manifested in devotion to one of the pantheon of gods) is very personal.
- There is no forgiveness; there is acceptance, and results (of one's behavior).

Transcendence (enlightenment) is explicit in Hinduism and may be explained in this way:

When, however, one is enlightened with the knowledge by which nescience is destroyed, then his knowledge reveals everything, as the sun lights up everything in the daytime.

(BHAGAVAD-GITA (B), TEXT 20: 16)

IMMEDIATE AFTER-CARE

The family is responsible for washing and preparing the body, and most families prefer that others do not touch the body. If family is unavailable, the eyes should be closed, limbs straightened, and the body wrapped in a plain sheet without emblems of other religions. Autopsies are permitted, but resisted.

FUNERAL AND BURIAL PRACTICES

Funeral ceremonies should occur within 24 hours of death. Cremation is the means of disposing of the body, and embalming is undesirable. If possible, the oldest son should break the skull of the deceased so that the soul is easily released.

Buddhism

Buddhism began in the 6th century BC, both as a reform of Hinduism and as a response to the human condition, to the suffering epitomized by illness, aging, and death. The founder of Buddhism was Gautama Siddharta, the Buddha (which means "the awakened," "the enlightened").

TENETS OF BUDDHISM

Belief in the Four Noble Truths is central to Buddhism. These are:

- All sentient beings suffer. Birth, illness, death, and other separations are inescapably part of life.
- The cause of suffering is desire. Desire is manifested by attachment to life, to security, to others. Most specifically the desire "to be" (Carse, 1980).
- The way to end suffering is to cease to desire.
- The way to cease to desire is to follow the Eightfold Path: (1) right belief (2) right intent (3) right speech (4) right conduct (5) right endeavor or livelihood (6) right effort (7) right mindfulness (8) right meditation.

Following the path leads to cessation of desire and to nirvana, or emancipation from rebirth.

Buddhism teaches tolerance of others and acceptance of life (non-attachment). The moral code of Buddhism is similar to the Ten Commandments of the Bible (Waddell, 1972). The principle of karma (or *kamma*) is basic to the practice of Buddhism. Karma is popularly interpreted as a moral precept: do right and you will be reborn into a higher state; do wrong and rebirth will be to a lower state. Karma is neither reward nor punishment, but simply cause and effect. In practice, life's misfortunes are often attributed to sins in this or in a previous lifetime.

DIVISIONS OF BUDDHISM

There are two primary divisions in Buddhism, *Theravada Buddhism*, which is practiced most often by people from Thailand, Cambodia, Laos, Burma, and Sri Lanka; and *Mahayana Buddhism*, or the "greater vehicle," which is practiced most often by people from Vietnam, China, Japan, and Tibet. Mahayana Buddhism includes the Zen Buddhism of Japan, the Lamaism of Tibet, and a uniquely Chinese form of Buddhism. In Theravada Buddhism, nirvana is achievable only through complete renunciation (non-attachment) and through living as a monk. The Buddha is "revered, not as a god but as one who has shown the way" (Bradley, 1963, p. 116). In practice, among the laity, the reverence is like that shown to a god. In some branches of Mahayana Buddhism, nirvana is possible for non-monks, and among lay persons there appears to be a greater belief in (often multiple) gods, in heaven, and in hell. Monks are more apt to view these as states of mind.

Belief in magic is common among some Buddhists, especially people from the Theravada countries of Thailand, Cambodia, and Laos, and also among Tibetans. Magico-religious practices are well-integrated into Buddhism, and include use of amulets, spells, and the presence and power of spirits.

The Buddha did not discuss the presence or absence of God; nor did he answer questions about death. On the question of immortality, the Buddha gave the "fourfold denial":

A saint is after death,
A saint is not after death,
A saint is and is not after death,
A saint neither is nor is not after death.

(QUOTED BY CARSE, 1980)

Buddhist scholars thus see four possibilities regarding life after death; the less scholarly, the majority of Buddhists, are likely to believe in rebirth with station, according to deeds.

A key issue in dying for many Buddhist patients and families is to maintain consciousness so that patients may "fill their minds with wholesome thoughts." Wholesome thoughts include awareness of the transient nature of what we view as existence, contemplation of past "good efforts," and being willing to "let go of life without clinging and grasping" (Ratanakul, 1991, p. 396). A quiet place for dying is preferred to a noisy or busy unit. A monk or lay religious leader may chant or lead chants to help promote a peaceful or insightful state of mind at death (Green, 1989a). Incense may be burned and amulets, including images of the Buddha, may be present as the person dies and afterward.

Some of the spiritual needs around which this chapter is structured may seem to apply less directly to Buddhists than to others. Meaning, for example, may be seen as illusion, while Emptiness, or the Void, are seen as real (The Diamond Sutra, p. 29). Emptiness is not in any way the nihilistic emptiness sometimes ascribed to this belief by non-Buddhists (Suzuki, 1968), but rather the "universal causal relatedness" of existence (Carse, 1980, p. 139). Relatedness is not to God, but to the "all." Hope is leavened with acceptance and sometimes passivity, but hope for a better life now, a better next-life, and for a better life for (one's) children is strong. Further, Buddhism is explicitly based on the hope of cessation of suffering. What then is there to transcend? For lay persons, a form of forgiveness, i.e., improved karma, is possible through merit. Practitioners of Zen Buddhism, on the another hand, live "beyond . . . the limitations of time, relativity, causality, morality, and so on" (Suzuki, 1956, p. 265).

Immediate Aftercare

Organ transplant and autopsy are permitted. Non-Buddhists may touch the body, and there is no particular belief about how the body should be treated.

Funeral and Burial Practices

Funeral and related practices vary according to the branch of Buddhism and to individual inclinations. Cremation is preferred by some and burial by others. Ideally, in many cases, the body should be kept at home for a day or more so that proper ceremonies may be conducted. The temple is another site for ceremonies. Most ceremonial activity is conducted at home, in a temple, or at grave or cremation sites, and less at funeral home chapels. Funeral ceremonies may be held a day or so after the death, and subsequent, but related ceremonies held again in a week or a month, or at other intervals. In some cases, ceremonies are delayed until the family saves enough money to conduct a proper ceremony.

Thus shall ye think of all this fleeting world:
A star at dawn, a bubble in a stream;
A flash of lightening in a summer cloud;
A flickering lamp, a phantom, and a dream.

THE DIAMOND SUTRA (OF THE BUDDHA), P. 74

References

Bhagavad-Gita (a). Translated by Swami Prabhavananda & C. Isherwood. (1951). New York: Mentor Religious Classics.

Bhagavad-Gita (b). Translated and interpreted by A.C. Bhaktivedanta Swami Prabhupada. (1972). New York: The Bhaktivedanta Book Trust.

The Bible. Revised Standard edition.

Bradley, D.G. (1963). *A Guide to the world's religions.* Englewood Cliffs, New Jersey: Prentice-Hall.

Carse, J.P. (1980). *Death and existence.* New York: John Wiley and Sons.

Cavendish, R. (1980). *The great religions.* New York: Arco. *The Diamond sutra and sutra of Hui Neng.* Translated by A.F. Price & W. Mou-Lam. (1969). Berkeley: Shambala.

Green, J. (1989a). Death with dignity: Buddhism. *Nursing Times.* 85(9), 40–41.

Green, J. (1989b). Death with dignity: Hinduism. *Nursing Times.* 85(6), 50–51.

Gordon, A. (1975). The Jewish view of death: Guidelines for mourning. In E. Kubler-Ross (Ed.), *Death: The Final Stage of Growth* (pp. 38–43). Englewood Cliffs, New Jersey: Prentice-Hall, Inc.

Heller, Z.I. (1975). The Jewish view of death: Guidelines for dying. In E. Kubler-Ross (Ed.), *Death: The final stage of growth* (pp. 38–43). Englewood Cliffs, New Jersey: Prentice-Hall, Inc.

The Koran. Translated by N.J. Dawood (1990). New York: Penguin Books.

Ponn, A.L. (1991). Judaism. In C.J. Johnson & M.G. McGee (Eds.) *How different religions view death* (pp. 205–227). Philadelphia: The Charles Press.

Rahman, F. (1966). *Islam.* New York: Holt, Rinehart, and Winston.

Ratanakul, P. (1991). Buddhism: Discussion of dying with dignity. In M. Abivan (Facilitator), Dying with

Dignity. (pp. 395–397). *World Health Forum. 12*(4), 375–399.

Scherman, N. (1984). *The complete art scroll Siddur.* New York: Mesorah Publications.

Steinberg, M. (1975). *Basic Judaism.* New York: Harcourt Brace Jovanovich Publishers.

Suzuki, D.T. (1956). *Zen Buddhism.* Garden City, New York: Doubleday Anchor Books.

Suzuki, D.T. (1968). *On Indian Mahayana Buddhism.* New York: Harper Torchbooks.

Waddell, L.A. (1972). *Tibetan Buddhism.* London: Dover Publications.

Sociocultural Care

We have all heard the lines from Rudyard Kipling's "Ballad of East and West":

Oh, East is East and West is West, and never the twain shall meet,
Till Earth and Sky stand presently at God's great Judgement Seat.

Most take this to mean that differences between dissimilar worlds or cultures are too great for understanding or meeting—at least until judgment day. But Kipling had more to say on the matter.

But there is neither East nor West, Border, nor Breed, nor Birth,
When two strong men stand face to face, tho' they come from the ends of the earth!

(KIPLING, 1930)

Of course there are differences, sometimes vast differences, among cultures. And sometimes it seems that they will not be resolved until, as Kipling said, we stand at "God's great Judgment Seat." Yet through strength, knowledge, understanding, tolerance, and good will, we can often meet across great cultural distances.

Great variations exist among all cultures, both in individual behavior, family structures, and community behavior. The purpose of this chapter is to give providers of care to the terminally ill a start toward a better understanding of the sociocultural differences among distinct groups in our society—some things to look for, or some pitfalls to avoid. The central goal in transcultural nursing is not to completely understand all cultures with whom we come into contact, but rather to:

- be sensitive to and aware of the beliefs and practices of individuals, families, and populations; and
- to learn to fit the care with those beliefs and practices.

The concept of culture includes the common "values, norms, beliefs, and practices of a particular group" (Pickett, 1993, p. 104). Culture is affected by ethnicity, socialization, religion, and other forces (Spector, 1991), including common experiences. Interested readers are referred to Spector (1991) and Leininger (1978) for a more detailed discussion of this concept.

In seeking to understand cultural values, it is important to remember that we live in a time of significant social upheaval. This may be represented, for example, by the fact that the cen-

Charles Kemp: TERMINAL ILLNESS: A GUIDE TO NURSING CARE. © 1995 J. B. Lippincott.

tral role of the family in many cultures is not only recognized but continually reaffirmed by our political and cultural institutions and yet, in many instances, family systems, regardless of ethnicity or culture, are barely functional.

In order to understand another and to learn to adapt oneself to his or her beliefs, it is necessary first to know oneself and to understand one's own culture. Each one of us is a product of our own conscious and unconscious psychological makeup and we carry this psychological "baggage" with us to every encounter—including patient-care encounters. We also carry with us conscious and unconscious cultural values that affect how we interpret what we see, hear, smell, and feel.

An overview of cultural views of health problems is helpful in assessing patients and families from diverse cultures. There are a number of tools available to accomplish this, but few are as functional and elegant as the work of Tripp-Reimer, Brink, and Saunders (1984). Answers to some or all of the following (slightly modified) questions to address to patients, developed by these authors, provide important insight into the different cultural perceptions of patients or family regarding health problems:

- What do you think caused your problem?
- Do you have an explanation for why it started when it did?
- What does your sickness do to you; how does it work?
- How severe is your sickness? How long do you expect it to last?
- What problems has your sickness caused you?
- What do you fear about your sickness?
- What kind of treatment do you think you should receive?
- What are the most important results you hope to receive from this treatment?

Tripp-Reimer, Brink, and Saunders suggest other questions, but given the realities of time constraints in providing care, the above are likely to be sufficient.

Information in regard to particular patients and families may be found in more than one of the sections of this chapter; for example, refugees and illegal immigrants are covered in one section but additional information for particular patients in this category can also be found in the culture-specific sections.

Native Americans

There are approximately two million Native Americans living in the United States, and the number is growing (World Almanac, 1992). There are more than 300 tribes speaking at least 200 languages, and there are significant similarities as well as differences among them. One of the unfortunate similarities is that, as a whole, Native Americans have poor morbidity and mortality rates, as well as other negative health indicators (Lewis, 1990).

Native Americans are, in some ways, less assimilated into the prevailing culture of the United States than are other minority groups, and many of them exhibit at most a marginal interest in the mainstream culture. Their life here today, when compared with memories of their past traditions, culture, and history, are a potent reminder of what has been lost; and of what is unlikely to ever be fully regained.

The extended family is the primary social unit among Native Americans. The tribe to which a family belongs is usually important in both individual and family life. Native Americans may view the health care system, and Western culture as a whole, as separate from Native American life, and thus undesirable—especially, for some, at the end of life.

Many Native American religious beliefs and practices are animist, and spirits and other supernatural phenomena are as real to many Native Americans as are microorganisms to other people. They may often view health problems as caused by spiritual forces—as much or more than they are caused by other agents. Diagnosing and healing are thus often sought from traditional, or spiritual, healers (Spector, 1991). There is also a belief that healing may be accomplished through ceremony, herbal remedies, or both.

Alcoholism is a common social ill among Native Americans. This is sometimes attributed to differences in alcohol metabolism (see Hanley, 1991), but may also be viewed in the context of unmet spiritual and cultural needs, such as hope, meaning, and relatedness. Alcoholism relates to terminal illness both as a contributing factor to the leading causes of death (Spector, 1991) and as a complicating factor in providing care.

Stoicism is a deeply-held value. Some Native Americans will deny pain or other problems; even, in some cases, in response to direct questions. History-taking may be viewed as intrusive and irrelevant. Cultural values of tribal or group interdependence, and their estrangement from the health care system, are often such that there is significant delay in seeking care. Communication problems existing between the United States' health care system and Native Americans include the following:

- Difficulty in speech communication: Native Americans are accustomed to speaking in a tone of voice whose volume level is much lower than that usually expected in clinic, hospital and other health care institutions.
- Differences in behavioral habits: Native Americans are accustomed to expecting a degree of intuitive ability in their interlocutors; in their culture, people do not look directly into others' eyes; and they are unaccustomed to seeing others take notes on their responses during an interaction (Spector, 1991).

Some Native Americans, especially the more traditional-minded, view death as a companion, and as an integral link in the chain of life. Attitudes or approaches vary among tribes; some are very accepting of death and others view dying people and death with fear (Lewis, 1990). Some wish their family members to die at home; others prefer a hospital setting. Suffering is a "major value in Indian culture" (Lewis, 1990, p. 28) and dying and grief may be met with stoicism and silence. Thus, the idea of sharing feelings may be rejected by the patient.

Asian Americans

The term "Asian American" is a good illustration of how people of enormous variation often are lumped together as one homogeneous group. Asian Americans include Cambodians, Chinese from China and "overseas" Chinese (or those who emigrate to the United States from previous locations of immigration), Indians, Japanese, Koreans, Lao (lowland and tribal), Filipinos, Taiwanese, Thais, Vietnamese— including Amerasians, or those of mixed Vietnamese-American descent—and others.

Some Asian Americans emigrated as businessmen, some as educators, and some as peasants; some are now businessmen and businesswomen, educators, or laborers. Some are Theravada Buddhist, some Mahayana Buddhist, some Shinto, some Catholic, some Protestant, some Hindu, some Muslim, and some (Chinese and Vietnamese) are influenced by a combination of Buddhism, Taoism, Confucianism, and ancestor worship (Ta & Chung, 1990). Asian Americans speak many different languages, and, in some cases, significant intolerance exists between different groups. Some disputes, e.g., that existing between Chinese and Vietnamese, can be traced back to events that occurred over a thousand years ago; some disputes are very recent. These differences are seldom revealed to health-care professionals. Despite the many differences, however, there are some similarities, and generalizations exist that often apply across different Asian cultures. These last are especially relevant in the case of first-generation immigrants and refugees.

Asian Americans, in comparison to most cultural groups in the United States, are taciturn (or customarily disinclined to speak) in extra-familial situations. Equanimity is highly valued among them. Pain, especially emotional pain, may be not be expressed, or may be indirectly expressed through such means as excoriating skin or dermabrasion. Withdrawal is far more common than complaint. Withdrawal also occurs when people are offended; and it is seldom helpful to try to talk about the offense with the person who withdraws. In general, if you want to know if there is a problem, you must ask about that specific problem; and by the same token, if you want to know the effects of a particular medication or treatment, you must ask specifically about what you want to know about. General questions such as "How are you?" and "How is it going?" almost always ellicit a meaningless response such as, "Fine, thank you." Sharing deep feelings, especially those that may be negative, is uncommon.

"Yes" or "no" questions are often a source of misunderstanding and should be avoided. A "yes" answer may mean either agreement, acknowledgment that the question is heard, or simply that the person would rather say "yes" than "no."

The family unit tends to be more important operationally among Asian Americans than it is in Western cultures, and whenever possible, the family should be included in decision making. Failure to do so may mean failure of the treatment, or that no decision will be made. Women are sometimes unable to make a decision without consulting their husbands. Mothers-in-law, despite appearances to the contrary, frequently wield tremendous power. Children are often pampered, but are expected to obey instantly and without argument. The choices and the freedom given to native-born American children are astonishing to most first-generation Asians. Using children to translate for adults should usually be avoided.

Asian Americans often are viewed as passive and accepting of fate. In fact, when nothing

can be changed, they tend to accept the situation. But when there is hope for change, Asian-Americans tend to be remarkably tenacious.

Chinese civilization and its religious-cultural concepts have influenced almost all Asian cultures (although some non-Chinese deny this) and their views of health and illness. The Chinese concept of balance (*yin-yang*, or the principle of the masculine and the feminine; the creative and the receptive, etc.) is universal, although it may be expressed through saying a food, drink, illness, or treatment is "hot" or "cold." Hot and cold here refer to yin or yang, respectively, and to intrinsic properties, not to temperature. Balance may also be related to the bodily "humors" such as blood, bile, and phlegm. Southeast Asians, and Chinese in particular, believe in troublesome "winds" in the body. Attempts to confer with patients about yin and yang, and so on, are unlikely to be successful. Magico-religious amulets, strings, statues, and other items are common among some, and their power or validity should not be discounted. Spirit possession is a reality for many Cambodians, Lao, Thai, and Vietnamese (author, 1985). Herbal remedies, Chinese and others, are widely available in the United States and may be used along with, or in place of, Western medicines (Wilson & Ryan, 1991).

Terminal illness for Asian Americans often brings unusually overwhelming nostalgia and sadness, especially in the case of refugees. Dreams of flying home are common. The stark reality is that they will die in a strange land that often seems uncaring and disrespectful. Hospitals and treatments are stranger still. For many Southeast Asians, talking about the possibility of dying brings bad luck (Lang, 1990).

Some family members, especially if the family is not well-educated, are likely to stay away from the terminally ill person for fear of contracting the disease, or for other reasons. This can be very distressing for the staff involved with such a case. Generally, however, the family usually stays close by the patient at all times. Failure to do so may also be due to problems of transportation or to misunderstanding about what is permitted. Communication with Western staff members may be limited by language and/or cultural reluctance to express personal feelings (Wilson & Ryan, 1990).

African Americans

The history of our nation has been such that, for a variety of reasons (by some, still bitterly debated), African Americans tend to be poorer, die sooner, and have a higher prevalence of AIDS, especially among women and children, than do most other cultural populations in the United States (Cherry & Giger, 1991). Many African Americans share in common feelings of resentment toward and opposition against racism, perceived as a collective and central issue of life. Interaction with others is sometimes inhibited by the natural effects of this perception, compounded and reinforced by the still-existing though attenuated prejudices in our society; by others' lack of knowledge about African Americans, their history, and their culture; and by racial politics that seek constantly to exploit racial divisions.

Assimilation, especially in economic terms, into the dominant, mainstream culture has been a very slow process in the case of African Americans. Many native-born African Americans today are in a state of tremendous transition and self-definition. Other African Americans came to the United States relatively recently, after generations spent in other, diverse cultures, bringing with them other particular traditions and cultural values (from the West Indies, from South and Central America, etc.).

Since the Civil Rights Movement began, over 25 years ago, many African Americans have moved up the socioeconomic-political ladder while others, except for the presence of an appliance or two, remain essentially where they were, 150 years ago. There also exists some friction in relations between African Americans and other ethnic groups, including recent arrivals whose ability to establish businesses and find jobs is resented by some. As is the case, however, for many sociocultural groups adapting to life in the United States, a rise in social (i.e., economic) status usually serves to level many seemingly diverse characteristics; in terms of attitudes toward health care and technology, for example, middle-class African Americans tend to be very similar to any other middle-class group.

Protestantism—often Baptist, or one of a number of other smaller, or fundamentalist denominations—is a common religion. Religious faith and church congregations and institutions have traditionally been extremely important in the African American community, and often functioned as their only viable political force in or outside the community. While still a powerful force, Christianity now has a rival in the Muslim faith. The number of African American Muslims (both from the traditional Muslim faith and members of the Muslim-inspired Nation of Islam) is growing, and they provide a strong moral voice in the African American community. The Pan-Africanism movement is endeavoring to build a universal African culture among African Americans through rediscovery and reaffirmation of traditional cultural practices and ideals and, for example, recently introduced *Kwanzaa*, a system of life values celebrated during the Christmas season, from December 26 through January first.

One of the most cited obstructions to the advancement of African Americans has been the persistence of the "single parent, female head of household" family structure (most predominantly among the poor), which presents a challenge to everyone involved in a terminal illness situation. A common family scenario involves a dying parent, cared for by a daughter, who is also a single parent—an extreme burden on both mother and children. Even when families are intact, socioeconomic factors often prohibit working members of the family from being present during the dying process.

Another common situation, however, is an older woman caring for her husband and several live-in grandchildren. One of the positive aspects of this situation is that there are many family members living communally, with a strong tradition of family caring for family. This is an example of an instance of the "interdependent, multigenerational kinship system," which may include "quasi-kin" (Brown, 1990, p. 70).

The family care that is given is often very good, but at times affected by finances. Personal care and hygiene issues are often a high priority for African Americans caring for a sick family member. The extended kinship system is essential in providing quality care.

Healing practices among African American groups include faith-healing (of the kind practiced by some more mainstream Americans, particularly those living in the "Bible belt" areas) and voodoo and related practices among some immigrants from the Caribbean and tropical Africa, and African Americans living in the New Orleans area and in the deep (rural) south. As with any other group, there are also folk remedies practiced by many African Americans. Although these vary according to several factors, they also include well-known varieties, like chicken soup, oil of camphor, etc. Buttermilk, for example, is often used in place of liquid food supplements like Ensure.

Public and communal grief are openly expressed at traditional African American funerals, which, in some areas, are termed "home-goings." As with other African American services, people in the congregation respond spontaneously and out loud to the sermon. The choir may sing softly in the background during the sermon and prayers. There is a gradual increase in emotion as the funeral progresses, and when the moment for the solo arrives, deep emotion is expressed by many. It is, in fact, difficult not to feel a deep communal grief at these funerals—regardless of one's own ethnicity. They seem to go beyond the African American experience alone, and to touch, in a real way, all of humanity's experi-

ence of suffering and grief. In the southern United States, there are usually printed programs for the funeral, and these include a photograph of the deceased. Funerals are most often held on Saturday or Sunday, and thus there may be a four- or five-day delay in burial.

Hispanic Americans

Like Asian Americans, there is a large variety of Hispanic Americans and they tend to be grouped together by many non-Hispanics. The fact that most speak Spanish, or a dialect of Spanish, and that many are Catholic, makes them more similar as a group than are Asian Americans. Within the broad group, however, significant differences exist. Native-born Hispanic Americans often disdain new immigrants—known as "wet-backs." Mexican and Central American groups segregate themselves from one another, although an outsider would be unaware of the dividing lines. Each Hispanic group, Puerto Ricans, Cuban Americans, etc., has their own distinct culture.

Hispanics tend to be reluctant to acknowledge, report, or describe pain. At the same time, moaning, especially for women, is acceptable and may not necessarily be indicative of severe pain or loss of control (Calvillo & Flaskerud, 1991, p. 20). Carrying on with activities of daily living and stoicism are highly valued. Self-control (*controlarse*) includes (Calvillo & Flaskerud, 1991):

- ability to withstand the stress of adversity (*aguantarse*)
- acceptance of fate (*resignarse*)
- cognitive coping, i.e., working through a problem (*sobreponerse*)

Thus, we see another example of what seems to be paradox: Working through problems and acceptance of fate are both valued. If the first does not work, then there is always the second.

The widely recognized concept of *macho* also influences approaches to dying and death.

Unfortunately, the concept is frequently viewed only as a foolish male arrogance. It is more functional to see macho as indicative of a strong sense of honor that affects the way in which Hispanic men approach life and death.

The basis of health and illness is thought by some Hispanics to be a balance between hot and cold, and wet and dry (Spector, 1991). These are intrinsic properties of various substances and there are differences of opinion about what is "hot," what is "cold," etc. Emotional or spiritual health problems, such as *susto*, a problem of the soul, may cause serious disability. As discussed earlier, not all people subscribe to these beliefs and not all subscribers can articulate them. It is not uncommon to have family members with varying beliefs, especially across generations, e.g., one person invested in modern technological care and another in traditional healing. Fortunately, this does not often present a problem: most Hispanic Americans, especially in the context of multigenerational families, are comfortable with pluralistic health care.

Traditional beliefs include preventing or treating illness through prayer, amulets, medals, candles, statues, or pilgrimages. *Curanderos*, or folk healers practice in many communities. Healing through Curanderos is usually some combination of prayer, counseling, supernatural forces, herbs, and other means. *Herbalistas* are found in most communities. Many homes, especially in rural areas, have shrines with statues, candles, and pictures of saints.

A recent influx of new immigrants—both legal and illegal—from Cuba, Brazil, etc. has helped promote the growth of *Santeria*, a cult that combines spiritualism, African folk religion, and Catholicism. Santeria healers, called *Santeros*, are seldom accessible to people outside the cult.

Sickness, including dying, is usually a family affair and many people are likely to be around the patient's bedside (Soto & Villa, 1990). Religion, a part of daily life, is also part of the dying process. Catholics will want a priest to provide the rite of anointing of the sick. Pictures of saints or saint candles may be present; for example, St. Peregrine (patron of cancer patients), St. Joseph (patron of the dying), or Our Lady of Lourdes (patron of illness), as well as the Virgin of Guadelup, or Our Lady of San Juan. Most parishes have an active auxiliary, and members are likely to be involved.

Public expression of grief is expected, especially among women (Salcido, 1990). Families and the social networks are materially supportive during bereavement. Among the poor, the financial disaster of death is mitigated by ongoing, extended family support.

Mainstream Culture

Dominant values of the mainstream culture— for the most part middle, upper-middle and upper class Americans—include: striving for optimal health, belief in democracy, individualism, achieving and doing, valuing cleanliness, attending to timeliness, and belief in technology (Leininger, 1978). A less widely recognized, but powerful value is the belief that choices should always be available. Thus, there are many options open to these classes. There is a widespread belief that there is always an answer or solution. This, of course, is irrational, but it does serve (for better or for worse) to push the limits of medicine and to give hope.

Cognitive coping is valued. There is a strong tendency to think in terms of the "why" of the problem rather than the "what," i.e., to focus on treating the cause of pain vs. the pain itself. It is assumed that there is a reason for and a meaning to everything.

Self-control is extremely important to many. Thus, in the context of dying, some live in agony, controlled by the pain, rather than make effective use of opioids to control the pain, because they don't want to "lose control" or to "be controlled by drugs." The loss of control inherent in advanced illness is difficult to accept. Some are reluctant to express emotions, except, at times, anger. In a very real sense, terminal illness repudiates many of the values of these socioeconomic classes of the mainstream culture, particularly for white, Anglo-Saxon Americans, and it is not uncommon to hear such a patient say, "I can't believe this is happening to me."

The nuclear family is the primary social unit; members of the larger family are often scattered across the country. Geographic distance and increasing numbers of single-parent families means that there is often little substantive family support. When the family is seriously involved, almost all the work falls on one person, most commonly, just as in the other cultures discussed above, on the wife, daughter, or daughter-in-law. Perhaps from a sense of guilt, or from unresolved, interpersonal feelings toward the parent who is dying, sons, and to a lesser extent, daughters who live out-of-town can be a highly disruptive force in efforts to provide quality, palliative care. Demands for additional testing and treatment are common when such individuals visit the patient. Careful explanation of care may help prevent disruption.

While many changes have occurred in recent years, especially among hospice users, the dying process often remains oriented for these classes toward technology or institutions, rather than toward patient and family.

New Age Culture

One of the effects of the consciousness-raising revolution of the 1960s has been the growth of what is often referred to as "new age" beliefs or culture. These beliefs are found mainly among members of the mainstream culture discussed above. New age beliefs have distinct religious and philosophical aspects. Two forces were primarily instrumental in the growth of new age philosophy:

- Many members of the privileged classes in the West realized that, no matter how much material wealth could be amassed and put to use, life was still empty.
- The availability of drugs like LSD meant that anyone willing to take the risk of ingesting a psychedelic, or "mind manifesting" substance, was open to the unique opportunity of having a spiritual—or at least an extreme—experience.

While psychedelic drug use has declined, and far fewer people are "dropping out," there are significant numbers of people who subscribe in some degree to related beliefs and practices. Nearly all the countless schools, belief systems, cults, and other manifestations of the New Age culture share at least some distrust of mainstream institutions, including religion, science, and health care. Belief tends to center around personal religious experience (seldom mainstream Protestant or Catholic) and humanistic ideals. The existence of God is acknowledged, though not given the importance it has in traditional religions. There is usually an acceptance of alternative religious and healing practices. Meditation, diet, and alternative healing through a variety of massage, herbal, and other remedies are common in the context of terminal care, especially among patients with AIDS.

While many hospice ideals are readily accepted by New Age cultural proponents, there is frequently a tendency to resist some of the technology or aggressive aspects of palliative care. Dying may be seen as an opportunity for spiritual growth and experience. Friends may be deeply involved in the process. The patient's autonomy is paramount. The work of Stephen Levine (1982) is helpful in understanding this perspective.

Spiritual needs are directly addressed in new age philosophy. Meaning abounds and hope is pervasive. Relatedness often focuses on human relationships more than on God. Acceptance is more prevalent than forgiveness. Transcendence of fear, pain, and other problems of the human condition is what this is all about. "His restlessness and fear fell away with his identification with the body. His long teaching from cancer had opened him to life, to death" (Levine, 1978, p. 5).

Refugees

Refugees represent a growing sociocultural population with a number of characteristics that are often common across cultures. One such characteristic is a lack of awareness of choices. Most people in the world have very limited choices in food, housing, education, and health care. If a particular medication or treatment is not effective, or has undesirable side effects, some people will assume that there are no other options. It is very common among refugees to report neither problems nor treatment failures.

More often than not, refugees present with immense psychosocial and often spiritual distress. The degree of distress is often related to degree of trauma, e.g., concentration camp experience, torture, multiple deaths of relatives (R.F. Mollica, personal communication, April 24, 1992). However, even when there is no history of exceptional trauma, the process of displacement and efforts to adjust to new circumstances are significantly stressful (Jones, 1986). Post-traumatic stress disorder serves as a prototypical model for refugee mental health, with symptoms emerging years after displacement (Mollica, Caspi-Yavin, Bollini, Truong, & Lavell, 1992).

Characteristics of refugees that impact their health and their response to terminal illness (Author, 1992) include:

- Displacement: Refugees leave their homeland to exist in a foreign, and often hostile culture. It is difficult to die a stranger in a strange land.

- Loss/grief related to the past: Refugees lose their past. Old ways of life, people, and things are destroyed by war and, with the onset of terminal illness, will clearly never be regained.
- Loss/grief related to the present: To function in the new land, a refugee must undergo immense, wrenching, and incessant change. Whatever old ways are retained are seldom functional in the new circumstances of advanced disease.
- War/trauma experience: Terminal illness is likely to bring up suppressed memories of atrocities and of other terrible events.
- Shortage of community resources: Not only do refugees have difficulty accessing existing community resources, there may also be a shortage of indigenous resources. A fact of refugee community life is that nearly everyone is operating at personal and familial limits, with few reserves left over for others.

Terminal illness often brings great sadness for refugees and there are few, if any, means of sharing or dealing with the sadness and loss. Nowhere else is the concept of ministry of presence as important as when working with terminally ill refugees.

In addition to whatever beliefs, practices, or perspectives exist specific to displaced persons, refugees are also almost always from cultures different from those of both mainstream and minority America. Cultural and language barriers thus compound the issues inherent in the life of a refugee. Those from rural areas are often users of folk remedies; some of which are efficacious, and some not.

The Very Poor

The very poor, known in political science as the "underclass," are those people who have been poor for several generations and who seem unlikely to change in subsequent generations.

Many, especially those living in densely populated urban ghettos, are welfare recipients. The very poor are distinct from people who are poor, jobless, homeless or otherwise disadvantaged, but who are able to envision for themselves a realistic potential to improve their circumstances. Defining characteristics of this population are hopelessness and little self-awareness of the possibility of a realistic potential for change.

The skills of people who have long been very poor are specific to their circumstances, and are thus in many ways inconsistent with the skills needed to interact effectively in the health care system. Making an appointment, arriving on time, refilling a prescription before the bottle is empty, carrying identification, and many other behaviors that seem basic and logical to providers may be unfamiliar and difficult to accomplish for many of these patients.

Everything takes more time to do for people for people in these circumstances. Finding their way, through private or public transportation, to health care facilities may require enormous effort. Clinic appointments in the facilities provided for the very poor often require spending an entire day—especially if lab tests are part of the appointment. Picking up prescriptions—paper or medicine—usually requires at least several hours' wait. Opioids are usually unavailable (legally) in the areas where this population lives; and possession of opioids in the home or apartment can draw the attention of criminals. Whatever the health-care related activity, it almost always requires more time—and carries additional costs in terms of personal dignity—for the very poor to accomplish than for anyone else in our society. Thus, essentially every factor—extrinsic (the system) and intrinsic (attitudes)—works to minimize health and health care. Compliance is also often a problem, and while there are notable exceptions, modest objectives for teaching should be considered.

Of course, people who are "very poor" are (or should be) entitled to the same levels of competence and caring as anyone else. At times, because of socioeconomic, educational, institutional, and other limitations, the challenges to clinicians in providing quality care are greater with patients who are very poor than with other patients.

Referrals and teaching present particular challenges. Referrals to community or institutional resources is often of little use because patients or their families may have difficulty contacting and accessing resources, or because resources may not respond as expected to people in this population. It may thus be necessary to provide advocacy and to help people through "the system." Teaching is often a challenge because of experiential, cultural, educational, and other differences that exist between the nurse and the patient. At least in the early stages of care, limited goals are appropriate. Based on patient and family abilities to learn and utilize information, goals can be expanded.

Overall, an increase in frequency and duration of services may be necessary, even when the situation seems stable, and more vigilance is required. Medications and other necessary supplies and basic necessities—like rent money—may run out seemingly without warning, and this requires frequent monitoring on the part of the practitioner. In the same manner, deterioration in the patient or family status may occur without notification to the nurse.

In short, to work effectively with members of this population, it is necessary to learn patience in working around limitations, whether those limitations are the patient's or those of the institutions.

Health Care Providers

Health care providers can be viewed as a significant and distinct sub-culture, perhaps the most homogeneous of any discussed in his chapter. The culture is generally rigid, and many roles are gender-related, although, as with other cultures, some of the barriers are breaking down.

Cultural values of health care providers include a strong belief in technology and "silent suffering" in response to pain. Health care providers may have goals different from those of patients, such as seeking to reduce pain rather than to relieve it (Calvillo & Flaskerud, 1991). Providers may hold the "major American cultural values" (Leininger, 1978), including:

- seeking optimal health;
- belief in democracy/individualism;
- achieving and doing;
- valuing cleanliness;
- attention to timeliness; and
- belief in technology.

While these may seem logical and natural to some, they may not be the values of all patients and all families. On a one-to-one basis, cultural differences may be easier to deal with individually than institutionally. What may seem completely logical and natural to middle and upper-middle class health care providers may be incomprehensible to others.

The problem-solving orientation of health care professionals may come into conflict with other cultures. The psychology of the West and of middle-class, mainstream culture health care providers, includes the idea that problems should be solved and that people can "deal with it." This culture-specific belief is not shared by everyone.

References

Brown, J.A. (1990). Social work practice with the terminally ill in the Black community. In J.K. Parry (Ed.) *Social work with the terminally ill: A transcultural perspective* (pp. 67–82). Springfield, Illinois: Charles C. Thomas.

Calvillo, E.R. & Flaskerud, J.H. (1991). Review of literature on culture and pain of adults with focus on Mexican-Americans. *Journal of Transcultural Nursing* 2(2), 16–23.

Cherry, B., & Giger, J.N. (1991). Black Americans. In J.N. Giger & R.E. Davidhizar (Eds.), *Transcultural nursing* (pp. 147–182). St. Louis: Mosby Year Book.

Hanley, C.E. (1991). Navaho Indians. In J.N. Giger & R.E. Davidhizar (Eds.), *Transcultural nursing* (pp. 215–238). St. Louis: Mosby Year Book.

Jones, E.R. (1986). How to Reach Out to Refugees. *Journal of Christian Nursing.3* (2). 14–17.

Kemp, C.E. (1985). Cambodian refugee health care beliefs and practices. *Journal of Community Health Nursing.* 2(1), 41–52.

Kemp, C. (1992). Health services for refugees in countries of second asylum. *International Nursing Review.* 40(1), 21–24.

Kipling, R. (1930). The ballad of East and West. In *Barrack room ballads.* London: Standard Book Company.

Lang, L.T. (1990). Aspects of the Cambodian death and dying process. In J.K. Parry (Ed.) *Social work with the terminally ill: A transcultural perspective* (pp. 205–211). Springfield, Illinois: Charles C. Thomas.

Leininger, M. (1978). The significance of cultural concepts in nursing. In M. Leininger (Ed.) *Transcultural nursing: Concepts, theories, and practices* (pp. 121–137). New York: John Wiley & Sons.

Levine, S. (1978, December). Approaching death. *Hanuman Foundation Dying Project Newsletter, 2.*

Levine, S. (1982). *Who dies?* Garden City, New York: Anchor Books.

Lewis, R. (1990). Death and dying among the American Indians. In J.K. Parry (Ed.) *Social work with the terminally ill: A transcultural perspective* (pp. 23–32). Springfield, Illinois: Charles C. Thomas.

Mollica, R.F., Caspi-Yavin, Y., Bollini, P., Truong, & T., Lavelle, J. (1992). Validating a cross-cultural instrument for measuring torture, trauma, and post-traumatic stress. *Journal of Nervous and Mental Disease.* 180(2), 111–116.

Pickett, M. (1993). Cultural awareness in the context of terminal illness. *Cancer nursing.* 16(2), 102–106.

Salcido, R.M. (1990). Mexican-Americans: Illness, death and bereavement. In J.K. Parry (Ed.) *Social work with the terminally ill: A transcultural perspective* (pp. 99–112). Springfield, Illinois: Charles C. Thomas.

Soto, A.R., & Villa, J. (1990). Una platica: Mexican-American approaches to death and dying. In J.K. Parry (Ed.) *Social work with the terminally ill: A transcultural perspective* (pp. 113–127). Springfield, Illinois: Charles C. Thomas.

Spector, R.E. (1991). *Cultural diversity in health and illness* (3rd ed.). Norwalk, Connecticut: Appleton & Lange.

Ta, M. & Chung, C. (1990). Death and dying: A Vietnamese cultural perspective. In J.K. Parry (Ed.) *Social work with the terminally ill: A transcultural per-*

spective (pp. 191–203). Springfield, Illinois: Charles C. Thomas.

Tripp-Reimer, T., Brink, P.J., & Saunders, J.M. (1984). Cultural assessment: Content and process. *Nursing Outlook.* 32(2), 78–82.

Wilson, B., & Ryan, A.S. (1991). Working with the ter-minally ill Chinese-American patient. In J.K. Parry (Ed.) *Social work with the terminally ill: A transcultural perspective* (pp. 145–158). Springfield, Illinois: Charles C. Thomas.

World Almanac. (1992). *The world almanac.* New York: Pharos Books.

Grief and Bereavement Care

And the king was deeply moved, and went up to the chamber over the gate, and wept; and as he went, he said, 'O my son Ab'salom, my son, my son Ab'salom! Would I have died instead of you, O Ab'salom, my son, my son!' "

2 SAMUEL 18:33

Grief is experienced "whenever the continuity of our lives has been destroyed" (Carse, 1980, p. 8). Grief is "suffering in response to loss" (Eakes, 1990, p. 243); and is conceptually defined as a "dynamic, pervasive, highly individualized process with a strong normative component" (Cowles & Rodgers, 1991, p. 121). Grief is thus:

- changing and non-linear (dynamic);
- composed of phases requiring *work* to move through (process);
- uniquely experienced by individuals (individualized);
- manifested physically, psychologically, socially, and spiritually (pervasive); and
- while experienced uniquely, usually composed of relatively predictable problems, extending over a relatively predictable period of time (normative).

When a significant other dies, grief may be related to factors in addition to that of the loss of the person. Life role, financial status, living arrangements, and having someone to depend on are common, associated losses (Poncar, 1989).

The terms grief, bereavement, and mourning are sometimes used interchangeably and there is disagreement about their precise meanings (Bohnet, 1986). For our purposes, bereavement and mourning can be defined as "being in a state of grief," i.e., grieving.

Characteristics of Grief

Grief following the death of a loved one may be expressed by denial, shock, inertia, loss of affect, intense yearning, (feelings of) losing control, anger, guilt, insomnia, sadness, depression, and spiritual despair (Carter, 1989; Hogan & Balk, 1990; Steele, 1990). It should also be noted here that a person for whom grief is felt is usually one who has been loved in the con-

Charles Kemp: TERMINAL ILLNESS: A GUIDE TO NURSING CARE. © 1995 J. B. Lippincott.

ventional sense of warm, loving feelings. At times however, tremendous grief or related feelings may be experienced in relation to a person for whom the griever felt primarily anger, rejection, or other negative emotion. Grief after death is felt not just for a person as a love object; it can also be felt for love unexpressed, anger unresolved, etc.

Seeking help, holding on (to the deceased), withdrawal, and inertia and aimlessness are common themes in grief (Carter, 1989; Switzer, 1970). Hallucinations (visions), or a strong sense of the presence of the deceased, are not uncommon. Family conflict is common, as is increased prescription and other drug use (Cooley, 1992). Physiologic manifestations of grief include anorexia, gastrointestinal disturbances, menstrual irregularities, fatigue, and shortness of breath (Gonda & Ruark, 1984; Gyulay, 1989a; Lindemann, 1944). Morbidity and mortality is greater among persons who are bereaved than among persons who are not (Shneidman, 1980).

Several theorists have proposed stages, or phases, in grief and Kubler-Ross' stages of dying are sometimes used to conceptualize grief. Common to several important models are the phases of avoidance, confrontation, and reestablishment (Cooley, 1992). Such phases are helpful to the extent that they may help (1) make sense of a global or overwhelming situation, and (2) keep the focus on the process rather than on each separate problem. These phases do not, however, reliably predict grief-related behaviors.

Like any other human behavior or experience, grief and mourning may be carried to extremes in behavior or in length. What constitutes "extremes" is subject to debate. Nuss and Zubenko (1992, p. 350) suggest that depression lasting more than a year after the death may "reflect the exacerbation of a premorbid psychiatric disorder." Shneidman (1980, p. 173) reports that acute mourning lasts "at least around one year." In sudden, traumatic death—e.g., by murder or suicide—acute grief is likely to last longer (Gass & Chang, 1989). Obsessive-compulsive behavior, depression, interpersonal sensitivity, global symptoms and their intensity, anxiety, hostility, and somatization may continue for more than three years in some cases, e.g., when a child dies (Moore, Gillis, & Martinson, 1988). There is a growing recognition among some experts that for some, grief may be "possibly limitless in regard to time" (Cowles & Rodgers, 1991, p. 121). Rather than thinking of getting over grief, it may be more helpful to think in terms of "living beyond it" (Gyulay, 1989b). What is normal, then, is not well-defined, and extreme grief may simply be the case for some.

Grief may also precipitate great personal or spiritual growth. Few would choose this means of growth, but the opportunity to choose to *not* grieve does not exist; the only choice is how to respond to the grief. Thus, out of the pain of countless deaths and losses have emerged countless, unnamed people with a greater appreciation of self and life.

Anticipatory Grief

Anticipatory grief has long been thought to have beneficial effects on later grief (Herth, 1990; Rando, 1986) or to help persons move toward acceptance of death (Curry & Stone, 1991). This idea is in part related to the knowledge that unexpected death may result in greater grief than the expected death of someone after an extended illness (Hazzard, Weston, & Gutterres, 1992). There is evidence, however, that anticipatory grief is positively correlated with depression and stress in survivors. Anticipatory grief may thus be seen as a "potential risk factor for poor early bereavement adjustment" (Levy, 1991, p. 24) and therefore not necessarily a process to encourage. The emotional distress experienced prior to a death is often difficult; for some people, it may prove helpful in confronting later events. It should not, however, be thought of as a means of intervention.

Dysfunctional Grief and Assessment Parameters

A variety of terms have been used to give a name to grief, or similar concepts, that exceed normative boundaries (whatever they may be) and are related to poor outcomes, especially persistent depressive symptoms. These include: pathological grief, abnormal grief, morbid grief, unresolvable grief, chronic grief, and complicated grief (Lindgren, Burke, Hainsworth, & Eakes, 1992; Wolfelt, 1991). Among the types of dysfunctional grief are:

- absent grief, characterized by no expression of grief, or by psychic numbing;
- distorted grief, characterized by distortion, usually exaggeration, of one or more components of grief—anger or guilt are the most common;
- converted grief, similar, if not the same as a conversion disorder in which there is a "loss of, or alteration in physical functioning . . . not limited to pain" (American Psychiatric Association, 1987, p. 259); and
- chronic grief, which is unending grief that may even intensify over time.

Among the reasons for dysfunctional grief are social learning within families or cultures (e.g., that grief and death are best denied), uncertain loss (e.g., children who disappear), traumatic loss (e.g., by murder), and multiple losses (e.g., several loved ones dying at one time or within a short time). Personal attributes that may be seen as indicators of increased risk for poor outcomes in grief (Cooley, 1992; Nuss and Zubenko, 1992; Parkes 1978) are shown in Figure 6.1.

While the presence of one or more of these factors does not necessarily lead to a poor outcome, they do alert the practitioner to a higher degree of risk, and thus may function as assessment parameters. Additionally, bereaved persons should be assessed for physical problems related to, or exacerbated by, grief.

Interventions

Intervention in grief begins with primary prevention before death. Involving the family in caring for the person who is dying is important to all involved before death, and to the family after death. To know that they are/were helpful is something solid to which people can cling. Resolving or attempting to resolve con-

---

FIGURE 6.1
PERSONAL ATTRIBUTES SHOWING INCREASED RISK OF DYSFUNCTIONAL GRIEF

- Little time to prepare for the death
- Highly dependent or ambivalent relationship with the deceased
- Previously inadequate coping skills
- Dependence on emotion-focused coping strategies alone (vs. emotion-focused *and* problem-solving)
- Young age, e.g., adult with young children at home
- Perceived lack of social support
- Few financial and/or social supports, e.g., older, isolated persons
- No history of working outside the home
- Previous poor physical and/or mental health status, including alcohol and drug misuse

flicts is immensely beneficial. Managing symptoms, keeping the family informed of changes and their significance in the patient's condition, and providing reassurance and comfort are nursing actions that are helpful before and after the death (Hampe, 1975; Poncar, 1989).

Bereavement care is likely to accomplish the most during the first few months of mourning, before defense mechanisms have hardened. Many hospice programs plan the first bereavement contact for about two weeks after the death. This is when the usual rush of support immediately following the death decreases; and two to four weeks lies within the parameters of length of time during which to provide crisis intervention (Poncar, 1989). Holidays, birthdays, and other significant times are when the need for support tends to be highest. The first anniversary of the death is usually very difficult for survivors. Subsequent anniversaries are also significant. Intervention, then, includes action or problem-solving for these times.

There are certain tasks of bereavement (Castiglia, 1988; Cooley, 1992; Harr & Thistlethwaite, 1990; Parkes, 1978), and these tasks help to guide interventions. Consistent with the process and development of grief, the tasks are not subject to the mourner completing one and then moving on to the next. There is not a "next" task. Mourners typically move from one to another, address several at once, move back to a previous task, go deeper into feelings or understanding, do nothing, move on to another, and so on. The seven "tasks of bereavement" are discussed one-by-one in the following section. Making progress in these tasks means making progress in the process of grief. The long-term goals of grief work are:

- gradual reintegration into life and adjustment to life without the person who died; and
- prevention of prolonged changes in psychosocial patterns, especially prevention of depression.

TELLING THE "DEATH STORY"

There is an almost universal need among the bereaved to describe and redescribe events and feelings around the death. (Cooley, 1992). Every detail is gone over again and again—often past the time that family and friends are willing to listen. The need to tell this story more than others want to hear it may play some part in the common problem of diminished social support. The need to tell the story also conflicts with the desire to avoid the pain of grief. Interventions related to the mourner's need to tell the story include:

- Actively listening to the story: Among the specific directions for listening to the story are helping the mourner sequence the events in time and place, promoting acuity in perceiving the events, and separating what is real from what is not.
- Teaching family members and other sources of the mourner's social support system about this common need.
- Suggesting to the bereaved person that he or she write the story, and then being sure to read it.

EXPRESSING AND ACCEPTING THE SADNESS

There are several impediments common to initially expressing and accepting the sadness of grief. Some people will be aware of their feelings, but fear a psychological catastrophe if the feelings are expressed and acknowledged. "If I start to cry, I'll never stop." Another problem is a family or social norm of not expressing feelings. "In our family, we don't wallow in misery," or "I have to be strong for her/him/them." It is common among some to accept the practice of pseudo comfort that really only encourages people to be quiet and to repress their feelings: "There, there, it's going to be all-right." Expressing feelings may also be inhibited by institutions. Most hospitals are set up for efficiency—perhaps amenable to, at the most, quiet crying, but not to the deep anguish that may be felt.

For those stuck playing a role of "not hurting," a simple statement of what might be felt can help; "I'm so sorry. This must hurt terribly." Too many words can get in the way. Constant response to a person's attempts to fill the pain with words is not helpful. Silence may ease the expression of feelings. The old "psych nurse" technique of changing the setting to change the behavior may also facilitate the emergence of feelings. Take the person for a walk, sit in the car with him or her, or otherwise change the situation. Say, "It's OK to feel what you're feeling."

The loneliness of grief is not unexpected by most mourners. What is often surprising is the power of it overall, and the unexpectedness of the "small moments" of intense pain that appear amidst all the things once taken for granted (Yalom, 1988).

EXPRESSING AND ACCEPTING GUILT, ANGER, AND OTHER FEELINGS PERCEIVED AS NEGATIVE

In the immense stress of dying, death, and grief lies an illogical and almost universal trap for survivors: regret, which is concentrated often in the illusion that, after a lifetime of imperfection, "I/he/she/we/it should have been perfect!" Decisions, behavior, and words said are obsessively reviewed and inevitably found lacking. Regrets are inescapable and accepted by most people. Excessive guilt and anger are more problematic for many and are commonly associated with dysfunctional grief (Wolfelt, 1991).

Guilt is an integral part of grief (Lindemann, 1944) and "has its origin in a separation fear," i.e., anxiety (Switzer, 1970, p. 119). Dynamics of guilt-anxiety include regression; unconscious hostility toward the deceased;

violation of the relationship, i.e., past mistakes; and inability to perform the expected social role (of the bereaved). Problems in expressing guilt include the shame felt about whatever real or perceived transgressions are related to the guilt and a conscious or unconscious fear of punishment.

Acknowledging and expressing guilt is the first step in resolving it. Since shame and/or a fear of punishment are barriers in expressing guilt, a non-judgmental relationship is essential to this expression. While some rumination on perceived causes and feelings of guilt is productive, greater progress is made in the process of exploring the moral code associated with the guilt. Many people struggle to live under unrealistic moral codes. Changing such beliefs is extremely difficult and is not practical under most circumstances. Many people, however, can come to see which aspects of their values are realistic and which are unrealistic.

Once guilt is expressed, and to some extent understood, the process of acceptance of self or behavior can begin. Some (intellectual) acceptance may occur through expressing the guilt. Persons experiencing difficulties with guilt need to do additional work. Apologizing or otherwise communicating with the person who died can be done through writing a letter to him or her. It is helpful to the writer to read the letter aloud to the nurse. The concept of atonement (perhaps through helping others) may also be a part of acceptance. In essence, the nurse helps the survivor:

- accept feelings of guilt;
- recognize realistic and unrealistic reasons for guilt;
- find means to apologize or otherwise atone for the guilt; and
- begin to forgive self.

Anger may range from the barren bitterness of unfulfillment to the poignancy of a loving relationship lost:

After he died I was smelling his clothes and there was
no smell of him anywhere and I was really mad that
he . . . that . . . I mean, what if you were here trying
to smell me. Because he didn't even leave any scent.

(LEVINE, 1988).

For some, anger is more difficult to deal with than guilt. Indeed, guilt may be felt over feelings of anger toward the deceased. More often than not, hostility is turned inward and experienced as anger, depression, or guilt; or it may be turned outward toward others, rather than toward the idealized deceased (Switzer, 1970). For many, it feels normal to feel guilty and abnormal to feel angry. Anger is nevertheless a common component of grief and is "a product of guilt anxiety" (Switzer, 1970, p. 127).

As with guilt, the first step in resolving anger is to acknowledge and express it. While some anger toward others or self may be appropriate, the issue most in need of intervention is that which lies in the realm of the relationship with the deceased. The reality of relationships is that there is always some degree of ambivalence in them, often including hostility and aggression (Switzer, 1970). Thus, to acknowledge and express anger, it may be necessary to first de-idealize both the deceased and the mourner's relationship with them.

Anger was addressed earlier in chapter 1, under psychosocial needs of the individual. While much of that discussion applies to this one as well, anger in grief can also be addressed separately. Interventions include advising and helping the mourner to:

- maintain awareness of their own responses to anger, whether it is expressed directly or indirectly;
- directly express the anger about whatever object is perceived as at fault;
- identify and explore the underlying feelings, e.g., separation anxiety, frustration, betrayal, etc.; and

- deal with those underlying feelings. While separation anxiety is a broad issue encompassing multiple settings, it can be addressed here in terms of the person feeling bad about being apart from the one who died. The separation, however, is not just from the person, but also from roles (forever lost), hopes (never to be fulfilled), and other key aspects of self, not the least of which is a deep awareness of mortality.

REVIEWING THE RELATIONSHIP WITH THE DECEASED

While this occurs in part through other tasks, and extends throughout the person's life, some support specific to this task may be helpful. Reviewing the relationship with the deceased is similar to a life review, but focuses on the relationship. Besides talking or writing in general about the relationship, several key issues should generally be reviewed. Elements of this task, or direction, to encourage in working with the mourner include:

- Exploring the early days of the relationship: For spouses or life partners, how they met, courtship remembrances, and similar matters are important, and are seldom discussed with others. For parents, siblings, children (adult or child) of a parent who died, and similar persons, talking about early remembrances is vitally important. Since much conflict has its roots in early relationships, it is well to cover negatives as well as positives. A very productive direction to take is to address the question of what was hoped for and unfulfilled in the relationship.
- Exploring what would have been had the death not occurred: While painful, this is an important issue to confront in the process of healing.

EXPLORING POSSIBILITIES IN LIFE AFTER THE DEATH

Behind or within the pain of grief lies the forbidding question, "What now?" In the early days after the death, the answer often appears to be, horribly, this—this pain, this despair, this emptiness. Thus the task of exploring possibilities is filled with dread. Existing for some time in grief's suffering is a necessary precursor to looking to the future with anything other than dread. How long that time might be is impossible to estimate, and there is no specific point at which that task takes precedence over others. Rather, there (usually) is a gradual awareness that the future will not necessarily be without hope.

As the person comes to understand that life can go on and perhaps be good in some respects (and for some, this understanding seems to do an injustice to the memory of the deceased), the ability to think of the future increases. Along with this growing awareness is progress in other tasks and a concomitant increase in energy. Care should be taken that in the first flush of progress, the person does not attempt to do too much or to make extensive plans. Gradual progress with periods of regression and progression is the norm.

Some people will go on to form new, intimate relationships. Men are quicker than women to seek intimacy (Yalom, 1988). Either may fall into relationships that are emotionally damaging, especially if alcohol or drug use is involved. Specific interventions in promoting "going on with life" include:

- Help the mourner to identify goals and hopes that, following the loss, are achievable—and those that are not.
- Give the mourner the opportunity to re-grieve over the reality of life going on, or over other issues.
- Give the mourner the opportunity to explore possibilities for the future. There is no rush to know the future. Some of the person's ideas or hopes may be non-productive or illogical. The nurse is probably the only person willing to listen to such ideas. It does not hurt to fantasize about joining the Peace Corps or going back to college; and a few people actually take such steps. The freedom to express such ideas can allow the mourner the freedom to develop more practical plans.
- Teach the mourner problem-solving techniques, if needed. It is essential that the mourner begin by solving a small problem. Few people in these situations have the psychological reserves to fail and to try again. Since emotion-based coping is positively correlated with dysfunctional grief, rational problem-solving may help decrease the likelihood of complications.
- Social support is a key element in resolving grief, and directive assistance can be given in locating and using appropriate resources. Bereaved persons often feel less welcome than they did before the death at church, or with other former sources of social support. Although the nurse helps the mourner deal with his or her responses to this perceived rejection, more direct assistance can also be given. The experience of grief is so powerful and global to the bereaved that it may seem to them that everyone can see his or her needs and pain, and the failure of others to respond to the needs and pain is felt as rejection, or as a lack of caring. A common response for them then is to withdraw. The nurse can respond to, or prevent, such withdrawal by encouraging the person to go back to church or to their former sources of support, to *ask* for help, to ask *again* if help is denied; and to look elsewhere if help is again denied. Bereavement groups, while generally a temporary source of support (Yalom, 1990), can function as a kind of gateway to exploring a new life. These groups, and similar support, can be found through churches, synagogues, hospices,

the American Cancer Society, and other such organizations. Information on developing a group is given in the next chapter.

UNDERSTANDING COMMON PROCESSES AND PROBLEMS IN GRIEF

Many people have little or no understanding of the power of grief; the flood of emotions is thus a terrible surprise. The duration of grief is also a surprise for many. Providing normative information is thus extremely important in bereavement care. Having such information does not change any of the experiences of grief; it does, however, give the mourner a kind of voice in the background that says, "This is grief; it is not the beginning of breakdown." Information should be given verbally, and in writing. Readers are invited to utilize the "Summary of Grief Responses" at the end of this chapter for this purpose.

Working through these normative "levels" of grief leads to finding a way to reorganization—or adjustment to the environment, or life—without the deceased. In addressing grief, it is essential that the nurse remember that complete resolution, i.e., complete acceptance and lack of pain, may not be achieved. Most people get better, but many never return to their former level of functioning. Some, thankfully, achieve a higher level of functioning.

BEING UNDERSTOOD OR ACCEPTED BY OTHERS

The depth of the emotion of grief, as well as its intrinsic characteristics, result in isolation. Indeed, there is a time to be alone, to mourn, and to refrain from embracing. Just as the person who is dying must at some time be alone, so must the bereaved. So our purpose here is not to get the family and others to intervene in or to change the process, but rather to promote understanding of some of what the

bereaved person is going through. Although this does not "solve" the problem of isolation, it does, ironically enough, render the mourner's situation less "lonely" than it could be. The "Summary of Grief Responses" at the end of this chapter gives direction for family and friends.

Funerals and Other Rituals

There is universal need for funerals or similar rituals and every religion provides a structure for them. Rando (1984) provides a definitive discussion of the purposes and benefits of funerals. These are summarized in Figure 6.2.

A variety of options exist in funerals and related rituals. Funerals, planned within the context of the various faiths and denominations of the faiths, are the most common rituals. Memorial services or gatherings are increasingly common. Whatever the choice of the person who is dying and/or the family, the key issue is that a choice should be made, before the death whenever possible. Making choices and arrangements after the death is a difficult burden for mourners. Moreover, the process of making choices prior to death can be helpful in the psychosocial and spiritual care of the patient and family. At some point in patient and family discussions, suggest that they make plans. Most will have already thought of this, but many will not have known how to bring up such a sensitive subject.

Health care providers are seldom involved in funerals, except through their attendance at times. We should, from time to time, attend the funerals of our patients. We too benefit from participating in these ancient rituals.

Summary of Grief Responses

It is impossible to predict how an individual will respond to the death of a loved one. The following are common in grief, yet not all are experienced by all who mourn. They do not

---

FIGURE 6.2
PURPOSES AND BENEFITS OF FUNERALS

- Provide the last rite of passage for the person who died.
- Confirm and reinforce the reality of the death and the separation of the living and the dead.
- Assist in acknowledging and expressing feelings of loss and facilitating mourning.
- Stimulate recollections of the deceased and help validate the deceased person's life.
- Allow participation of the community in memorializing the person who died.
- Provide the comfort or other benefits of ritual.
- Provide means for the community to give and receive social and spiritual support.
- Begin the process of helping the bereaved back into the community.
- Help in the search for meaning.
- Affirm the social order: The community goes on despite death.
- Remind the living of their own and others' mortality.
- Furnish means and method in disposing of the body.

---

occur in a particular order and should not be thought of as stages that, once accomplished will not again arise.

Common psychological responses to grief include:

- Numbness or denial: This didn't happen. "It couldn't have happened. Maybe I can do something that can undo it."
- Guilt: "It's my fault." (Countless variations on) "If only I had, or I should have; why didn't I . . . I was not a good husband, wife, daughter, son, etc., etc." Old omissions and commissions are remembered.
- Anger: "How could he/she leave me like this?" "Why did she/he do this to me?" "Damned doctors (or nurses, hospital, etc.)." "This is an example of God's love?"
- Sadness: Behind the denial, guilt, and anger is the deep sadness. "He's (she's) gone; I am alone, and it will never be okay. I will never feel good again."
- Ambivalence: Love and anger get mixed up and go back and forth.
- Anxiety: Nervousness, or sensitivity to what others say and do or don't do, becomes a problem for many. Some feel like they are losing control. Tears come with little or no provocation.
- Unfairness: "It's just not fair!"
- Intense yearning: "I wish, I wish—Oh how I wish!"

Common physical responses to grief include:

- deep and total fatigue;
- insomnia, or in some cases, increased sleep;
- appetite disappears and food doesn't taste the same—which is okay, because food seems to get stuck in one's throat most of the time anyway;

- digestive and related problems appear;
- menstrual irregularities occur;
- muscles ache;
- chest pain may occur; and
- nothing feels good or right.

Common spiritual responses to grief:

- Anger toward God is common.
- Alienation from God, or spiritual emptiness, are also common.
- Life loses its meaning.
- Hope seems an illusion.

The purpose in listing these is not to try and shield the mourner from their experience, and so from pain. Some, most, or all of the above responses will be experienced, no matter what. This is the essence of grief. As time passes and the pain is confronted, however, the good days begin to outnumber the bad. Healing is not forgetting. It is remembering and going on in life.

What can be done? There is no medicine or action to take that will prevent the pain of grief. There are, however, some things that help people go through the process:

- Knowledge about grief helps the mourner know that what he or she is experiencing is normal.
- Knowing that countless others have also gone through it tells the mourner that there comes a time when it begins to get better— even when such a time seems impossibly far away.
- Everyone has faced terrible times in the past. Recognition of this fact, and the recollection of how one went through those times, may help in going through the time of grief as well.
- For those for whom the death of the loved one is the first great tragic experience of their lives, looking for new means of coping may be required. Some old friends may fall away, and that is a bitter pill to swallow. Encouraging the mourner to join a bereavement group helps many.

- Facing the fact that, when help is most needed, it is often most difficult to find can discourage the best efforts to cope with grief. The best advice for mourners is to encourage them to ask for help again and again, reminding them that—difficult as it seems—many people in their situation face the same isolation, and the same difficulty in finding help.
- Help the mourner evaluate the pros and cons of potential actions and decisions. For example, it is usually a good idea to avoid major decisions, especially those that involve large sums of money, while one is going through the process of grief. And acting on spontaneous impulses focused on finding some relief, or escape, from the pain—like a spur-of-the-moment vacation, or excessive intake of alcohol, or of tranquilizers or other drugs, etc.—may prove counter-productive.
- Remind the mourner that countless experiences like theirs have shown that no true remedy—neither "happiness," nor complete knowledge and security about the inevitability of their loved one's death, nor anything else on this earth—exists that can banish the pain and suffering of grief. However, these same experiences also confirm that, somewhere along the way, something will happen, and it *will* get better.

References

American Psychiatric Association. (1987). *Diagnostic and statistical manual of mental disorders* (3rd ed., revised). Washington, DC: Author.

Bohnet, N.L. (1986). Bereavement care. In M.O'R. Amenta & N.L. Bohnet (Eds.), *Nursing care of the terminally ill* (pp. 247–262). Boston: Little, Brown and Company.

Carse, J.P. (1980). *Death and existence: A conceptual history of human mortality.* New York: John Wiley & Sons.

Carter, S.L. (1989). Themes of grief. *Nursing Research.* 38(6), 354–358.

Castiglia, P.T. (1988). Death of a parent. *Journal of Pediatric Health Care.* 2(3), 157–159.

Cooley, M.E. (1992). Bereavement care: A role for nurses. *Cancer Nursing 15*(2), 125–129.

Cowles, K.V. & Rodgers, B.L. (1991). The concept of grief: a foundation for nursing research and practice. *Research in Nursing and Health. 14*(2), 119–127.

Curry, L.C., & Stone, J.G. (1991). The grief process: a preparation for death. *Clinical Nurse Specialist. 5*(1), 17–22.

Eakes, G.G. (1990). Grief resolution in hospice nurses. *Nursing and Health Care. 11*(5), 243–248.

Gass, K.A. & Chang, A.S. (1989). Appraisals of bereavement, coping, resources, and psychosocial health dysfunction in widows and widowers. *Nursing Research. 38*(1), 31–36).

Gonda, T.A., & Ruark, J.E. (1984). *Dying dignified*. Menlo Park: Addison-Wesley.

Gyulay, J.E. (1989a). Grief responses. *Issues in comprehensive pediatric nursing. 12*(1), 1–32.

Gyulay, J.E. (1989b). Editorial. *Issues in Comprehensive Pediatric Nursing, 12*(4), iii–iv.

Hampe, S.O. (1975). Needs of the grieving spouse in a hospital setting. *Nursing Research, 24*(2), 113–119.

Harr, B.D., & Thistlethwaite, J.E. (1990). Creative intervention strategies in the management of perinatal loss. *Maternal-child nursing journal, 19*(2), 135–142.

Hazzard, A., Weston, J., & Gutterres, C. (1992). After a child's death: factors related to parental bereavement. *Journal of Developmental and Behavioral Pediatrics, 13*(1), 24–30.

Herth, K. (1990). Relationship of hope, coping styles, concurrent losses, and settings to grief resolution in the elderly widow(er). *Research in Nursing and Health. 13*(2), 109–117.

Hogan, N.S., & Balk, D.E. (1990). Adolescent reactions to sibling death: Perceptions of mothers, fathers, and teenagers. *Nursing Research, 39*(2), 103–106.

Levine, S. (Facilitator). (1988). Conscious living/dying (Cassette Recording No. SL1-27-8811). Delray Beach, Florida: Hanuman Foundation.

Levy, L.H. (1991). Anticipatory grief: Its measurement and proposed reconceptualization. *Hospice Journal, 7*(4), 1–28.

Lindemann, E. (1944). Symptomatology and management of acute grief. *American Journal of Psychiatr,. 101*, 141–148.

Lindgren, C.L., Burke, M.L., Hainsworth, M.A., & Eakes, G.G. (1992). Chronic sorrow: A lifespan concept. *Scholarly inquiry for nursing practice, 6*(1), 27–40.

Moore, I.M., Gillis, C.L., & Martinson, I. (1988). Psychosomatic symptoms in parents 2 years after the death of a child with cancer. *Nursing Research, 37*(2), 104–107.

Nuss, W.S., & Zubenko, G.S. (1992). Correlates of persistent depressive symptoms in widows. *American Journal of Psychiatry, 149*(3), 346–351.

Parkes, C.M. (1978). Psychological aspects. In C.M. Saunders (Ed.), *The management of terminal disease* (pp. 44–64). London: Edward Arnold.

Poncar, P.J. (1989). The elderly widow: Easing her role transition. *Journal of Psychosocial Nursing, 27*(2), 6–11.

Rando, T.A. (1984). *Grief, dying, and death*. Champaign, Illinois: Research Press Company.

Rando, T.A. (Ed.) (1986). *Loss and anticipatory grief*. Lexington, MA: D.C. Heath.

Shneidman, E. (1980). *Voices of death*. New York: Harper and Row.

Steele, L.L. (1990). The death surround: Factors influencing the grief experience of survivors. *Oncology Nursing Forum, 17*(2), 235–241.

Switzer, D.K. (1970). *The dynamics of grief*. New York: Abingdon Press.

Wolfelt, A.D. (1991). Toward an understanding of complicated grief: A comprehensive overview. *American Journal of Hospice & Palliative Care, 8*(2), 28–30.

Yalom, I., & Vinogradov, S. (1988). Bereavement groups: Techniques and themes. *International Journal of Group Psychotherapy, 38* (4), 419–446.

Yalom, I. (1990). Response to discussion of bereavement groups: Techniques and themes. *International Journal of Group Psychotherapy, 40*(1), 105–107.

Developing a Bereavement Group

Group support is a commonly accepted and effective means of preventive intervention for persons who are bereaved (Davis, Hoshinko, Jones, & Gosnell, 1992). In the absence of existing or accessible services, it is sometimes necessary to develop a bereavement group. Typically, such a group meets eight to ten times and then disbands. To develop a bereavement group, it is necessary to understand or learn concepts of (1) group dynamics, and (2) grief and bereavement care.

General techniques for groups include "establishing norms, encouraging process review, and making here-and-now interventions" (Yalom, 1988, p. 425). More specific techniques used in a bereavement group include: operationalizing the curative factors of universality; cohesiveness; instilling hope; imparting information; altruism; interpersonal learning; catharsis; and existential factors. The corrective recapitulation of the primary family group, interpersonal learning, development of socializing techniques, and imitative behavior may occur to a lesser extent. For a complete discussion of these concepts, or curative factors, see Yalom, 1985. Each technique mentioned above

is discussed in the following paragraphs. How they are implemented/operationalized will vary among group leaders.

- Establishing norms is accomplished initially by a brief explanation by the group leader, and throughout the bereavement group meetings by reinforcing, modeling, or encouraging behavior consistent with norms. Norms of bereavement groups include the following:
1. Self disclosure is essential to bereavement and other groups. From self disclosure arises cohesiveness, universality, hope, learning, and other essential processes.
2. A precondition of self-disclosure is trust within the group and confidentiality without.
3. Members look to one another as the experts on grief and coping. While the leader may occasionally offer suggestions or observations related to bereavement, it is far better that members be the source of altruism and information. The greatest trap for a leader who knows about grief, but not group process, is to act as a primary source of information.

Charles Kemp: TERMINAL ILLNESS: A GUIDE TO NURSING CARE. © 1995 J. B. Lippincott.

4. Members take significant responsibility for the content and process of the group. While this norm can seldom be developed as fully as in a psychotherapeutic group, the greater the group responsibility, the greater the group progress.

- Encouraging process review is the heart (and hardest part) of leading a group. Process review looks at what is happening beneath the words or in what is happening or not happening because of the words. Examples of process questions are: "What were you feeling when (person's name) was describing her husband's last days?" "What do you think might have been unsaid tonight?" "What has been going on with you since last week?" "What was the hardest part of sharing this with the others in the group?"

- Making here-and-now interventions is a part of the process of groups. A group that is cohesive—in which universality, altruism, hope, and process review are operational—*is* a here-and-now intervention. The group is an opportunity for members to share feelings and aspects of self as they might wish they had at another time. The here-and-now interventions are not advice given in the group, but the process within (and as a consequence without) the group.

- Universality is the realization that group members are not alone and unique in their responses to grief. Isolation is a powerful dynamic in grief, and to hear that others feel that isolation, pain, and myriad other responses is liberating. Self-disclosure by group members leads almost inevitably to operationalizing universality. This process can begin with the introduction of group members to one another. There are many "go-round" formats. Among the topics to suggest are that each person state (always with the freedom not to do so): the name of the person who died, relationship with the deceased, feelings about being in the group,

primary feelings since the death, cause of death, and so on. Universality is facilitated through the course of the group by group members identifying aspects of similarity in their experience. Even when events and feelings are dissimilar, universality still exists in the power of the experience.

- Cohesiveness is the feeling of togetherness in the relationship of the group as a whole to its members. Cohesiveness develops over time as members struggle together with pain, anger, guilt, and other issues that in other circumstances tend to be isolating but which, in the accepting atmosphere of a group, are unifying. Writing summaries of each meeting and sending them to members several days before the next meeting may increase cohesion and promote process (Yalom 1988).

- Hope is necessary for any therapeutic endeavor to succeed. Hope is instilled in several ways. First, group members see that others are surviving bereavement. Second, members are seeking help by being in a group, and such an effort indicates hope, or the ability to hope. Finally, the leader demonstrates hope by her or his presence and behavior.

- Imparting information, especially on normative aspects of grief, is part of any bereavement group (Cooley, 1992; Silverman, 1976). Giving information is the primary focus of some groups, especially when the leader is inexperienced in leading groups or when the group is sponsored through a large organization. In such groups, typically, a concept (determined by curriculum) is presented by the leader, or by an outside expert, in the first half of the meeting time and then in the second half, it is discussed by group members. It is more productive for members to give information to one another.

- The expectation that mourners do something to help another person can be burdensome for the mourners. However, in the midst of the suffering, guilt, anger, etc. of grief, a bereavement group provides the rare opportunity for members to do good for others simply by being (in the group).

- Catharsis, the expression of strong feeling, is a basic part of the therapeutic process. A bereavement group provides a safe place to express feelings that might not be accepted elsewhere. Guilt and/or anger are common. The powerful feelings associated with grief make catharsis almost inevitable. Focusing on process review and here-and-now interventions promotes catharsis. Ultimately, catharsis itself is less valuable than the universality of the feelings and the group's acceptance of the person who expresses the feelings.

- Existential factors can be summarized as facing the basic facts of life and death, and taking responsibility for the response to these realities. Accepting the reality of a loved one's death, of facing life alone, and even of finding new relationships, are difficult existential issues. As with other aspects of grief, it is unreasonable to expect that all of life's existential issues would be faced in a bereavement group. As previously noted, the group serves as a gateway, not as the final answer to a new life.

Other factors relevant to planning and implementing a bereavement group include: qualities of the leader, the site of group meetings, and termination. Requisites for group leaders include: (1) knowledge and experience in group process, and (2) knowledge of grief. Although it is beneficial for practitioners such as nurses, doctors, social workers, and chaplains to be supportive of survivors participating in the group, practitioners who gave care to the deceased should generally not act as group leaders for survivors. Practitioner leaders may find themselves objects of idealization, anger, or monopolization.

One of the most common sites for bereavement group meetings is a church or other house of worship to which group members belong, but community centers or other civic locations with which members of the group might already be familiar, or might in the future be able to develop an affiliation, are also suitable. An office is less desirable, but sometimes it is the only reasonable choice. Comfort and security are essential.

In reference to "termination," it is necessary to admit how paradoxical it seems to emphasize, for a bereavement group, that it is helpful for its members to be able to come to an end—here is yet *another* loss. At the same time, talking about termination is an opportunity to bring into consciousness the concept of "anticipated regret," i.e., "What will be regretted when this group ends, and what can be done about these anticipated regrets now?" (Yalom, 1988, p. 431). For some members, there is even an element of recapitulating part of a primary relationship in this concept: it is a chance, however symbolic, to do a better job of saying "good-bye." Other group members will continue to see and support one another after the group disbands. Like many other such self-support efforts, post-termination activities may not continue indefinitely.

As is standard for any serious therapist, supervision is strongly recommended. The key to effective leadership of bereavement groups is ability in group process.

References

Cooley, M.E. (1992). Bereavement care: A role for nurses. *Cancer Nursing, 15*(2), 125–129.

Davis, J.M., Hoshinko, B.R., Jones, S., & Gosnell, D. (1992). The effect of a support group on grieving individuals' levels of perceived stress. *Archives of Psychiatric Nursing, 6*(1), 35–39.

Silverman, P.R. (1976). The widow-to-widow program: an experiment in preventive intervention. In E.S. Shneidman (Ed.), *Death: Current perspectives* (pp. 356–363). Palo Alto: Mayfield.

Yalom, I. (1985). *The theory and practice of group psychotherapy* (3rd ed.). New York: Basic Books.

Yalom, I. & Vinogradov, S. (1988). Bereavement groups: Techniques and themes. *International Journal of Group Psychotherapy, 38*(4), 419–446.

Ethical Issues in Terminal Care

All the major ethical issues, or dilemmas, are brought into full focus in the process of providing terminal care. The "most fundamental" moral or ethical principle is respect for persons (American Nurses Association [ANA], 1985, p. i). From this principle follows the more specific principles of:

- respect for autonomy—the patient's right of self-determination;
- beneficence or benevolence—doing good or meeting needs;
- nonmaleficence—doing no harm;
- veracity—truth-telling;
- confidentiality—respecting privileged information;
- fidelity—keeping promises; and
- justice—treating fairly.

Each of these principles is a concrete and nonacademic issue in caring for persons who are dying. "Every nursing activity, however ordinary" (Levine, 1989, p. 128) is an opportunity to express the very highest ethical principles. Ethical principles may be thought of as duties—though not duties in the sense of something onerous that must be done (although giving care is onerous at times)—but as what may be expected of another in a human relationship (Dunstan, 1978).

Clinical issues, such as pain control, loss of control, and sexuality, have been identified as ethical issues (Caruso-Herman, 1989; Foley, 1991; Lisson, 1989). However, *all* clinical decisions entail a value, or ethical judgment. Clinical issues, then, are best addressed as goals of therapy and in terms of broader principles, such as beneficence, nonmaleficence, etc. For purposes of clarity, this chapter is structured around the principles given in the *Code for Nurses with Interpretive Statements* (ANA, 1985).

Operationalizing ethical principles or duties requires making value judgments. While making such judgments is a problem for many nurses (Lisson, 1989), they must be made. Nurses no longer have the dubious privilege of pretending not to judge their own and others' actions.

Ethical principles should also be considered in a cultural context because ethical and moral values are not the same in all cultures (Battin, 1991). Autonomy, for example, is not valued in all cultures or in all sociopolitical systems, and

Charles Kemp: TERMINAL ILLNESS: A GUIDE TO NURSING CARE. © 1995 J. B. Lippincott.

its meaning is intensely debated in Western cultures. From at least some perspectives, autonomy is central to such questions as abortion and euthanasia. The latter is discussed at the end of this chapter, under the section "Decisions Near the End of Life."

Autonomy

Autonomy, or the individual's freedom of self-determination, is "basic to respect for persons" (ANA, 1985, p. i) and is central to ethical, professional practice. While competence—the mental capacity to make a decision—is necessary in order to practice autonomy, practically speaking, autonomy may also be limited by economic, political, legal, and other issues (Thompson & Thompson, 1985).

Decision making, especially to forgo or withdraw treatment, is the primary issue in terminal care and autonomy (Otte & Allen, 1987). To reach the conclusion that one is dying and will therefore decide to forgo further curative treatment moves a person from the primarily dependent role of "patient" to the far more autonomous role of "the person who is dying" (Van Eyes, 1991). Decisions should be made by competent, or "normal choosers" (Beauchamp & Childress, 1989, p. 69) and the following factors are inherent in decisions: (1) intentionality, (2) understanding, and (3) decisions made without "controlling influences that determine the action," i.e., voluntarily, or with free consent (Beauchamp & Childress, 1989, p. 69). The central issues within the principle of respect for autonomy are competence, informed consent, and voluntariness (intention either does or does not exist).

COMPETENCE

The capacity to "perform a task" is the "single core meaning" of competence (Beauchamp & Childress, 1989, p. 80). In the context of termi-

nal care decisions, the primary task to perform is to understand the risks and benefits of treatment and thus make a rational decision about what treatment to forgo and when to forgo it. Competence operates along a continuum and may change, for example, with the onset and resolution of hypercalcemia, depression, and other physical or psychological problems. Competence is not global: a person may be mentally, but not physically competent; or vice versa (Latimer, 1991).

INFORMED CONSENT

To realize competence it is necessary that the patient be fully aware of all "information that a reasonable person, in a comparable situation, would need to make a similar decision" (Fowler, 1989, p. 960). (Note that making the decision, not the conclusion reached, is where the similarity lies.) Informed consent thus includes the patient's ability to perform the task of understanding and deciding and the professional's provision of the necessary information. Further, the patient must not just be *able to understand*, but must *actually* understand the information. Therefore, as always, the nurse determines patient response—in this case, to the reception of information.

VOLUNTARINESS

The extent of freedom from operating "under the control of another agent's influence" determines the extent of voluntariness (Beauchamp & Childress, 1989, p. 107). Influence may include coercion, manipulation, and persuasion. "Another agent" may include another person who exercises power, who controls or manipulates information, or who otherwise influences the patient; the "agent" may also be a drug addiction, a compulsion, or, in the view of some, physiological or psychological factors (Fowler, 1989).

Beneficence

Beneficence (or benevolence) is commonly defined as doing good (ANA, 1985). More completely defined, beneficence requires: (1) providing benefit to another, and (2) "a balancing of benefits and harms" (Beauchamp & Childress, 1989, p. 194).

Beneficence may also be defined as meeting needs and as the highest duty in health care, and indeed, in all human endeavors (D. Foster, personal communication, February, 1992). When we examine competent terminal care, we see that it is focused completely on the patient's needs. The cornerstone of care in advanced disease—relieving suffering (Scanlon & Fleming, 1989; Van Eys, 1991)—epitomizes this view of beneficence. Beneficence is best considered as an action of "mercy, kindness, or charity" (Beauchamp & Childress, 1989, p. 194) that is taken with regard to the greatest good and the least harm. The question of balancing good and harm is a central question in terminal care: what treatment is appropriate and when should treatment be discontinued?

There is not a clear distinction between beneficence and nonmaleficence (Otte & Allen, 1987). However, differences between these two principles are obscured by examining them as one principle (Beauchamp & Childress, 1989). At least one noted ethicist makes the definitive

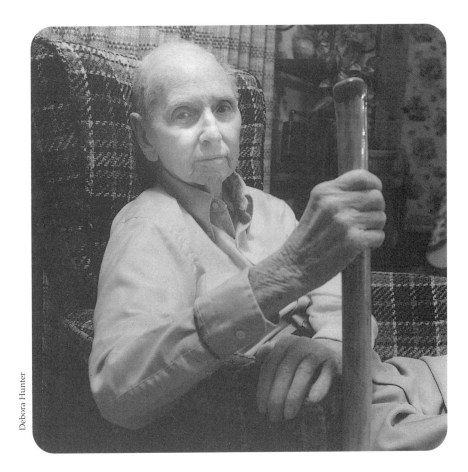

Debora Hunter

statement that "the notion that there is no morally significant difference between omission and commission is just wrong" (Callahan, 1992, p. 52). Beneficence includes removing harmful conditions, preventing harm, and doing good (Fowler, 1989). All of these are clearly actions; something done. Nonmaleficence, on the other hand, is something harmful *not* done, e.g., futile surgery on a patient who will certainly die. In the crucible of terminal care decisions, there is often a profound difference between beneficence and nonmaleficence. That difference may be difficult to see at the time of care.

Nonmaleficence

Nonmaleficence encompasses not inflicting physical, psychological, social, spiritual, or any other harm, "including harm to the dignity of the patient" (Fowler, 1989, p. 961). While nonmaleficence is most often viewed in terms of physiological interventions, it should also be considered in psychological, social, and spiritual care. An "assault of truth," for example, may be a maleficent act (Latimer, 1991, p. 330). The duty of nonmaleficence, to do no harm "on balance" (American Medical Association [AMA], 1992, p. 2230) may come into conflict with wishes or duties of patients, families, and/or nurses in terminal care situations in one of several ways. The most obvious is the situation in which requests may be made, or actions considered or taken, to end the life of the patient (this is discussed in a later section). The question of what treatment is best, when it should be provided, and when it should be discontinued, are major issues in many situations.

For whom and when, for example, are intravenous fluids beneficent and for whom and when are they maleficent? How are the questions of quality of life and sanctity of life balanced in a society, and within a profession, that places an extremely high value on both (Amenta & Bohnet, 1986)?

Veracity

Veracity includes not lying and not deceiving (Beauchamp & Childress, 1989). The question of "what" to tell, and "how" to tell patients and families has long troubled health professionals who care for the terminally ill (Saunders, 1978a). Truth-telling affects not only the moral relationship between the patient and the nurse, but also significantly influences the patient's quality of life (High, 1989). While in the past, nurses often operated as if in primary relationship with physicians, or with hospital hierarchies, and in secondary relationships with patients (Bernal, 1992), the primary relationships are now indisputably with patients. The *Code For Nurses with Interpretive Statements*, as well as various other standards, clearly states that the nurses' responsibility is to the patient. The patient—not the nurse, physician, family, or anyone else—is responsible for determining whether information is to be given (see also the discussion of voluntariness above).

Traditionally, and appropriately, the physician is the person who first tells the patient the diagnosis and prognosis. When such information is not given in a reasonable period of time, and a patient asks about diagnosis or prognosis, the nurse may experience conflict about the best course of action. In such cases, the nurse should be guided by the "universal moral principles" (ANA, 1985) cited in the nurses' Code and discussed in this section: The truth should be told. How the truth is told, and its extent, may vary, but given the choice between lying and telling the truth, one should opt for the truth, except in the most extraordinary circumstances, such as protecting a person from external threats (i.e., political persecution, etc.). Telling the truth may be personally uncomfortable and may result in difficulties at work. Nevertheless, the principles of beneficence, autonomy, and veracity take precedence over the desire to avoid conflict.

Confidentiality

The nurses' duty is to "hold all information in confidence" except that which is "pertinent to a client's treatment and welfare." This information is shared "only to those directly concerned with the client's care" (ANA, 1985, p. 4–5). The Nurses' Code also specifies that the duty of confidentiality is "not absolute when innocent parties are in direct jeopardy."

Evidence exists that confidentiality is "widely ignored and violated in practice" (Beauchamp & Childress, 1985, p. 330), both among individuals and institutionally. Respecting privileged information is an extremely important ethical issue facing nurses in terminal care. Some information is so sensitive that hearing it may be considered more a "priestly" function than one of health-care professionals. Indeed, caring for persons with terminal illness, and the ethical issues woven throughout it, is a situation in which there often exists more of the theological than not (Childress, 1990; Levine, 1978)—especially when nurses are doing a good job.

As with other ethical principles, confidentiality can present difficult dilemmas. How much "direct jeopardy" warrants overriding confidentiality, and where do legal obligations fit? If, for example, a competent patient hints at suicide, what actions might the nurse take? If the same patient presents with behavior indicating a high risk for suicide, what actions might be appropriate?

Fidelity

Fidelity can be interpreted as fundamentally "a covenant . . . of faithfulness" between human beings (Ramsey, 1970, p. xii). A more specific, but less edifying definition is "keeping promises" (ANA, 1985, p. i). In either case, fidelity means more than "doing what one says one will do." Fidelity includes the implicit or explicit contracts or covenants that exist by virtue of one person seeking health care from another (Beauchamp & Childress, 1989). Practicing fidelity means doing what one says one will do, and also holding true to the ethical principles of nursing. As with veracity, the principle of fidelity may bring the nurse into "morally troubling" conflict (Beauchamp & Childress, 1989, p. 347). A basic dilemma, or conflict, is choosing actions when the patient's welfare is in conflict with institutional or other demands. Again, the purpose of nursing is the patient's welfare, and thus conflicts will arise.

To provide competent terminal care is to confront our helplessness in the face of death and suffering. This is painful work. And in doing it we answer the question of what covenants we keep with our fellow human beings. We say, "Yes, we will watch with you." This work is one of the highest acts of fidelity.

Justice

The practice of justice includes delivering care without discrimination or prejudice "in every situation" (ANA, 1985, p. 4). The principle of distributive justice often refers to the allocation of scarce resources, whether in giving care to an individual or participating in, or planning, a program. Major theories of justice (Beauchamp & Childress, 1989) include egalitarian (equal access), libertarian (rights to liberty), and utilitarian (mixed criteria to maximize public utility). Utilitarian theories are commonly practiced in Western health care systems. The philosophy of terminal and hospice care is explicitly just in both the treatment of individuals and of humanity (Saunders, 1978b).

The practice of justice does not ignore injustice, and nursing acknowledges this: the nurse seeks to promote the acceptance of justice by others (ANA, 1985).

Decisions Near the End of Life

The ability of advanced knowledge and technology to maintain life, coupled with increased societal concern about quality of life, brings the issue of decisions that must be taken near the end of life into sharp focus. The immense public interest in the Karen Ann Quinlan case, in Dr. Jack Kevorkian's "suicide machine," and in the publication of the best-selling book, *Final Exit* (Humphry, 1991) indicate that the issue is vital.

Requests made or actions considered or taken to control the character of care or to end the life of the patient may include (AMA, 1992):

- Withholding or withdrawing life sustaining treatment: This may include the often difficult-to-define "extraordinary measures"—resuscitation—or more usual measures, such as intravenous fluids or oxygen. The increasing use of advance directives helps patients plan and helps surrogate decision makers and health care personnel make the often momentous decisions connected with modern health care.
- Providing palliative treatment that may have fatal side effects: This is sometimes termed "double-effect euthanasia" (AMA, 1992). The principle of double effect is a "meta-ethical or procedural principle," and is most often encountered in situations of intractable symptoms, like pain or suffocation, when the "compelling moral obligation is relief of distress" (Latimer, 1991, p. 331). The ANA's nurses' Code is clear on this matter: Nurses may provide interventions to relieve suffering "even when the interventions entail substantial risks of hastening death" (ANA, 1985, p. 3).
- Euthanasia, i.e., action taken to end a life for merciful purposes: euthanasia includes:
  1. involuntary euthanasia—performed on a competent person without that person's consent;

  2. nonvoluntary euthanasia—performed on an incompetent person;
  3. voluntary euthanasia—performed on a competent person at that person's request. The terms "active" and "passive" euthanasia are less commonly used in current debates (AMA, 1992).
- assisted suicide: The difference between assisted suicide and euthanasia is the degree of health professional participation (Brock, 1992). In the former, the professional facilitates the death and in the latter, they directly cause death.

A key issue in all the above is the question of whether the action causes death in a person who would not otherwise die at the time of the action. Withholding or withdrawing treatment are increasingly accepted measures when treatment would extend both life and suffering; and when the person or his/her proxy desire that treatment be withdrawn. Suicide itself is more widely accepted as rational and moral (Clouser, 1991) today, and in the United States, assisted suicide is viewed by some experts as "not in itself morally wrong" (Battin, 1991, p. 305).

Euthanasia and assisted death are clearly actions that cause death before it might naturally occur (Callahan, 1992; AMA, 1992). Euthanasia and assisted death are issues of intense debate in industrialized nations (Crigger, 1992). Nursing, however, is clear about the issue: "The nurse does not act deliberatively to terminate the life of any person" (ANA, 1985, p. 3).

While a full appraisal of the debate on euthanasia and assisted death (hereafter referred to as euthanasia) is beyond the scope of this work, it may be helpful to explore a few of the key issues that exist within the fundamental question of euthanasia. These are posed below as questions. There are no easy answers to any of them, and ultimate responsibility, here as elsewhere, rests with the individual;

however, considerations relevant to the practitioner in terminal care are discussed.

- Does euthanasia incontrovertibly violate the principle of nonmaleficence? And if it does not, is the fear expressed by some—that sanctioning euthanasia could put its practitioners, and society, on a potentially destructive "slippery slope" that could end with violation of the most fundamental ethical principles—well-founded?
- Does the availability of sanctioned euthanasia result in the termination of suffering among the terminally ill who choose this option? And is the suffering of family members also similarly affected? Significant research findings (Klagsbrun, 1991) leave little doubt about an affirmative answer to the first question, but the second question is less tractable in terms of measurable results; the case for cause and effect here is much more complex, and family suffering could be affected by the availability of sanctioned euthanasia both positively and negatively, in relation to any number of factors.
- Is euthanasia, radical though it may be, nevertheless almost a moral imperative in some cases of extraordinary circumstances and suffering? Most of us in this work have been witness to terrible suffering. There are memories that are a dagger in the heart. Nevertheless, there are those who, struggling to develop competency in caring for people who are dying, would question whether the number of unmanageable patients is great enough to warrant a change in the centuries-old moral traditions of our culture (Brescia, 1991).
- Can guidelines on sanctioned euthanasia be consistently interpreted and implemented? There are reports (Keown, 1992) that, in the Netherlands for example, guidelines are interpreted and implemented in various ways, and, at times, ignored.

- Does the availability of sanctioned euthanasia increase individual autonomy? Some (ten Have and Welie, 1992) find that the power of the physician is increased. Others (Brock, 1992) assert that patient autonomy is not diminished.
- Euthanasia can decrease the often crippling financial costs of advanced disease—might this mean that the commitment to care diminishes? Some find that there is little evidence for concern (Brock, 1992), while others posit a realistic danger that euthanasia, like other aspects of the health care system, would be used unequally in the case of the poor and of others without adequate medical coverage (Scofield, 1991).
- Would sanctioned euthanasia affect efforts for improvement in the competent care of the terminally ill? Unquestionably, suicidal ideation often stems from uncontrolled symptoms and other suffering (Foley, 1991; Holland, 1993), and beneficence—manifested as absolute dedication to relieving pain and suffering—is a moral imperative in terminal care.

Summary

Terminal care is fraught with non-academic ethical issues and dilemmas. The nurse is confronted with decisions that profoundly affect the lives of patients, their families, themselves, and their colleagues. The ANA Nurses' Code addresses the fundamental ethical principles, but these issues are not easily addressed; nor are the dilemmas easily resolved. The struggle with these life and death questions is, however, one of the most fundamental and significant struggles in all our lives, and nurses' efforts to act and react intelligently, responsibly, and morally within that struggle are imbued with an undeniable nobility. Despite the difficulties and the uncertainty involved, there is no contradiction in considering ourselves fortunate in living these experiences.

References

Amenta, M.O'R., & Bohnet, N.L. (1986). *Nursing care of the terminally ill.* Boston: Little, Brown and Company.

American Medical Association, Council on Ethical and Judicial Affairs. (1992). Decisions near the end of life. *Journal of the American Medical Association, 16*(267), 2229–2233.

American Nurses Association. (1985). Code for nurses with interpretive statements. Kansas City, MO: Author.

Battin, M.P. (1991). Euthanasia: The way we do it, the way they do it. *Journal of Pain and Symptom Management, 6*(5), 298–305.

Beauchamp, T.L., & Childress, J.F. (1989). *Principles of biomedical ethics* (3rd ed.). New York: Oxford University Press.

Bernal, E.W. (1992). The nurse as patient advocate. *Hastings Center Report, 22*(4), 18–23.

Brescia, F.J. (1991). Killing the known dying: Notes of a death watcher. *Journal of Pain and Symptom Management, 6*(5), 337–339.

Brock, D.W. (1992). Voluntary active euthanasia. *Hastings Center Report, 22*(2), 10–22.

Callahan, D. (1992). When self-determination runs amok. *Hastings Center Report, 22*(2), 52–55.

Caruso-Herman, D. (1989). Concerns for the dying patient and family. *Seminars in Oncology Nursing, 5*(2), 120–123.

Childress, J.F. (1990). The prophetic and the priestly. *Hastings Center Report, 20*(6), 18–19.

Clouser, K.D. (1991). The challenge for future debate on euthanasia. *Journal of Pain and Symptom Management, 6*(5), 306–311.

Crigger, B-J. (1992). Dying well? A colloquy on euthanasia and assisted suicide. *Hastings Center Report, 22*(2), 6.

Dunstan, G.R. (1978). Discerning the duties. In C.M. Saunders (Ed.), *The management of terminal disease* (pp. 181–188). London: Edward Arnold.

Foley, K. (1991). The relationship of pain and symptom management to patient requests for physician-assisted suicide. *Journal of Pain and Symptom Management, 6*(5), 289–297.

Fowler, M.D. (1989). Ethical decision making in clinical practice. *Nursing Clinics of North America, 24*(4), 955–965.

High, D.H. (1989). Truth telling, confidentiality, and the dying patient: New dilemmas for the nurse. *Nursing Forum, 24*(1), 5–10.

Holland, J.C. (1993). Principles of psycho-oncology. In J.F. Holland, E. Frei, R.C. Bast, D.W. Kufe, D.L. Morton, & R.W. Weischselbaum (Eds.), *Cancer medicine* (3rd ed.) (pp. 1017–1032). Philadelphia: Lea & Feiberger.

Humphry, D. (1991). *Final exit.* Eugene, Oregon: The Hemlock Society.

Keown, J. (1992). On regulating death. *Hastings Center Report, 22*(2), 39–43.

Klagsbrun, S.C. (1991). Physician-assisted suicide: a double dilemma. *Journal of Pain and Symptom Management, 6*(5), 325–328.

Latimer, E.J. (1991). Ethical decision-making in the care of the dying and its application to clinical practice. *Journal of Pain and Symptom Management, 6*(5), 329–336.

Levine, S. (1978, March). Practice at work. *Hanuman Foundation Dying Project,* p. 2–5.

Levine, M.E. (1989). Beyond dilemma. *Seminars in Oncology Nursing, 5*(2), 124–128.

Lisson, E.L. (1989). Ethical issues in pain management. *Seminars in Oncology Nursing, 5*(2), 114–119.

Otte, D.M., & Allen, K.S. (1987). Ethical principles in the nursing care of the terminally ill adult. *Oncology Nursing Forum, 14*(5), 87–91.

Ramsey, P. (1970). *The patient as person.* New Haven: Yale University Press.

Saunders, C.M. (1978a). Appropriate treatment, appropriate death. In C.M. Saunders (Ed.), *The management of terminal disease* (pp. 1–9). London: Edward Arnold.

Saunders, C.M. (1978b). The philosophy of terminal care. In C.M. Saunders (Ed.), *The management of terminal disease* (pp. 193–202). London: Edward Arnold.

Scanlon, C., & Fleming, C.M. (1989). Ethical issues in caring for the patient with advanced cancer. *Nursing Clinics of North America, 24*(4), 977–986.

Scofield, G.R. (1991). Privacy (or liberty) and assisted suicide. *Journal of Pain and Symptom Management, 6*(5), 280–288.

ten Have, H.A.M.J., & Welie, J.V.M. (1992). Euthanasia: Normal medical practice? *Hastings Center Report, 22*(2), 34–38.

Thompson, J.E., & Thompson, H.O. (1985). *Bioethical decision making for nurses.* Norwalk: Appleton-Century-Crofts.

Van Eyes, J. (1991). The ethics of palliative care. *Journal of Palliative Care, 7*(3), 27–32.

Stress and Health Care Providers

It is no surprise that it is stressful to work with people who are dying. Numerous books, studies, articles, and countless dissertations document the sources and responses to stress among health care providers (e.g., Flaskerud, 1992; Kash & Holland, 1989; Paradis, 1987; and many others).

Physical Manifestations and Sources of Stress

Physical manifestations of stress reactions, or "burnout," include fatigue, headache, appetite changes, sleep pattern disturbances, and nausea and vomiting. Psychological manifestations include feelings of helplessness, hopelessness, apathy, and irritability (Belle, 1988; Massie, Heiligenstein, Lederberg, & Holland, 1991). Typical responses to stress include detachment or over-attachment to patients, working increased or decreased hours (anything but a happy medium), and problems in personal relationships (Ray, Nichols, & Perritt, 1987). Alcohol and drug use, depression, and suicide are the more common pathological responses by health care professionals to stress (Massie, Heiligenstein, Lederberg, & Holland, 1991).

A major source of stress in working with people who are dying is the regular contact with the most fundamental human fear—fear of death—as well as with suffering, hopelessness, meaninglessness, and uncertainty. Other sources of stress include the psychological/social isolation that may attend this unique work (others' everyday concerns may seem trivial), and, in the case of those who work with patients with AIDS, mortal danger to self and loved ones (Driedger & Cox, 1991). Less recognized, but very powerful sources of stress in caring for people who are dying are the system in which the care is given (Vachon, 1987b), and interpersonal conflicts with other health care or administrative personnel.

Personality variables play an enormous and difficult-to-delineate role in the perception of and response to stress. Major personality traits related to stress response are motivation, personal values, and personality and coping style (Vachon, 1987a).

Regardless of the specific sources of stress for a particular person or group, the undeniable fact is that stress exists and it will not go away.

Charles Kemp: TERMINAL ILLNESS: A GUIDE TO NURSING CARE. © 1995 J. B. Lippincott.

(Is there anyone working in hospice, oncology, AIDS care, etc. who does not occasionally fantasize about a job in which there is no stress, no pain, no meaning?) What can be done about stress—what *must* be done—is to modify the response to stressors. There are organizational measures for dealing with stress. But in the final analysis, it is the responsibility of each individual to deal with her or his stress.

Strategies for Dealing with Stress

The first step in a healthy response to stress is to recognize and accept that stress exists and that everyone who works with the dying is at risk for negative effects of stress. Whether one is feeling the effects of stress or not, measures should be taken to prevent its negative effects. It is important to remember that people do not always feel stress as such. Rather than recognize their feelings for what they are, some may experience them instead as the desire to have a few more drinks (and a little more often), to enter into an impulsive relationship, to get angry more often (to themselves, justifiably, of course), or as a host of other behaviors that seem to them, if not perfectly correct, then at least as viable as any other kind of truthful response.

Education and experience are correlated with decreased burnout (Driedger & Cox, 1991). In other words, expertise, or competence, is an effective means of decreasing anxiety and stress. Competent practitioners do better work and tend to feel better about themselves and their work (Vachon, 1987a); and so do their patients. The first and most important competence is clinical competence. Clinical competence comes from three sources: education, experience, and personal qualities of the practitioner. It is essential that all three aspects be enhanced. Too many practitioners limit themselves by depending on their extant or experiential competencies.

Among the other important competencies is the ability to communicate and understand other people's communications, particularly in stressful situations. The ability to deal with other people's (and one's own) anger is especially important (Degner, Gow, & Thompson, 1991). Increasing one's knowledge about dying and grief is important. Social-cultural competencies, such as learning about cultures other than one's own, are also essential in our multicultural society. Practitioners working with patients with AIDS, for example, benefit themselves and their patients by learning about lifestyles that may be different from their own.

Social support is an important, positive factor in working effectively with people who are dying (Driedger & Cox, 1991). Basically, this work is almost impossible to do alone. Spouses or life companions, family members, and colleagues are the most common sources of support (Eakes, 1990). While other sources exist, it is not uncommon, though this seems surprising, to find situations where support from colleagues is lacking, or inadequate. Staff meetings or support groups are a common means of generating social/organizational support among peers. How and by whom these groups are led is critically important. One of the curiosities of hospice and other programs is the frequency with which support groups for nurses and other staff are led by non-nurses. The question of who participates in support groups is one that should be carefully considered. The presence of supervisory or administrative staff is often inhibiting. Certainly, at a minimum, there should be regular, multidisciplinary team or case conference meetings, which, if effectively conducted, can provide some needed social support.

The freedom to express feelings—a component of some social support systems, but not of others—is important. Formal case conferences, for example, are not usually appropriate forums for expressing strong feelings. Team meetings may be more appropriate, and team support groups are often the most appropriate. A consistent need to express grief and/or anger, etc. probably indicates a high level of stress and unmet needs. Whatever the setting, it is important that every practitioner have a person or persons in whom she or he can confide any of their feelings about the work. Expressing feelings, however, as a sole means of dealing with stress is unlikely to be successful. "Coping is most effective when balanced between cognitive, or problem-solving, and emotion-based strategies" (Vachon, 1987a).

Spiritual support is another logical and often neglected aspect of dealing with the stress inherent in working with people who are suffering and dying (Belle, 1988). Whether or not one is aware of them, spiritual values are intrinsic to human life (Jung, 1953). While it is inappropriate to urge personal spiritual values on patients or other staff, it is equally inappropriate to exclude those values from our own needs and practices in a workplace where dying and death are the order of every day.

The search for spiritual support has become increasingly more complicated in our Western societies. Inspirational, or self-help books, programs and organizations abound, but the seeker—especially when the need is greatest, as is the case in working with the dying—can ultimately remain more perplexed than nourished. As discussed in chapter 3, when an individual feels the need of a spiritual support beyond what has sustained them in the past, one alternative is to explore traditional models. Regardless of one's experience and outlook, the fact is that, throughout human history, people have come together in places of worship to find meaning, hope, relatedness, or simply common cause with one another. The spiritual healing power of tradition and ritual alone, particularly when it touches chords in our early memory and experience, is sometimes overlooked.

Setting reasonable goals is another factor essential to minimizing or managing stress. If a practitioner works toward explicit or implicit patient goals—like keeping all symptoms well-managed, and all family relationships reconciled—and simultaneously toward practitioner goals—like remaining understanding in all circumstances, and always meeting all needs—then failure, frustration, and high stress are the inevitable outcome. If, on the other hand, goals are individualized and reasonable, in terms of each patient and of self, then failure, frustration, and stress are decreased.

Collaborative relationships with patients and families are important to many practitioners in dealing with grief and stress (Eakes, 1990). This sort of relationship is characterized by balance between over- and under-involvement with patients and families. Over-involvement is characterized by a pattern of nurse-patient relationships consistently based on emotion. Such relationships actually reflect nurses relating to their own responses to patients, rather than to the patients themselves (Travelbee, 1971). Under-involvement is characterized by a pattern of interacting with patients and families as though they were problems, or situations in need of diagnoses, or burdens. Paradoxically, a pattern of deep involvement with individual patients/families is advocated by some as a means of humanizing practice (Martin & Julian, 1987).

Another aspect of nurse-patient relationships that reduces grief and stress is achieving a sense of closure when the patient dies (Eakes, 1990). Whether through spending time with a family after the death, attending the funeral, or by other means, it is generally helpful to find some way of achieving a sense of closure in nurse-patient relationships.

Lifestyle management, i.e., measures taken to live in a healthier manner, is a key aspect of modifying the response to stress. Physical exercise, improved diet (including moderation in caffeine intake), adequate sleep, conscious pacing of life in general (and of practice in particular), separating work from home, and judicious use of drugs and alcohol are the basic measures taken to improve lifestyle. (Vachon, 1987a). All the above should be implemented in everyone's life; and, of course, not many of us come this close to perfection. Using a prescription, however, of "one at a time, steadfastly, and with reasonable personal goals," all of these measures can be achieved.

While individuals need to take primary responsibility for coping with their own stress, it is important that organizations also address the issue. The most important organizational or "environmental" coping mechanism is for staff to feel that they belong to a team (Vachon, 1987a, p. 212). From the traditions of the Marine Corps to those of the hospice, *esprit de corps* plays a central role in helping people to act effectively in situations that are beyond the normal capacities of most people. Building a team usually requires mindful effort on the part of formal or informal leaders. Efforts to incorporate group dynamics, motivational techniques, and other aspects of team-building is effort well-spent. Other organizational measures to reduce or help staff better cope with stress include: responding to and acting on staff problems as much as possible, working to create a milieu that is conducive to coping with stress, care in staff selection, and administrative policies congruent with human needs (Vachon, 1987a).

Although they are not specific to stress reduction, factors that lead to job satisfaction vs. dissatisfaction (Herzberg, 1975, p. 367) should also be considered in the exploration of stress as it relates to terminal care. Factors leading to "extreme satisfaction" in work are, in descending order:

1. achievement (e.g., successful outcome of care);
2. recognition, especially of achievement;
3. the work itself;
4. responsibility; and
5. advancement.

Factors leading to "extreme dissatisfaction" in work, from most to least dissatisfaction, are:

1. organization policy and administration;
2. supervision;
3. work conditions;
4. salary; and
5. relationship with peers.

Incorporating these factors into the organization decreases the perception and/or effects of stress. Failure to incorporate them decreases satisfaction and increases stress.

References

Belle, J.L. (1988). Supporting the deliverers of care: Strategies to support nurses and prevent burnout. *Nursing Clinics of North America, 23* (4), 843–850.

Degner, L.F., Gow, C.M., & Thompson, L.A. (1991). Critical nursing behaviors in care for the dying. *Cancer Nursing, 14*(5), 246–253.

Driedger, S.M., & Cox, D. (1991). Burnout in nurses who care for PWAs. *AIDS Patient Care, 5*(4), 197–203.

Eakes, G.G. (1990). Grief resolution in hospice nurses. *Nursing and Health Care, 11*(5), 243–248.

Flaskerud, J.H. (1992). Psychosocial aspects. In J.H. Flaskerud & P.J. Ungvarski (Eds.), *HIV/AIDS: A guide to nursing care* (2nd ed.) (pp. 239–274). Philadelphia: W.B. Saunders Company.

Herzberg, F. (1975). One more time: How do you motivate employees? In *Harvard Business Review on management* (pp. 361–376). New York: Harper and Row.

Jung, C.G. (1953). Psychology and alchemy. In J. Jacobi & R.F.C. Hull (Eds.), *C.G. Jung: Psychological reflections* (pp. 338–339). Princeton, New Jersey: Princeton University Press.

Kash, K., & Holland, J.C. (1989). Special problems of physicians and house staff. In J.C. Holland & J.H. Rowland (Eds.), *Handbook of psycho-oncology: Psychological care of the patient with cancer.* New York: Oxford University Press.

Martin, C.A., & Julian, R.A. (1987). Causes of stress and burnout in physicians caring for the chronically and terminally ill. In L.F. Paradis (Ed.), *Stress and burnout among providers caring for the terminally ill and their families.* New York: The Haworth Press.

Massie, M.J., Heiligenstein, E., Lederberg, M.S., & Holland, J.C. (1991). Psychiatric complications in cancer patients. In A.I. Holleb, D.J. Fink, & G.P. Murphy (Eds.), *Clinical oncology* (pp. 576–586). Atlanta: American Cancer Society.

Paradis, L.F. (Ed.) (1987). *Stress and burnout among providers caring for the terminally ill and their families.* New York: The Haworth Press.

Ray, E.B., Nichols, M.R., & Perritt, L.J. (1987). A model of job stress and burnout. In L.F. Paradis (Ed.), *Stress and burnout among providers caring for the terminally ill and their families* (pp. 3–28). New York: The Haworth Press.

Travelbee, J. (1971). *Interpersonal aspects of nursing* (2nd Ed.). Philadelphia: F.A. Davis Company.

Vachon, M.L.S. (1987a). *Occupational stress in the care of the critically ill, the dying, and the bereaved*. Washington: Hemisphere Publishing.

Vachon, M.L.S. (1987b). Team stress in palliative/hospice care. In L.F. Paradis (Ed.), *Stress and burnout among providers caring for the terminally ill and their families* (pp. 75–103). New York: The Haworth Press.

II | Pain Management

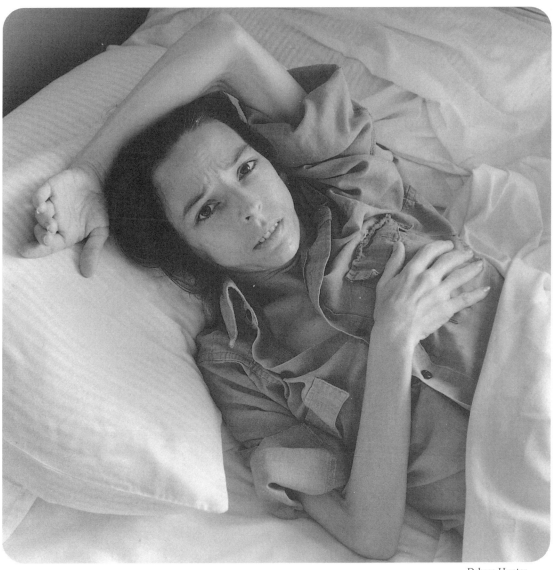

Debora Hunter

Introduction

Managing symptoms is the *sine qua non* of terminal care, and pain is the most problematic and feared symptom (Brescia et al., 1990). Pain is defined as "an unpleasant sensory and emotional experience associated with actual or potential tissue damage, or described in terms of such damage" (American Pain Society [APS], 1992, p. 2). The prevalence of pain in patients with advanced cancer ranges from 50%–80%, depending on tumor type, and research and other variables (Portenoy, 1989; Wachtel, Allen-Masterson, Reuben, Goldberg, & Mor, 1988). Although focused on cancer pain, the principles outlined in Part II of this book (chapters. 10, 11, and 12) are readily applied to pain in other diseases, including heart disease, AIDS, and multiple sclerosis.

While the causes of patients' suffering can be found in factors other than that of poorly managed pain care, lack of success in managing pain and other symptoms virtually guarantees failure in the "fourth phase of cancer prevention . . . preventing suffering." Success in managing pain increases the likelihood of "death with dignity" (MacDonald, 1991, p. 253).

In most patients with cancer, the problem of unmanaged pain is unnecessary and due to errors in, or lack of assessment of, proper treatment (APS, 1992; Grossman, 1993). As many as 30% of post-surgical patients with cancer may *never* be assessed for pain by a nurse (Storey, 1992) and in the remainder, assessment by nurses and/or physicians is likely to be inadequate. Despite significant advances in knowledge of treatment modalities, results remain poor—even in hospices—in many cases because the knowledge is not utilized (APS, 1992; Fife, Irick, & Painter, 1993; Grossman, 1993; Storey, 1992).

This section of the book offers clinical responses to the problem of pain. Chapter 10 provides basic principles of pain management, chapter 11 gives an overview of types of pain, pain syndromes, and assessment techniques, and chapter 12 covers methods of pain management.

But there is more to pain management than just clinical issues. Some of the social, cultural, and political issues that influence pain are briefly discussed in chapter 10. Underlying any potential changes in negative influences within the nurse's control is the issue of attitude toward pain management. If the nurse's attitude is one of acceptance of the health care system tradition—patients living in unnecessary pain—then, of course, many of that nurse's patients will live in unnecessary pain. If the nurse's attitude is one of rigorous assessment and management of pain, then far fewer of that nurse's patients will live in unnecessary pain.

Acting as an agent of change in any social system or culture is often uncomfortable. In the culture of our health care system, working toward change can be

extremely difficult. It can be significantly threatening to some health care professionals—nurses and doctors alike—to be challenged on questions such as
whether a patient should or should not have a particular degree of pain; or on
whether everything appropriate is being done to manage a patient's pain. Only
an unrelenting dedication to relieving pain will lead to success. In this endeavor,
as in so many worthy struggles in life, it is important to remind ourselves that
some people will oppose us, and that many more will never acknowledge the
validity of our efforts.

References

American Pain Society. (1992). *Principles of analgesic use in the treatment of acute pain and cancer
      pain* (3rd ed.). Skokie, IL: Author.
Brescia, F.J., Adler, D., Gray, G., Ryan, M.A., Cimino, J., & Mamtini, R. (1990). Hospitalized
      advanced cancer patients: a profile. *Journal of Pain and Symptom Management, 5*(4), 221–227.
Fife, B.L., Irick, N., & Painter, J.D. (1993). A comparative study of the attitudes of physicians and
      nurses toward the management of cancer pain. *Journal of Pain and Symptom Management, 8*(3),
      132–139.
Grossman, S.A. (1993). United States: Status of cancer pain and palliative care. *Journal of Pain and
      Symptom Management, 8*(6), 437–439.
MacDonald, N. (1991). Palliative care—The fourth phase of Cancer prevention. *Cancer Detection
      and Prevention, 15*(3), 253–255.
Portenoy, R.K. (1989). Cancer pain: Epidemiology and syndromes. *Cancer, 63*(11), 2298–2307. Pitts-
      burgh, PA: Oncology Nursing Press.
Storey, P. (1992). Cancer pain management: How are we doing? *American Journal of Hospice and
      Palliative Care, 9*(3), 6–8.
Wachtel, T., Allen-Masterson, S., Reuben, D., Goldberg, R., & Mor, V. (1988). The end stage can-
      cer patient: Terminal common pathway. *The Hospice Journal, 4*(4), 43–80.

Pain: Principles of Management

In years past, pain was considered only as a physiological phenomenon. Unfortunately, this view of pain is still held by some nurses and physicians. Pain, however, is a multidimensional phenomenon, with numerous influences on its magnitude.

Influences on Pain

Many factors—physiological, psychological, sociocultural, spiritual, and institutional—can positively or negatively influence the experience of pain (Arathuzik, 1991; Haviley et al., 1992; McGuire, 1992). While practitioners and researchers tend to focus on factors that exacerbate pain, it should be remembered that there also are factors whose absence or presence positively influence the pain experience. Factors that may influence pain and suffering (Coyle, 1991; McGuire, 1992; Walsh, 1990) include:

- other symptoms, such as nausea or dyspnea;
- fear of pain;
- other fears or anxieties, especially those surrounding death;

- previous success or failure in coping with pain;
- depression;
- spiritual well-being;
- family or other interpersonal support or conflict;
- hope or hopelessness (despair);
- the meaning of the pain to the patient, family, and staff; and
- preconceived notions on the part of practitioners, e.g., that there should be less pain than the patient is experiencing, or that pain *should* be experienced.

One of the worst situations is that in which pain is combined with other factors, and the other factors and the pain begin to reinforce and amplify one another. For example, pain leads to anxiety; anxiety to conflict; conflict to anxiety; anxiety to physical tension and increased pain; and so on, in an endless vicious cycle.

Charles Kemp: TERMINAL ILLNESS: A GUIDE TO NURSING CARE. © 1995 J. B. Lippincott.

Factors Leading to Inadequately Managed Pain

Despite significant advances in pain management, pain remains a serious and unnecessary problem for many patients with advanced disease (American Pain Society [APS], 1992; Schug, Zech, & Dörr, 1990; Sheehan, Webb, Bower & Einsporn, 1992; Storey, 1992; Ufema, 1992). Pain is a serious problem because it results in vast suffering, and the suffering is unnecessary because, while simple means exist to manage pain in approximately 90% of patients with pain from cancer (Schug, Zech, & Dörr, 1990), and alternative means exist to treat the pain in the other 10% (Foley, Bonica, & Ventafridda, 1990), pain treatment continues to be "inadequate" and "inconsistent" (Paice, 1991, p. 847). Sadly, the "most common reason for unrelieved pain . . . is the failure of staff to routinely assess pain and pain relief" (APS, 1992, p. 2). Other reasons for unrelieved pain are:

- The lack of knowledge that exists among nurses and physicians of currently accepted concepts of pain management (Lindley, Dalton, & Fields, 1990; Grossman, 1993; Paice, 1991).
- Social/cultural fears or myths (of staff and patients) concerning cancer pain and using opioids to manage the pain. The two most pernicious of these are that pain is inevitable and that using opioids is bad and will result in loss of control and addiction (Foley, 1989; McCaffery and Beebe, 1989). Staff fear of patient respiratory depression is also a factor (Coyle, 1991). Cultural values of stoicism and self-control contribute to the problem.
- Some patients, and, unfortunately, staff, believe that pain is a given in cancer. The idea of pain management may be foreign to such persons (Coyle, 1991).
- Social/legal impediments to using opioids,

i.e., administrative (non-medical) systems to monitor narcotics prescriptions (Grossman, 1993; Hill, 1989).
- Problems in communication among staff and between staff and patients (Ferrell, Eberts, McCaffery & Grant, 1991): Such problems can be disease-related, interpersonal, or cultural or linguistic. (See the discussion below on communication issues.)
- Certain disease characteristics are more likely to result in poor pain control. These include: neuropathic pain origins, rapid disease progression, and pain of rapid onset and brief duration (Portenoy, 1989).
- Patient characteristics associated with poor pain control include: expressing suffering and psychological difficulties through pain (Portenoy, 1989) and difficulty expressing feelings in general (D. Overton, personal communication, January 31, 1992).

PROBLEMS IN COMMUNICATIONS

Common staff problems in communicating with patients about pain are: (1) knowledge deficit about pain (it is hard to find out what is going on if one doesn't know what questions to ask—or even not to ask!); (2) poor interpersonal skills, e.g., anxiety, impatience, difficulty attending, and so on; and (3) language or cultural barriers (see chapter 4). Common patient problems in communicating include:

- Fear of the implications of pain, i.e., that increased pain heralds advancing disease, that increased pain means that feared narcotics will be used (Cleeland, 1990), or that painful procedures may result from complaints of pain (APS, 1992).
- Experience with health professionals failing to respond to pleas for help with pain. Many patients have been told, "We'll control your pain" and have then spent days, weeks, or months in pain. And many

patients have had their complaints of pain discounted by health professionals (Ferrell, Eberts, McCaffery & Grant, 1991). Other patients may try to "be good patients" who do not complain, and who are thus better liked by staff (Cleeland, 1990).

- Patients or family members who feel that the pain is deserved because of some misdeed, or that pain is somehow required of patients with cancer (Coyle, 1991).
- The presence of anxieties because of a belief that focus on pain may divert efforts to cure the disease (Cleeland, 1990).
- The presence of language or cultural barriers.

Principles of Effective Pain Management

The World Health Organization (WHO) (1986) provides an uncomplicated, three-step oral drug therapy to manage pain in patients with pain from cancer (see Managing Specific Pain Situations, in chapter 12). WHO guidelines for managing pain are essentially the same as those promoted since the mid-1960s by Dame Cicely Saunders and others. For the approximately 10% of patients whose pain is not manageable through the WHO therapy, other effective techniques exist (Foley, Bonica, & Ventafridda, 1990; APS, 1992). These are discussed further on. The following is a list of basic principles for effective pain management:

- Use medications or techniques that are appropriate to the severity and specific type of pain (see chapter 12).
- Give medications in amounts sufficient to control the pain and at intervals appropriate to the medication's duration of action. When changing medications, use equianalgesic conversions (see chapter 12).
- Use oral medications when possible. Controlled release morphine (CRM) is the first drug of choice for patients with chronic cancer pain. As noted elsewhere, oral medications are effective in about 90% of patients with cancer pain.
- Give medications around the clock (ATC) at regular intervals (prophylactically) so that a relatively constant titer is maintained, and the patient does not reexperience pain. Awaken the patient to receive medications on schedule. PRN orders are open to great variation in clinical judgment competencies (McCaffery & Beebe, 1989), and often to undermedication as well (Paice, 1991).
- Use adjuvant medications (nonsteroidal, anti-inflammatory drugs [NSAIDs], corticosteroids, anticonvulsants, antidepressants, phenothiazines).
- Assess for and treat side effects or complications; anticipate problems when a side effect is likely—e.g., constipation from narcotics, or nausea in a patient with a history of nausea. All patients and families should have instructions and means *on hand* to manage breakthrough pain. Morphine sulfate (not controlled release) or hydromorphone tablets or suppositories are choices for families not prepared to give injections.
- Assess for tolerance: As noted earlier, some patients are reluctant to complain. Regular assessment is thus necessary.
- Assess for and intervene in psychosocial and spiritual issues related to the pain.
- Do not look only to pharmacology or to any other single means of controlling pain (Herr & Mobily, 1992). A variety of effective psychological interventions exist, and there are also situations in which radiation, neurosurgery, or other interventions are the treatment of choice.
- Approach each patient as an individual who brings unique beliefs, strengths, and weaknesses to the immense experience of cancer pain.
- Teach the patient and family these principles of pain management.

Goals, Objectives, and Responsibilities in Pain Management

The goal of pain management in patients with chronic cancer pain is to "achieve continuous suppression of pain" (Babul, Darke, Anslow, & Krishnamurthy, 1992, p. 400). Complete eradication of pain without some sedation is difficult to achieve (Murphy, 1991). The effort is nevertheless directed toward the golden mean of a completely pain-free and completely alert patient.

The primary goals in treating patients with pain are:

- manage the pain and prevent further occurrence; and
- as much as is possible, determine the etiology and whether it indicates pathology that may further impact the quality of the patient's life (Walsh, 1990).

Pain is thus approached in two ways: as a problem in itself, and as a means of preventing or minimizing other problems. This second approach is often neglected, especially in palliative care. The consequences of neglecting the etiology of pain can include irreversible paralysis (see the section on Spinal Cord Compression in chapter 13), seizures (see the section on Increased Intracranial Pressure in chapter 13), circulatory collapse (see section on Pericardial Effusions in chapter 14), and other serious problems.

Nursing responsibilities, or the scope of practice in managing pain, established by the Oncology Nursing Society (Spross, McGuire, & Schmitt, 1991) are:

- describing the phenomenon;
- identifying aggravating and relieving factors;
- determining the meaning of the pain to the individual;
- determining etiology;
- determining definitions of optimal relief;
- deriving nursing diagnoses;
- assisting in determining interventions; and
- evaluating efficacy of interventions.

Another key responsibility is to "titrate prescribed analgesics and adjuvant drugs" (Wilkie, 1990, p. 339). Clearly, nursing's role in managing pain and other symptoms is expanding.

References

American Pain Society. (1992). *Principles of analgesic use in the treatment of acute pain and cancer pain* (3rd ed.). Skokie, IL: Author.

Arathuzik, D. (1991). Pain experience for metastatic breast cancer patients. *Cancer Nursing, 14*(1), 41–48.

Babul, N., Darke, A.C., Anslow, J.A., & Krishnamurthy, T.N. (1992). Pharmacokinetics of two novel rectal controlled-release morphine formulations. *Journal of Pain and Symptom Management, 7*(7), 400–405.

Cleeland, C.S. (1990). Assessment of pain in cancer: Measurement issues. In K.M. Foley, J.J. Bonica, & V. Ventafridda (Eds.). *Proceedings of the Second International Congress on Cancer Pain* (pp. 47–55). New York: Raven Press.

Coyle, N. (1991). Initial assessment and ongoing evaluation of cancer pain. *American Journal of Hospice and Palliative Care, 8*(6), 27–35.

Ferrell, B.R., Eberts, M.T., McCaffery, M., & Grant, M. (1991). Clinical decision-making and pain. *Cancer Nursing, 14*(6), 289–297.

Foley, K.M. (1989). Controversies in cancer pain. *Cancer, 63*(11), 2257–2265.

Foley, K.M., Bonica, J.J., & Ventafridda, V. (Eds.). (1990). *Proceedings of the Second International Congress on Cancer Pain.* New York: Raven Press.

Grossman, S.A. (1993). United States: Status of cancer pain and palliative care. *Journal of Pain and Symptom Management, 8*(6), 437–439.

Haviley, C., Gagnon, J., MacLean, R., Renz, J., Jones, O., De Witt, W., Nyberg, K., Burns, C., & Pohl, D. (1992). Pharmacological management of cancer pain. *Cancer Nursing, 15*(5), 331–346.

Herr, K.A., & Mobily, P.R. (1992). Interventions related to pain. *Nursing Clinics of North America, 27*(2), 347–369.

Hill, C.S. (1989). Pain management in a drug-oriented society. *Cancer, 63*(11), 2383–2386.

Lindley, C.M., Dalton, J.A., & Fields, S.M. (1990). Narcotic analgesics: Clinical pharmacology and therapeutics. *Cancer Nursing, 13*(1), 28–38.

McCaffery, M., & Beebe, A. (1989). *Pain: Clinical manual for nursing practice.* St. Louis: C.V. Mosby.

McGuire, D.B. (1992). Comprehensive and multidimensional assessment and measurement of pain. *Journal of Pain and Symptom Management, 7*(5), 312–319.

Murphy, T. (1991). Alternative drug delivery systems. *American Journal of Hospice and Palliative Care, 8*(6), 36–42.

Paice, J.A. (1991). Unraveling the mystery of pain. *Oncology Nursing Forum, 18*(5), 843–849.

Portenoy, R.K. (1989). Cancer pain: Epidemiology and syndromes. *Cancer, 63*(11), 2298–2307.

Schug, S.A., Zech, D., & Dörr, U. (1990). Cancer pain management according to WHO analgesic guidelines. *Journal of Pain and Symptom Management, 5*(1), 27–32.

Sheehan, D.K., Webb, A., Bower, D., & Einsporn, R. (1992). Level of cancer pain knowledge among baccalaureate nursing students. *Journal of Pain and Symptom Management, 7*(8), 478–484.

Spross, J.A., McGuire, D.B., & Schmitt, R.M. (1991). Oncology Nursing Society position paper on cancer pain. Pittsburgh, PA: Oncology Nursing Press.

Storey, P. (1992). Cancer pain management: How are we doing? *American Journal of Hospice and Palliative Care, 9*(3), 6–8.

Ufema, J. (1992). Pain control survey results: Not good. *American Journal of Hospice and Palliative Care, 9*(1), 11–12.

Walsh, T.D. (1990). Symptom control in patients with advanced cancer. *American Journal of Hospice and Palliative Care, 7*(6), 20–29.

Wilkie, D.J. (1990). Cancer pain management: State of the art nursing care. *Nursing clinics of North America, 25*(2), 331–343.

World Health Organization. (1986). *Cancer pain relief and palliative care.* Geneva: Author.

Pain: Classification and Assessment

Cancer pain syndromes, first elucidated by Kathleen Foley in 1975, provide a means by which pain can be classified and clinically understood (Ventafridda, 1990). Understanding pain syndromes and other characteristics of pain help determine: (1) etiologies and, thus, treatment; and (2) potential for complications of advancing disease.

Classification of Pain

The two general types of pain are acute and chronic. Acute pain results from tissue damage and usually resolves when the damage is resolved. Acute pain is generally associated with physical signs, such as tachycardia, hypertension, diaphoresis, mydriasis, and pallor (American Pain Society [APS], 1992).

Chronic pain is "pain that persists a month beyond the usual course of an acute disease or a reasonable time for an injury to heal or that is associated with a chronic pathologic process that causes continuous pain or the pain recurs

at intervals for months or years" (Bonica, 1990, p. 19). Chronic pain is seldom accompanied by the physical signs characteristic of acute pain. Chronic pain is more complex than acute, both in terms of pathophysiology (of the pain itself and in its effects on other symptoms), and of psychosocial and spiritual issues (Foley, 1987; Levy, 1985). Cancer pain can be acute, chronic, or intermittent (APS, 1992) and because of the global nature of the disease, it can also be a combination of these.

Pain is further classified physiologically as somatic, visceral, or neuropathic (deafferentation) pain (Payne, 1990):

- Somatic pain is described as constant, localized, aching, and/or gnawing: pain from bony metastases, for example, or following surgery (Foley, 1991), with bone pain being a common cause of severe pain in patients with cancer (Walsh, 1990).
- Visceral pain is described as constant, poorly localized, deep, and squeezing; it is sometimes referred to cutaneous sites. Abdominal or thoracic viscera are the origin of visceral pain, and examples include shoulder pain from diaphragmatic paralysis or liver/lung metas-

Charles Kemp: TERMINAL ILLNESS: A GUIDE TO NURSING CARE. © 1995 J. B. Lippincott.

tases, pancreatic pain, and pain from bowel obstruction (Foley, 1991; Portenoy, 1989).

- Neuropathic pain is described as "paroxysms of shooting or shock-like" pain, "on a background of burning, constricting sensation" (Payne, 1990, p. 22). While not referred, neurologic pain can "be projected to the appropriate dermatome" (Walsh, 1989, p. 330). Brachial plexopathy due to Pancoast's tumor or breast cancer, sacral plexopathy, postherpetic neuralgia, and phantom limb pain are examples of neuropathic etiologies (Foley, 1991; Portenoy, 1989).

These classes of pain are often mixed. Tumor infiltration of nerve and spine, for example, results in mixed somatic and neuropathic pain (Foley, 1991). Any of these classes of pain may also "be complicated by sympathetically maintained pain," which is described as "severe, burning . . . with dysesthesias and hyperpathia, as well as skin and bone changes (Payne, 1989, p. 2267). In most patients with advanced cancer, there is more than one site of pain and often more than one classification.

Somatic and visceral pain respond well to treatment by reduction of the tumor, opioids plus adjuvant medications, and sometimes neurosurgical or anesthetic treatment. Neuropathic pain does not respond as well to these treatments and is thus more challenging to treat (Coyle, 1991). Adjuvant medications, both tricyclic antidepressants and anticonvulsants—e.g., carbamazepine—assume a greater importance in neuropathic pain (Payne, 1989). The types of pain and their treatment are described in greater detail below.

Readers are referred to Foley (1991) and Portenoy (1989) for specific cancer pain syndromes; they are described below within broad terms.

Direct tumor involvement accounts for the source of about 75% of patients' pain (Coyle, 1991).

- *Invasion of bone:* The most common problems are the pain itself, neurological deficits, and pathological fractures. Bone pain is often worse at night (Walsh, 1989). Common sites are:
  1. Base of skull: Regional pain is usually the first symptom; cranial nerve involvement, other neurological signs, and changes in the range of motion of the neck are common.
  2. Vertebral bodies: The first and sometimes only symptom is pain. Central back pain (90%) with or without radicular pain is the most common. Neurologic signs and symptoms may follow, e.g., motor followed by sensory impairment (Ratanatharathorn & Powers, 1991). The outcome of untreated vertebral body metastases is spinal cord compression, which is discussed more completely under neurological problems. Quick action is required when vertebral involvement is suspected. Signs and symptoms are related to the (spinal) level of involvement, except that pain is sometimes referred, e.g., from L_1 or T_{12} to the ipsilateral iliac crest, or sacroiliac joint.
  3. Generalized involvement of bone: Multiple bone metastases are the most frequent cause of bone pain. Besides vertebrae, early metastases are commonly found in ribs and pelvis. Later metastases are found in the skull, femora, humeri, scapulae, and sternum. (Enck, 1991a).
- *Tumor infiltration of nerves*
  1. Peripheral nerves: Pain is constant or paroxysmal or both, aching or burning, and often in an area of sensory loss. Pain may be localized or radiating. Common tumor sites are chest wall, rib (intracostal nerves), retroperitoneal, and paraspinal areas. The latter may cause cord compression.
  2. Nerve plexi:
     A. Brachial plexopathy is most common in patients with lung or breast cancer. Severe regional pain (shoulder, arm, scapula, sometimes extending

to fingers) usually is the first symptom. Pain may be aching, with burning dysesthesias of the hand. Motor and sensory changes occur in the affected arm. Progressive pain and/or Horner's syndrome (unilateral ptosis, miosis, sinking eyeball, and anhidrosis and flushing of the affected side) indicate probable extension into epidural space. Patients with brachial plexopathy are at risk for cord compression.

B. Lumbosacral plexopathy is most common in patients with regional tumors or metastasis, e.g., gynecological, genitourinary, colorectal. Aching pain in the lumbosacral area, groin, or leg (usually ipsilateral), is the most common first symptom. Continuous or paroxysmal dysesthesias may also occur. Lower extremity weakness and sensory loss are common. Cord compression may occur.

3. Epidural spinal cord compression: Pain is the most common first symptom, followed by motor and sensory weakness.

4. Leptomeningeal metastases: Pain may be constant headache or lower back pain. Neurologic signs vary.

5. Brain metastases: The headache from increased intracranial pressure is "classically the worst headache ever experienced" (Levy, 1985, p. 395). Headache is usually experienced before getting out of bed and improves about an hour after arising. Accompanying symptoms are changes in mentation, nausea, and vomiting (Glover & Glick, 1991). A more complete discussion of increased intracranial pressure can be found in chapter 13.

• *Invasion, compression, distension, obstruction, or stretching of viscera* (Levy, 1985): Pain in viscera—e.g., pancreas, stomach, intestine—may be dull, boring, lancinating, or colicky, depending on site and other factors (Baines, 1990; Beazley & Cohn, 1991). Pain from hepat-

ic metastases is of two types: most patients have right upper quadrant body wall pain; some have poorly localized abdominal pain radiating to flanks and back (Waldman, Feldstein, Donohoe, & Waldman, 1988).

PAIN ASSOCIATED WITH CANCER THERAPY

• *Postoperative pain* (We are concerned here only with pain that may continue or recur well past surgery.)

1. Post-mastectomy: Pain in the arm, axilla, or chest wall may occur as late as several months after surgery and is described as tight and burning, exacerbated with movement.

2. Post-thoracotomy: Pain is at the surgical site and is often associated with tumor.

3. Post-radical neck: Pain may be constant and burning only, or accompanied by dysesthesia and intermittent shock-like pain. Radical neck surgery may damage motor nerves and result in aching neck or shoulder pain.

4. Post-amputation: Phantom limb pain that recurs after initial resolution may signal disease recurrence. Pain is usually burning and cramping.

• *Postchemotherapy pain*

1. Peripheral neuropathy: Vinca alkaloids and hexamethamelamine may result in burning pain in hands and feet. The pain usually resolves 4–6 weeks after therapy.

2. Steroid pseudorheumatism: Withdrawal of steroids can result in myalgia and arthralgia, but no objective signs of inflammation. Withdrawal of steroids significantly exacerbates bone pain.

3. Aseptic bone necrosis: Chronic steroid therapy, as well as other cancer therapy, may cause necrosis of the femoral or humeral head. The problem presents with pain, followed by progressive loss of function in the affected limb.

4. Mucositis: Methotrexate or 5-fluorouracil

can cause extremely painful mucositis that is not responsive to mouthwashes or topical agents (Levy, 1985).

- *Post-radiation pain* (The incidence of post-radiation damage is decreasing because of improved radiotherapy techniques [Levy, 1985].)
  1. Radiation fibrosis of nerve plexi (brachial or lumbosacral): Numbness or paraesthesia may occur from six months to twenty years after treatment. Sensory and motor weakness also occur.
  2. Radiation myelopathy: Although most patients with radiation myelopathy present with neurological deficits (paresis of one side and motor loss on the other), some have pain as an early symptom.
  3. Radiation-induced peripheral nerve tumors: Tumor may occur in the irradiated area as many as twenty years after radiation therapy.
  4. Radiation-induced bone necrosis: See aseptic bone necrosis above.
  5. Mucositis: See mucositis above.
- *Other:* Pain from cardiac tamponade, hypercalcemia, muscle spasms, myofascia, peptic ulcer, cystitis, osteoporosis, constipation, immobility, inflammation secondary to infection, decubitus ulcers, and post-herpetic neuralgia may be directly, indirectly, or not at all related to the cancer or cancer therapy (Twycross, 1978). See chapter 15 for a more complete discussion of decubitus ulcers and post-herpetic neuralgia; and chapter 27, on AIDS, for problems of opportunistic infections.

Assessment of Pain

Knowledge of pain syndromes, symptoms other than pain, and psychosocial and spiritual issues in terminal illness are interfaced with assessment parameters to develop an understanding of the nature and meaning of the patient's pain (McGuire, 1992). Since cancer pain is largely a subjective and multi-dimensional experience, communication between patient and nurse is of the utmost importance: The more difficulty in communicating, the more problems will exist in management (Cleeland, 1990).

Common staff problems in communicating with patients about pain are: (1) knowledge deficit about pain (It is hard to find out what is going on if one doesn't know what questions to ask, or isn't even aware of the need to ask!); (2) poor interpersonal skills, e.g., anxiety, impatience, difficulty attending, and so on; and (3) language or cultural barriers (see chapter 5).

The first assessment question should generally be something like, "Tell me about the pain." This general, unspecific question gives the patient the opportunity to say what is on his or her mind, and perhaps to give critical insight into the situation. Initially directing the patient's thoughts instead to specific questions may result in submerging key information—which the patient needs to communicate—in a sea of assessment questions. In addition, some specific assessment questions may be less relevant than what patients actually have on their minds. The final assessment question should be to ask the patient if he or she has any further thoughts about the pain or the pain control.

Nurses and physicians consistently and sometimes drastically underestimate patient pain (Cleeland, 1990; Storey, 1992). Patient estimations of pain, the "gold standard" (Bruera, Fainsinger, Miller, & Kuehn, 1992) are the best source of information. "Believe the patient's complaint of pain" (Foley, 1991, p. 563).

Comprehensive assessment parameters are listed below. Many patients have difficulty being specific. The practitioner must be patient and persistent in such cases. It is essential that pain be *systematically* assessed by all staff and that assessments be *systematically* communicated among staff (Cleeland, 1990; Lee, McPherson, & Zuckerman, 1992; McGuire, 1992). This measure alone has a salutary effect on pain (Faries, Mills, Goldsmith, Phillips, & Orr, 1991). Because cancer pain is "dynamic and ever-changing" (Cleeland, 1990, p. 540), it must be assessed regularly throughout care.

The assessment parameters given below are based on WHO Cancer Pain Relief (1986) guidelines, on the short-form McGill Pain Questionnaire (Melzack, 1987), the Memorial Pain Assessment Card (Fishman et al., 1987), and the Wisconsin Brief Pain Questionnaire (Cleeland, 1990; Daut, Cleeland, & Flanery, 1983). WHO guidelines are known to be effective (Schug, Zech, & Dörr, 1990) and the latter three are multi-dimensional and have good reliability and validity (McGuire, 1992). Pain assessment tools are included at the end of this chapter. These incorporate most of the parameters given below.

PAIN ASSESSMENT PARAMETERS

- *Location(s) and radiation:* It is important to help the patient be as specific as possible. Most pain assessment tools include frontal-view and back-view line drawings of a human figure. Patients shade in the areas on these drawings where they feel pain, and thus document information that is helpful in determining etiology. The practitioner can use a different color pencil, or clear overlays, to mark surgery, radiation, known metastases, or other significant sites. Use of graphics does not obviate the need to look at and touch the sites of pain indicated by the patient.

- *Severity:* There are several types of scales to help assess the severity of pain. A verbal rating scale (VRS), also termed a categorical scale, offers words such as "none," "mild," "moderate," "severe," and "overwhelming" for patients to choose from in describing the intensity of pain. A visual analogue scale (VAS) uses a straight 10 cm line with one end representing no pain and the other the worst possible pain (see Figure 11.1, VAS-Type Scale, in conjunction with Figure 11.2, Brief Pain Inventory). The patient marks the line at the place he or she most feels the pain. Recently, several drug manufacturers (Janssen Pharmaceutica and Knoll Pharmaceuticals) began providing colored VAS scales to practitioners.

- *Quality:* The patient's own words should be employed in documentation. Terms like dull, aching, sharp, shooting, burning, numb but feels bad, and so on, point to the classification, or origins, of the pain (see earlier discussion of types of pain). Unpleasant sensations other that pain per se should be documented.

- *Influencing factors (other than medications) and patterns:* What makes the pain better or worse? When is pain most severe; least severe; is it constant, does it comes and go gradually, or is it paroxysmal; is it worse at a particular time of day or night? Are there any Feelings (emotional or spiritual factors) that affect the pain?

- *Other physical symptoms, especially those that are new or increasing:* Motor, sensory, and range of motion changes are particularly important because they indicate probable neurological involvement. Nausea and vomiting may be associated with significant processes, such as increased intracranial pressure and hypercalcemia.

- *Impact of pain on (1) activity, (2) mood, (3) enjoyment of life, (4) sleep, (5) sociability, and (6) any other relevant aspect of life:* Pain impact or "pain-related disability" is one of the primary components in chronic pain classification attempts (Korff, Ormel, Keefe, & Dworkin, 1992).

- *Meaning of the pain to the patient (and at times, the family)*

- *Pain history:* Data should be gathered on whether pain occurred suddenly or developed gradually, and whether it developed after a particular event (e.g., changes in medications—especially analgesics and steroids—coughing spells, falls, etc.). What medications and/or treatments succeeded in controlling the pain, and what failed?

- *Effects of current medication(s):* Assessing the effects of medication(s) is a complex issue, sometimes needlessly complicated by polypharmacy (Walsh, 1990). Baseline data include:
  1. Name of medication(s)
  2. Effects

FIGURE 11.1
VAS-type scale

No pain ——————————————————————————— Worst possible pain

FIGURE 11.2. **BPI-type scales**

The brief pain inventory (BPI) makes the VAS easier for patients to understand by
using a line numbered 0–10 as shown below.

Pain assessment

No   Pain as bad
pain   0   1   2   3   4   5   6   7   8   9   10   as you can
                                                                               imagine

The patient assesses her or his pain on an average and at the time of assessment.

Relief assessment

No   Complete
relief   0%   10%   20%   30%   40%   50%   60%   70%   80%   90%   100%   Relief

The patient assesses her or his relief on an average and at the time of assessment.

3. Length of effects
4. Problems patient and family think result from the medication(s)
5. Patient and family feelings about the medication(s)
6. History of medication(s) taken for pain
7. Any over-the-counter, homeopathic, or herbal remedies used

Of course, not all of these parameters are assessed in every patient encounter. They should all, however, be included in every initial assessment. A short form, or tool, such a VAS scale, and specific questions based on the

patient's current and potential pain status, should be used for more frequent assessment.

Examples of forms that can be used as functional tools are shown in Figure 11.3 , Initial Pain Assessment; Figure 11.4, Flow Sheet—Pain (for monitoring pain on an hourly or other periodic basis); Figure 11.5, Patient/Family Teaching Point: Use of Daily Diary (guidelines on how to teach the use of the Daily Diary); and Figure 11.6, Daily Diary (for patient tracking of pain status—especially useful for patients at home).

It is not enough to ask the patient, "How are you feeling today?"

FIGURE 11.3. *Initial Pain Assessment Tool*

Date _____

Patient's Name _____ Age _____ Room _____

Diagnosis _____ Physician _____

Nurse _____

I. LOCATION: Patient or nurse mark drawing.

II. Intensity: Patient rates the pain. Scale used _____
    Present:
    Worst pain gets:
    Best pain gets:
    Acceptable level of pain:

III. QUALITY: (Use patient's own words, e.g., prick, ache, burn, throb, pull, sharp) _____
_____

IV. ONSET, DURATION, VARIATIONS, RHYTHMS: _____
_____

V. MANNER OF EXPRESSING PAIN: _____
_____

VI. WHAT RELIEVES THE PAIN? _____
_____

VII. WHAT CAUSES OR INCREASES THE PAIN? _____
_____

VIII. EFFECTS OF PAIN: (Note decreased function, decreased quality of life.)
    Accompanying symptoms (e.g., nausea) _____
    Sleep _____
    Appetite _____
    Physical activity _____
    Relationship with others (e.g., irritability) _____
    Emotions (e.g., anger, suicidal, crying) _____
    Concentration _____
    Other _____

IX. OTHER COMMENTS: _____
_____

X. PLAN: _____
_____

Note: Reproduced with permission from *Pain: Clinical Manual for Nursing Practice* by M. McCaffery and A. Beeb, 1989, St. Louis: The C.V. Mosby Company.

FIGURE 11.4. *Flow Sheet—Pain*

Patient _____ Date _____

*Pain rating scale used _____

Pain rating acceptable to patient: _____

Analgesic(s) prescribed: _____

Time	Pain rating	Analgesic	R	P	BP	Level of arousal	Other†	Plan & comments

*Pain rating: A number of different scales may be used. Indicate which scale is used and use the same one each time. For example, 0–10 (0 = no pain, 10 = worst pain).

†Possibilities for other columns: bowel function, activities, nausea and vomiting, other pain relief measures. Identify the side effects of greatest concern to patient, family, physician, nurses.

Note. Reproduced with permission from *Pain: Clinical Manual for Nursing Practice* by M. McCaffery and A. Beeb, 1989, St. Louis: The C.V. Mosby Company.

FIGURE 11.5
Patient/Family Teaching Point: Use of Daily Diary

To: _____ (patient's name)   Date: _____

Filling out a daily diary will help us understand how pain affects your daily activities. With this information, we can work together toward the best possible control of your pain.

   An explanation of the columns in the diary follows.

Pain rating. Use whatever pain rating you and the health team have decided is easiest for you to use. The scale you are to use is_____

Medication. Fill in the name of the medication and the amount you take at the time noted in the far left column.

Other pain relief measures. Fill in any measures that you might use to get good control of the pain. This might include your favorite hobby, listening to music, or use of heat or cold over the painful areas.

Major activity being done. It is important for us to know how well you sleep and if walking or other activities have an effect on your pain.

   Have the diary available when you see the nurse or doctor next. Remember: You are the only one who can tell us what your pain is like. The more you tell us about your pain, the more information we have to plan, with you, ways to make the pain better.

Additional comments: _____

_____

_____

If you have any questions or problems with the diary, contact:

_____ (RN or MD name)   Phone _____

_____ (Nurse's name)

Note. Reproduced with permission from *Pain: Clinical Manual for Nursing Practice* by M. McCaffery and A. Beeb, 1989, St. Louis: The C.V. Mosby Company.

FIGURE 11.6. *Daily Diary*

Name _____ Date _____

Time	Pain rating scale	Medication type and amount taken	Other pain relief measures tried or anything that influences your pain	Major activity being done: lying, sitting, standing/ walking
12 mid-night				
1 AM				
2				
3				
4				
5				
6				
7				
8				
9				
10				
11				
Noon 12				
1				
2				
3				
4				
5				
6				
7				
8				
9				
10				
11				

Comments: _____

_____

Note. Reproduced with permission from *Pain: Clinical Manual for Nursing Practice* by M. McCaffery and A. Beeb, 1989, St. Louis: The C.V. Mosby Company.

References

American Pain Society. (1992). *Principles of analgesic use in the treatment of acute pain and cancer pain* (3rd ed.). Skokie, IL: Author.

Baines, M.J. (1990). Management of malignant intestinal obstruction in patients with advanced cancer. In K.M. Foley, J.J. Bonica, & V. Ventafridda (Eds.). *Proceedings of the Second International Congress on Cancer Pain* (pp. 327–335). New York: Raven Press.

Beazley, R.M. & Cohn, I. (1991). Tumors of the pancreas, gallbladder, and extrahepatic ducts. In A.I. Holleb, D.J. Fink, & G.P. Murphy (Eds.), *Textbook of clinical oncology* (pp. 219–236). Atlanta: The American Cancer Society.

Bonica, J.J. (1990). Definitions and taxonomy of pain. In J.J. Bonica (Ed.). *The Management of pain* (2nd ed.) (pp. 18–27). Philadelphia: Lea & Febiger.

Bruera, E., Fainsinger, R.L., Miller, M.J., & Kuehn, N. (1992). The assessment of pain intensity in patients with cognitive failure: A preliminary report. *Journal of pain and symptom management, 7*(5), 267–270.

Cleeland, C.S. (1990). Assessment of pain in cancer: Measurement issues. In K.M. Foley, J.J. Bonica, & V. Ventafridda (Eds.). *Proceedings of the Second International Congress on Cancer Pain* (pp. 47–55). New York: Raven Press.

Coyle, N. (1991). Initial assessment and ongoing evaluation of cancer pain. *American Journal of Hospice and Palliative Care, 8*(6), 27–35.

Daut, R.L., Cleeland, C.S., & Flanery, R.C. (1983). Development of the Wisconsin Brief Pain Questionnaire to assess pain in cancer and other diseases. *Pain, 17*, 197–210.

Enck, R.E. (1991). Understanding and managing bone metastases. *American Journal of Hospice and Palliative Care, 8*(3), 3–4.

Faries, J.E., Mills, D.S., Goldsmith, K.W., Phillips, K.D., & Orr, J. (1991). Systematic pain records and their impact on pain control. *Cancer Nursing, 14*(6), 306–313.

Ferrell, B.R., Eberts, M.T., McCaffery, M., & Grant, M. (1991). Clinical decision-making and pain. *Cancer Nursing, 14*(6), 289–297.

Fishman, B., Pasternak, S., Wallenstein, S.L., Houde, R.W., Holland, J.C., & Foley, K.M. (1987). The Memorial Pain Assessment Card. *Cancer, 60*(5), 1151–1158.

Foley, K.M. (1987). Cancer pain syndromes. *Journal of Pain and Symptom Management, 2*(2), S13–S17.

Foley, K.M. (1991). Diagnosis and treatment of cancer pain. In A.I. Holleb, D.J. Fink, & G.P. Murphy (Eds.), *Textbook of clinical oncology* (pp. 555–575). Atlanta: The American Cancer Society.

Glover, D., & Glick, J.H. (1991). Oncologic emergencies. In A.I. Holleb, D.J. Fink, & G.P. Murphy (Eds.), *Textbook of clinical oncology* (pp. 513–533). Atlanta: The American Cancer Society.

Korff, M.V., Ormel, J., Keefe, F.J., & Dworkin, S.F. (1992). Grading the severity of chronic pain. *Pain, 50*(2), 133–149.

Lee, D.S., McPherson, M.L., & Zuckerman, I.H. (1992). Quality assurance: Documentation of pain assessment in hospice patients. *American Journal of Hospice and Palliative Care, 9*(1), 38–41.

Levy, M.H. (1985). Pain management in advanced cancer. *Seminars in Oncology. 12*(4), 394–410.

McGuire, D.B. (1992). Comprehensive and multidimensional assessment and measurement of pain. *Journal of Pain and Symptom Management, 7*(5), 312–319.

Melzack, R. (1987). The short-form McGill Pain Questionnaire. *Pain, 30*(2), 191–197.

Payne, R. (1989). Cancer pain: Anatomy, physiology, and pharmacology. *Cancer, 63*(11), 2266–2274.

Payne, R. (1990). Pathophysiology of cancer pain. In K.M. Foley, J.J. Bonica, & V. Ventafridda (Eds.). *Proceedings of the Second International Congress on Cancer Pain* (pp. 1–5). New York: Raven Press.

Portenoy, R.K. (1989). Cancer pain: Epidemiology and syndromes. *Cancer, 63*(11), 2298–2307.

Ratanatharathorn, V. & Powers, W.E. (1991). Epidural spinal cord compression from metastatic tumor: Diagnosis and guidelines for management. *Cancer treatment reviews, 18*, 55–71.

Schug, S.A., Zech, D., & Dörr, U. (1990). Cancer pain management according to WHO analgesic guidelines. *Journal of Pain and Symptom Management, 5*(1), 27–32.

Storey, P. (1992). Cancer pain management: How are we doing? *American Journal of Hospice and Palliative Care, 9*(3), 6–8.

Twycross, R.G. (1978). Relief of pain. In C.M. Saunders (Ed.). *The management of terminal disease* (pp. 65–98). London: Edward Arnold.

Waldman, S.D., Feldstein, G.S., Donohoe, C.D., & Waldman, K.A. (1988). The relief of body wall pain secondary to malignant hepatic metastases by intercostal nerve block with bipivicaine and methylprednisolone, *Journal of Pain and Symptom Management, 31*), 39–43.

Walsh, T.D. (1989). Cancer pain. In T.D. Walsh (Ed.), *Symptom control* (329–343). Boston: Blackwell Scientific Publications.

Walsh, T.D. (1990). Symptom control in patients with advanced cancer. *American Journal of Hospice and Palliative Care, 7*(6), 20–29.

World Health Organization. (1986). *Cancer Pain Relief and Palliative Care*. Geneva: Author.

Pain: Techniques of Management

Effective pain management in advanced cancer is based on knowledge of pain syndromes, thorough and ongoing assessment, knowledge of treatment modalities (especially opioids), and the strong commitment of staff to using all three of the above. Developing this fourth component of effective pain management—a strong commitment—is as much a matter of changing attitudes as it is of increasing knowledge. The essential attitude should be: Pain *can* be managed and opioids *are* safe to use.

Opioids, principally morphine, are the mainstay in managing cancer pain (Inturrisi, 1990; Schug et al., 1992). Indeed, oral medications (with morphine being the primary medication), used according to World Health Organization (WHO) guidelines (see Figure 12.1, WHO Three-Step Analgesic Ladder), control pain in approximately 90% of patients (Schug, Zech, & Dörr, 1990). While new drugs and technologies abound (Wilkie, 1990)—not to mention new marketing schemes for them devised by the pharmaceutical companies—the paramount issue in pain management is not new technology but learning to adapt to whatever method or combination of methods we know will do the job—an adaptation to what we know *works*.

Pharmacological Management of Pain: Medications

MILD ANALGESICS: NONOPIOIDS

Nonopioid analgesics include acetaminophen and non-steroidal anti-inflammatory drugs (NSAIDs) such as aspirin, indomethacin, ibuprofen, fenoprofen, and naproxyn. Aspirin and acetaminophen are the analgesics of first choice for mild pain and, contrary to common belief, are equal in analgesic, antipyretic, and anti-inflammatory properties in cancer pain (Beaver, 1990). Aspirin and other NSAIDs are a mainstay for metastatic bone pain (Foley, 1991). Even when bone pain is severe, NSAIDs added to opioids contribute significantly to pain relief. Adjuvant medications, principally corticosteroids and psychotropic drugs, increase analgesia and have other salutary effects, given in combination with mild analgesics (Walsh, 1990c).

Acetaminophen has fewer adverse effects than aspirin, except in patients with liver disease (a significant liability for patients with lung, breast, GI, and GU tumors: see Part IV, Metastatic Spread: Implications for Patient

Charles Kemp: TERMINAL ILLNESS: A GUIDE TO NURSING CARE. © 1995 J. B. Lippincott.

FIGURE 12.1
World Health Organization Three-Step Analgesic Ladder

FREEDOM FROM CANCER PAIN

STEP 3   Opioid for moderate to severe pain
± non-opioid
± avjuvant

When pain persists or increases, proceed to Step 3

STEP 2   Opioid for mild to moderate pain
± non-opioid ±
adjuvant

When pain persists or increases, proceed to Step 2

STEP 1   Non-opioid
± adjuvant

Note. From World Health Organization, (p. 9), 1990: Author.

Care) and/or alcoholism. Aspirin and the other NSAIDs have adverse effects on the gastrointestinal, hematopoietic, hepatic, and renal systems, especially with chronic use (Foley, 1991). All the mild analgesics share the liability of ceiling effect, i.e., analgesia does not increase and toxicity occurs at higher doses.

MILD ANALGESICS: OPIOIDS

Mild opioids include codeine, oxycodone, hydrocodone, and propoxyphene. These medications are useful primarily when added to an NSAID that is not completely effective in controlling mild to moderate pain (Beaver, 1990). There are also times when a low-dose, mild opioid, combined with a low-dose NSAID, can produce analgesia without the side effects that

result from a higher dose of either alone. Clinical experience points to oxycodone as more effective than codeine or propoxyphene. Codeine alone, or used routinely, is best avoided because side effects are significant (Walsh, 1990b) and because the analgesia of a typical dose does not exceed that of the NSAIDs (See chart at the end of this chapter). Propoxyphene has the liabilities of minimal analgesic effects in many patients, long half-life, tendency to accumulate with chronic use, and overdose complicated by convulsions (Foley, 1991). Fixed dose combinations of NSAIDs and mild opioids are best avoided because, while increasing the dose of the opioid may have no adverse effects, the ceiling dose of the NSAID is quickly reached (Rogers, 1991).

The side effects of the mild opioids are essentially the same in nature as those of the strong opioids, which are discussed later on in this chapter.

MIXED AGONIST/ANTAGONIST AND PARTIAL AGONIST OPIOIDS

Opioid agonist/antagonists include penta-zocine (Talwin), butorphanol (Stadol), and nal-buphine (Nubain). Buprenorphine (Buprenex) is a partial agonist. These are best avoided for patients with chronic cancer pain because they do not produce greater analgesia than other opioids and are associated with greater psy-chomimetic side effects than are other (agonist) opioids (Walsh, 1990b). They also precipitate withdrawal in opioid-dependent patients.

STRONG OPIOID ANALGESICS

The strong opioid analgesics that are most effec-tive for moderate to severe pain are morphine, hydromorphone (Dilaudid), levorphanol (Levo-dromoran), and transdermal fentanyl (American Pain Society [APS], 1992; Foley, 1989; Inturrisi, 1990; Walsh, 1990b). Although used to good effect by some, both heroin and methadone have lia-bilities that suggest that the previously cited med-ications are better choices. Meperidine (Demerol) is a poor choice for managing cancer pain because chronic use can result in CNS excitability leading to seizures, especially in patients with renal dys-function (Foley, 1989). However, IM meperidine is more effective than IM morphine or hydro-morphone for painful procedures or for other occasional "pain emergencies" because meperi-dine penetrates the blood-brain barrier more quickly and gives less sedation or respiratory depression after the procedure (APS, 1992). These pain emergencies should not be considered the same as breakthrough pain.

Opioid side effects limit the use of opioids in some cases (Foley, 1991). In many other cases, however, use is limited by unrealistic concerns about adverse effects, such as respi-ratory depression and addiction (Paice, 1991). The principal side or adverse effects of opioids (APS, 1992; Foley, 1991; Haviley et al., 1992; Paice, 1991) include:

- *Sedation* is usually an early (initiating) side effect of opioid use, decreasing 2–5 days after a consistent dose is established. Seda-tion may, however, increase several days after analgesia is achieved with medications that have a long half-life (Inturrisi, 1990). Sedation results from medication effects on the CNS, and may also be related to exhaus-tion from chronic pain. Interventions include: (1) accepting sedation for several days; (2) gradual decrease in dose of opi-oids; (3) caffeine beverages or other stimu-lants given until early afternoon; (4) decreasing or eliminating all sedating med-ications, except for those that are essential (Haviley et al., 1992; Walsh, 1990b). Seda-tion, or a decrease in consciousness emerg-ing as a new development when a medica-tion regime is established, may be a sign of changes in disease processes. Naloxone should not be used unless there is a "clear threat to life . . . in an individual with an otherwise reasonable prognosis," lest a "massive pain breakthrough" occur (Walsh, 1990b, p. 366).
- *Nausea and vomiting.* Like sedation, this is most often an initiating side effect of opi-oids, and usually lasts 2–3 days. If nausea and vomiting do occur, antiemetics, such as prochlorperazine (Compazine) or metoclo-pramide (Reglan) should be given on schedule (Walsh, 1990b) and gradually withdrawn after 3–5 days (increased time intervals between taking the medicine). Some patients respond to a change in opi-oid and others benefit from a change in reg-imen, e.g., from oral to controlled release; or route, e.g., from oral to rectal or continuous subcutaneous infusion (APS, 1992). Correct equianalgesic conversions are important—and a common source of error—when

changing routes or medications (see the section on Equianalgesic Conversions later on in this chapter). Practitioners must be alert to the possibility of nausea and vomiting originating in etiologies other than opioids, e.g., in bowel obstruction, hypercalcemia, increased intracranial pressure, etc.

- *Constipation* is part of chronic opioid use, especially when the patient is: also taking NSAIDs, is immobile, is ingesting inadequate fluids and fiber (Cushman, 1986), and is depressed. A bowel regimen consisting of adequate fluids, the avoidance of constipating foods, and a stool softener and mild laxative should be initiated *at the same time* opioids are started. Preventing constipation is discussed more fully in chapter 17, Gastrointestinal Problems and Interventions.

- *Confusion* may result from excessive dosing or from inadequately controlled pain.. Changes in the reduction of the amount of opioid given resolves confusion from these causes. Hallucinations, accompanied by sudden mood changes without confusion or thought disorder, develop in small numbers of patients. Symptoms respond to haloperidol and a change in opiate (Bruera, Schoeller, & Montejo, 1992). Confusion may also result from brain metastases, hypercalcemia, medications other than opioids, and other causes (see chapter 13).

- *Urinary retention* is a transient side effect, occurring most often in older patients. Catheterization may be required (Inturrisi, 1990).

- *Dry mouth* may be due as much to the anticholinergic properties of antidepressants as to opioids.

- *Pruritus* is a common, but not necessarily distressing side effect of opioids. Fentanyl and oxymorphone (Numorphan) cause less itching than do other strong opioids (APS, 1992). Most patients develop tolerance to pruritus (see Chapter 15).

- *Respiratory depression* is potentially the most dangerous side effect. Since respiratory depression seldom occurs in patients who regularly take opioids, its importance in patients with terminal cancer is "exaggerated" (Walsh, 1990b, p. 362). Tolerance to respiratory depression from opioids develops quickly with regular use (Foley, 1991). Respiratory depression occurs most frequently in patients with severe pain who receive large first-time doses (APS, 1992), especially of methadone or levorphanol (Foley, 1989); and in patients with rapidly changing respiratory status (Walsh, 1990b). Patients whose pain is newly relieved often fall asleep, which adds to depressant effects, as well as creates the possibility of airway obstruction by the tongue. Such patients should be closely observed 3–4 hours past the peak plasma level of the drug (APS, 1992). Adjusting opioid dose on the basis of respiratory rate, however, is "inappropriate" (Walsh, 1990b, p. 367).

- *Addiction or dependence* is feared by patients and professionals alike. The risk of addiction in medical-surgical patients of any kind is insignificant: In one study of 11,882 patients given opioids, four developed problems of addiction (Porter& Jick, 1980). Research at St. Christopher's Hospice showed that patients who regularly used heroin for pain control, and who discontinued the medication because the etiology of the pain was resolved, did not experience problems of addiction or dependence following discontinuation (Twycross, 1978). Several fears, or issues, are subsumed under that of "addiction":

1. Psychological dependence—a state of overwhelming craving for a drug and patterns of behavior that include going to extreme lengths to obtain the drug.

2. Physical dependence—a state in which discontinuation of a drug is accompanied by distress. Contrary to dramatic portrayals of drug addicts in agony, discontinuing oral opioids for patients with cancer results in "mild to moderate anxiety, tremulousness, and sweating" (Walsh,

1990b, p. 367). Gradual discontinuation of opioids decreases distress. "Clock-watchers" and other patients who are labeled as "a problem" with respect to analgesics are almost invariably patients whose pain is poorly managed, often with injections of inadequate amounts of medication given at intervals exceeding the duration of action of the medication. These patients are iatrogenically dependent and iatrogenically suffering.

3. Tolerance—a state in which ever-larger doses of medication are required to achieve the same effect; with the underlying fear that it doesn't take long to reach a point at which no dose is effective; i.e.,"They're saving the strong stuff for when the pain gets really bad." About 50% of patients with cancer pain take increasing amounts of opioids until death (Foley, 1991). However, after an initial rapid rise, there tends to be a much slower rate of increase (Twycross, 1978). Approximately 30% of patients maintain a stable dose and 20% decrease the dose over time, until death (Foley, 1991). Tolerance is first manifested by a decrease in duration of analgesia (APS, 1992). Tolerance is addressed by shortening the interval at which medications are given, increasing the dose, adding adjuvant medications, or switching to another opioid. Cross-tolerance between opioids is not complete, and the American Pain Society (1992) recommends that when switching opioids, the patient should be started on one-half the equianalgesic dose, then titrated upward, according to relief of pain. Failure to control pain with strong opioids initially is not a problem of tolerance, but an indication that more medication, adjuvants, or different techniques are needed. Switching medications under these circumstances is an exercise in futility, and using one-half the equianalgesic dose is an exercise in cruelty.

ADJUVANT MEDICATIONS

Adjuvant medications are used to potentiate the effects of opioids, to decrease side effects of opioids, to treat associated symptoms (Bruera, 1991), and to treat pain that responds poorly to opioids. Adjuvant medications include: tricyclic antidepressants, anxiolytics, corticosteroids, anticonvulsants, and phenothiazines.

Tricyclic Antidepressants

Amitriptyline (Elavil), desipramine (Norpramin), doxepin (Sinequan), imipramine (Tofranil), and nortriptyline (Pamelor) are among the more commonly used antidepressants in advanced cancer. Antidepressants have analgesic effects that are apparently independent of their antidepressant effects (Monks, 1990). Their analgesic effects are primarily in neuropathic pain from postherpetic neuralgia, diabetic neuropathy, cancer treatment, and brachial and lumbosacral plexopathy (APS, 1992; Foley, 1991). Antidepressants also affect the depression and anxiety that both accompany and influence the pain of advanced disease. The sedative properties of antidepressants (except for desipramine and nortriptyline) mean that they can be used for insomnia as well as for improving mood and pain. Doses are lower in patients with advanced cancer than for those whose primary diagnosis is depression. Effects are usually experienced in 24–48 hours vs. the 2–3 weeks required in patients with a psychiatric diagnosis of depression. The starting dose for amytriptyline is 25 mg and for elderly patients, 10 mg, both in a single bed-time dose. This may be titrated up to 75 mg (Foley, 1991). Side effects such as dry mouth, palpitations, blurred vision, constipation, and edema are often transitory (Monks, 1990). Tricyclic antidepressants are also used for pain in multiple sclerosis.

Anti-Anxiety Medications

While anxiolytic medications are often prescribed in terminal illness, they are not indicated in managing chronic pain, nor are they as useful as antidepressants in addressing issues associated with chronic pain. Although anxiety is common to patients with depression or pain, especially those with acute pain, the primary issue is often the depression rather than the anxiety: Resolve the depression and the anxiety also is likely resolved; resolve the anxiety and depression remains. Care should be taken to ensure that anxiety, rather than depression, is the primary problem.

Corticosteroids

Dexamethasone (Decadron), prednisolone (Cortolone, Delta-Cortef), and prednisone are examples of the corticosteroids commonly used for symptom control in patients with advanced cancer. Corticosteroids reduce pain through reducing inflammation and also improve appetite, increase strength, and generally improve the patient's sense of well-being (Bruera, 1991). Specific indications for corticosteroids include pain from bone metastases, brachial or lumbosacral plexopathy, and metastatic arthralgia. Corticosteroids are also used to ameliorate increased intracranial pressure, spinal cord compression, and superior vena cava syndrome (Walsh, 1990c). The side effects of chronic use should not be an issue in patients with advanced cancer. Several side effects should, however, be noted: (1) because it may cause sleep disturbances, prednisone should not be taken at night; and (2) rapid withdrawal exacerbates pain, hence withdrawal should be gradual (APS, 1992).

Anticonvulsants

Carbamazepine (Tegretol), phenytoin (Dilantin), clonazepam (Klonopin), and baclofen (Lioresal) are often effective in relieving neuropathic pain, such as: the dysesthetic component of postradical neck surgery (APS, 1992; Foley, 1991); lancinating pain, for example, from postherpetic neuralgia (APS, 1992); or carcinomatous neuropathies, i.e., tumor invasion of nerves (Loeser, 1990). Doses for both carbamazepine and phenytoin begin at 100 mg/day and

increase for carbamazepine over 8–10 days, up to 800 mg/day, and for phenytoin up to 300 mg/day (Foley, 1991). Serum levels of anticonvulsants, as well as CBCs, should be monitored. Neutropenia is a potential untoward effect of carbamazepine. Patients should thus be carefully monitored for infection, especially if blood work is not regularly done. Increased doses of corticosteroids and methadone may be required for patients taking phenytoin.

Phenothiazines

Methotrimeprazine (Levoprome) is the only phenothiazine with significant analgesic properties (APS, 1992). Methotrimeprazine is recommended for intermittent use, and in patients with bowel obstruction; 15 mg methotrimeprazine IM is equivalent to 10 mg morphine IM (Foley, 1991). Prochlorperazine (Compazine) is an effective antiemetic and is available in suppository as well as in oral and IM forms. Other phenothiazines are reported, but not proven, to have analgesic properties (Walsh, 1990c). Other pain-related indications for phenothiazines are extreme pain with anxiety, psychomotor agitation, insomnia not responsive to other measures, bladder or rectal tenesmus, and ureteral spasm (Monks, 1990).

Managing Specific Pain Situations

Adjuvant medications are not specified in most cases below because of variation in circumstances. However, consideration should be given to adjuvant medications in all patients. Anxiety and depression exacerbate pain, hence should always be addressed. Rescue medications should be available in all cases. As with other situations, troublesome side effects of opioids and other medications are treated prophylactically (Twycross, 1990; Walsh, 1990b).

- Mild to moderate somatic or visceral pain is treated with non-opioids, such as acetaminophen, or NSAIDs, e.g., aspirin plus an adjuvant medication; or mild opioids, especially oxycodone plus an adjuvant medication.

- Moderate to severe somatic or visceral pain is treated with opioids combined with adjuvant medications. Radiation, chemotherapy, and other measures to correct the etiology are the first choice, but for a variety of reasons, they are not always possible (Stillman, 1990).

- Neuropathic pain often requires an anticonvulsant (carbamazepine, phenytoin) as an adjuvant, and anesthetic or neurosurgical procedures may be indicated (Coyle, 1991). The "burning component" of neuropathic pain responds better to antidepressants than to opioids (Stillman, 1990). Tricyclic antidepressants usually produce results in several days, but may take as long as several weeks (Gonzales, 1992). Mexiletine (Mexitil) has shown effectiveness in neuropathic pain (Wilkie, 1990).

DIFFICULT TO MANAGE PAIN

- Severe bilateral or midline lower body pain, e.g., of pelvis, not relieved by opioids and not eligible for radiation therapy (radiation is a first choice if possible) is responsive to spinal opioids (Hassenbusch et al., 1990).

- Patients with cachexia or dysphagia can sometimes take suppositories. If not, or if analgesia is unsatisfactory, consider continuous subcutaneous infusion of an opioid with bolus capability; or if bolus is not possible, Dilaudid HP (10 mg/mL) or morphine HP can be given for pain flare-ups.

- Steroid pseudorheumatism is the appearance of myalgias, arthralgias, and other symptoms after steroids are reduced. Increasing steroids relieves the symptoms (Portenoy, 1989).

- Myofascial pain is characterized by local aching, and the resulting muscle stress or splinting from adjacent pathology. If opioids are not effective, measures such as "spray and stretch techniques, trigger point injections, and physiotherapy" may be effective (Portenoy, 1989, p. 2306). Massage and heat may also help, and muscle relaxants may be useful (Levy, 1985).

- Headache from increased intracranial pressure responds to corticosteroids. Progressive intracranial malignancy can be managed by 12 mg of dexamethasone PO QID. Prophylactic cimetidine may be indicated (Levy, 1985).

- Lymphedema, or soft tissue swelling with pain, can occasionally be reduced with diuretics (Levy, 1985).

- Intestinal colic from obstruction occurs in approximately 75% of patients with inoperable obstruction. Stimulant laxatives, metoclopramide, and domperidone should be discontinued (Baines, 1990). Antispasmodics, antiemetics, and analgesics are standard treatment (Mercadante & Maddaloni, 1992). Medications may have to be delivered by continuous subcutaneous infusion, in which case, hyoscine 0.8 mg/24 hours, increasing slowly to 2 mg/24 hours, may be effective (Baines, 1990). Hyoscine can also be taken sublingually.

- Rectal or bladder spasm pain is partially or completely relieved with belladonna and opium suppositories (Levy, 1985).

- Body wall pain secondary to malignant hepatic metastases is safely and effectively treated with intracostal nerve block (Waldman, Feldstein, Donohoe, & Waldman, 1988).

CHILDREN AND OLDER ADULTS

Pain in infants and children has traditionally been undertreated (Berde, 1991). Children and babies older than six months experience approximately the same clinical effects from opioids as do young adults (APS, 1992; Berde, 1991). Infants less than six months are at higher risk of apnea from opioids than others, hence must be very closely monitored. Oral opioids are effective for most children (Berde, 1991). After oral, continuous IV infusion and continuous subcutaneous infusion are the preferred routes of administration of medications (Inturrisi, 1990). Patient controlled analgesia (PCA) appears to be effective for children seven or older (Berde, 1991).

Assessment is a major challenge in treating children with pain, especially those younger than four years. Parents are often utilized in obtaining a pain history and giving information on words or terms their children use for pain. However, depending on parents to assess pain is as unsatisfactory as depending on anyone else other than the patient: Accuracy is unlikely. Behavioral clues in children with chronic pain are as unreliable as in adults. Children may even use a game or other types of play as a means of distraction to cope with pain. *Some children deny pain rather than take intramuscular or even subcutaneous injections.* A number of self-report tools and scales are in use. Among them are the following, which appear to produce effective results (McGrath, Mathews, & Pigeon, 1991, p. 515): the Faces Scale, Poker Chip Tool, visual analogue scales (VAS), and "pain thermometers." Most children older than four use self-report tools satisfactorily; and children older than eight are able to use numerical scales (Hester, Jacox, Miaskowski, & Ferrell, 1992). Readers should consult the pediatric literature for specifics on children and pain. The Hester et al. (1992) article is a good starting point.

Pain is incorrectly considered by some as not as great a problem among older adults as it is among younger adults (Brescia et al., 1990). Older adults have greater sensitivity to opioids than do younger adults and are at greater risk from accumulation and toxicity from medications with a lengthy plasma half-life, such as methadone and levorphanol. The primary difference between older and other adults is that older adults *complain* less of pain.

PATIENTS WITH A HISTORY OF SUBSTANCE ABUSE

Patients with a history of substance abuse or addictive disease (i.e., chronic or excessive use of alcohol or prescription or illegal drugs) present unique challenges in pain management. Problems may arise with patients over-using opioids or other medications to alleviate psychological distress to the detriment of pain management. Binges of opioid consumption may result in toxic side effects and subsequent poor pain status (McCorquodale, De Faye, & Bruera, 1993). Mixing opioids, tranquilizers, hypnotics, and other medications commonly used in terminal illness with one another and/or with alcohol can result in confusion, sedation, and death.

Problems also arise with this category of patient from different practitioner perspectives and goals. Pain specialists may view drug use as a means of coping with pain and addiction specialists may view it as a primary addiction (Savage, 1993). Others may tend to underprescribe because of concern about initiating or perpetuating addiction (McCorquodale, De Faye, & Bruera, 1993).

Assessment of a patient's potential for or actual misuse of opioids or other medications (Wesson, Ling, & Smith, 1993) includes the following:

- Does a history of misuse exist? This can be a difficult question to address because dishonesty with others and self is part of addiction. In addition to a frank history of substance use, practitioners should be alert to patient resentment of questions about substance use, their rationalization of misuse, and a history of weekend binges.
- Are medications taken reliably? Assessment of reliability includes assessment of records, monitoring consumption, and reports from others.
- Is the patient in control of use? A pattern of using all medications before time to refill

can indicate a problem of control. Claims that medications were lost should be viewed with suspicion.

- Does the patient seek drugs? A characteristic of addiction is a consistent effort to maintain supply, coupled with anxiety when the supply is depleted. Obtaining prescriptions from more than one source indicates probable difficulties.

Care is challenging when a patient is in pain and there is the possibility, or even the certainty, that the patient has the potential or is actually abusing drugs, either singly or in combination. Managing pain in such a situation includes: (1) frank communication with the patient and family, including a written care plan; (2) avoidance of medications with the highest abuse potential (especially Dilaudid); (3) use of medications with less abuse potential (especially sustained-release morphine tablets and methadone); (4) regular and careful monitoring of consumption (counting the tablets); (5) limiting prescription-writing to one physician only; and (6) utilizing a specialist in addictions (McCorquodale, De Faye, & Bruera, 1993; Wesson, Ling, & Smith, 1993). The nurse should also remain aware of the potential for family involvement, either as drug-use facilitators for the patient or as actual users themselves.

Routes and Administration

Oral medications, given in sufficient amounts, at regular and appropriate intervals, and with diligent attention to preventing side effects, are remarkably effective in controlling pain. Patients unable to swallow tablets can often take suspensions. Hydromorphone tablets can be crushed and put into suspension (APS, 1992). While intervals between medication doses are based on duration of action, the peak drug effect for most opioids (morphine, hydromorphone, oxycodone) occurs in 1.5–2 hours (except for controlled release opioids). There-

fore, if analgesia is not achieved in that time, and if side effects of non-controlled release opioids are mild, the patient can safely take a second dose (APS, 1992).

Controlled release morphine, e.g., MS Contin and Roxanol SR, provide longer duration of action than do immediate release morphine sulfate, hydromorphone, and other opioids. MS Contin's duration of action is 12 hours, but eight-hour intervals are required for some patients (Ferrell, 1991). Roxanol's duration of action is eight hours. For home care patients in particular, this means greater convenience and fewer mistakes. Hospitalized patients also prefer the less frequently given controlled release morphine over immediate release (Shepard, 1990). Controlled release morphine is also available in suspension and has efficacy, duration of action, and adverse effects similar to the better-known tablets (Boureau et al., 1992). Rescue medications should be available, whether for hospitalized or home care patients. Converting from immediate release opioids to controlled release is a significant issue, and is covered in the section on Equianalgesic Conversions.

The oral route is significantly less expensive than others; for example, patient controlled analgesia (PCA) (Ferrell & McCaffery, 1991). There are, however, other effective routes and situations in which they are indicated, including:

- Rectal suppositories (morphine, hydromorphone, levorphanol) are effective and less expensive than the high-tech routes discussed below (Kinzbrunner, Policzer, Miller, & Neiber, 1990). Patients with dysphagia or those who are unable to tolerate oral medications, are good candidates for rectal suppositories. Correct placement (approximately 1.5 inches deep) is essential to achieve consistent analgesia (Mather, 1991; McCaffery & Beebe, 1989). Some medications in oral form, including oxycodone, morphine, hydromorphone, and methadone, can be given rectally. Tablets are crushed, dissolved in 5 mL hot water, the solution cooled to body temperature, and then given via any clean small lumen rubber or other flexible tubing (McCaffery & Beebe, 1989). Note that controlled release tablets convert to immediate release in solution (McCaffery & Beebe, 1989).

- Intramuscular injection is most appropriate for acute pain, e.g., for postsurgical, myocardial infarction, etc. Appropriate uses of IM injections in chronic cancer pain are occasionally: (1) prior to painful procedures; and (2) for severe breakthrough pain. IM injections are not appropriate for managing chronic cancer pain. Liabilities of IM injections include the pain of administration, difficulty in reaching a steady-state of analgesia, and potential for muscle or soft tissue fibrosis, or sterile abscesses.

- Subcutaneous injection, e.g., of high potency hydromorphone (Dilaudid HP) is appropriate for cachectic patients under the circumstance given above.

- Intravenous infusion is most appropriate for newly admitted patients with out-of-control pain, or for patients whose pain or side effects are not managed by oral or other means, e.g., patients with cachexia, dysphagia, and bowel obstruction (Portenoy, 1990). The IV bolus gives the most rapid onset of effect of any routes, and is thus used to bring pain under control. The peak effect of intravenous morphine is reached in 15–30 minutes, and thus if analgesia is not experienced by the time of peak effect, and if side effects are not problematic, another bolus may be given (APS, 1992). Continuous IV infusion (CIVI) gives effective ongoing analgesia with minimal side effects in most patients with cancer (Portenoy, 1990), but presents more problems in patient care management than oral methods. IV infusions (usually pumps) are used successfully by some for home care patients. Again, patient care management is more challenging and IV complications can often be more of a problem at home than in the hospital.

Far too often, attempts to manage pain and other symptoms in ways other than through intravenous and other high-tech methods are completely inadequate (Ferrell & McCaffery, 1991). See also the following sections in this list on patient-controlled analgesia and intraspinal analgesia.

- Continuous Subcutaneous infusion (CSCI) of opioids via pump is used most appropriately for cachectic and dysphagic patients for whom IVs are difficult to start or maintain. Patient-controlled analgesia may also be delivered subcutaneously. A combination of CSCI, with provisions for extra or rescue doses, is best. Unless an IV line is already established, CSCI is superior to CIVI for home care (Bruera, 1990). Common medications are morphine and hydromorphone (Kerr et al., 1988), with hydromorphone HP giving the highest potency:volume ratio. The infusion site should be changed weekly unless local signs (redness and swelling) appear sooner (Bruera, 1990). Dose escalation occurs for most home care patients about every seven days, once analgesia reaches a steady state; others, however, require escalation at smaller or greater intervals (Bruera, 1990). See also the following section in this list on patient-controlled analgesia.

- Epidural or intrathecal intraspinal infusion uses less opioid (usually fentanyl or morphine) than systemic administration. Intraspinal infusion is used most appropriately for patients who are unable to tolerate opioids, or achieve relief, especially of regional pain below T_1, by other routes (APS, 1992; Enck, 1991; Murphy, 1991). Medications are delivered epidurally in single dose, intermittently by schedule or demand, or by continuous infusion; and intrathecally in a single dose. While complications are not a major liability, cost and insuring that staff have necessary expertise are significant issues (Ferrell & McCaffery, 1991; Murphy, 1991).

- Patient-controlled analgesia (PCA) pumps can deliver medications intravenously, subcutaneously, or epidurally. They are used successfully in surgical, oncology, and other settings, including the home; and new systems are rapidly being developed (Sawaki, Parker, & White, 1992). While the effectiveness of PCA vs. expert oral management of pain remains an issue of debate (Ferrell & McCaffery, 1991), it is clear that in at least the 10% of patients with cancer whose pain is not controlled with oral medications, PCAs are an option. Recall, however, that the problems in this 10% category are often found in the neuropathic nature of the pain, and thus opioids are less effective, regardless of the route. PCAs do have two qualities that make them more attractive to some: (1) some patients have a significantly greater sense of control over the pain and other aspects of their situation (Paradis, 1992); and (2) the high-tech nature of PCAs is comforting to some. For these patients, PCAs can be symbolic of the power of technology, and proof that caregivers have not surrendered. (Others may experience the high-tech nature of PCAs as intrusive.) Problems of PCAs include: cost (Sawaki, Parker, & White, 1992), which averages more than $4,000/month (Ferrell & McCaffery, 1991); need for staff expertise; and potential for complications, most of which occur in PCAs that incorporate predetermined interval demand doses (PCA-DD) and continuous background infusion (PCA-CI-DD) (Fleming & Coombs, 1992)—which are the features needed to adequately manage pain. Another problem is the question of what happens with patients who develop cognitive failure (Bruera, 1990).
- Transdermal fentanyl (Duragesic) is especially useful for patients whose pain is relatively stable. Adverse side effects include, but are not limited to, cardiovascular depression and stimulation, respiratory depression, and muscle rigidity (Stanley, 1992). Fentanyl takes 12–16 hours to produce a significant therapeutic effect, and 48 hours to produce steady-state blood concentrations (APS, 1992). Other medications are therefore required until analgesia is achieved.
- Unconventional, or developmental means of administering opioids include: intracerebroventricular, buccal/ sublingual, topical/transcutaneous, and intranasal (Mather, 1991).

Equianalgesic Conversions

Opioids have equivalent analgesic (equianalgesic) properties among routes and medications, but these vary according to medication and route. Converting from one medication or route to another carries significant potential for error. For chronic cancer pain, 30 mg of oral morphine is approximately equivalent to 10 mg IM morphine. Giving 10 mg of oral morphine in place of 10 mg IM morphine guarantees pain.

To make conversions, use equianalgesic charts (see Tables 12.1–12.4) to determine the appropriate initial dose, then titrate to effect. Examples:

- 10 mg morphine IM every four hours is equivalent to 30 mg morphine PO every four hours; 20 mg morphine IM every four hours is equivalent to 60 mg morphine PO every four hours.
- 60 mg morphine PO or 20 mg IM is equivalent to 15 mg hydromorphone PO or 3 mg IM.
- 75 mg meperidine IM is equivalent to 20 mg methadone PO or 10 mg IM.

To change from continuous IV opioids, e.g., morphine, to oral, determine how much morphine is taken in 24 hours, use the IM equivalency to convert that amount to the oral equivalent for 24 hours, and divide the 24 hour dose

TABLE 12.1.
ANALGESICS FOR MILD TO MODERATE CANCER PAIN

Analgesic	PO dose range (mg)	Duration of action (h)	Maximum 24 h dose (mg)	Comments
Acetysalicylic acid (aspirin, etc.)	500–1000	3–4	4000	Give with caution to patients with renal dysfunction, hematologic disorders, or in combination with steroids. GI upset may occur. Do not give to children under 12 years. Rectal suppositories available for children and adults.
Acetaminophen (Tylenol, etc.)	500–1000	3–4	4000	Give with caution to patients with renal dysfunction or anemia. Minimal GI side effects. Rectal suppositories available.
Ibuprofen (Motrin, Nuprin, Advil, etc.)	200–400	4–6	2400	200 mg gives greater analgesia than aspirin 650 mg. Fewer side effects than aspirin.
Naproxen (Naprosyn)	250–500	6–8	1250	Side effects similar to aspirin. Slower onset and longer duration of action.
Choline magnesium trisalicylate (Trilisate)	1000–1500	12	2000–3000	Fewer side effects than aspirin. No effect on platelets.
Diflunisal (Dolobid)	1000 initial dose, then 500	8–12	1500	Precautions similar to those for aspirin. Initial loading dose shortens onset time

Note: Data from American Pain Society, 1992; Foley, 1991; Haviley, et al., 1992; Inturissi, 1990.

by six (for regular morphine) to determine how much oral morphine to give every four hours (APS, 1992, p. 12). To determine the amount to give for single IV boluses (when pain is not controlled), use half the IM dose (APS, 1992).

Equianalgesic data on rectal opioids are not well established. Based on clinical experience, McCaffery and Beebe (1989) suggest that rectal and oral doses may be similar in effect. Mather (1991) reports that the bioavailability of rectal morphine is somewhat greater than oral; and that the bioavailability of rectal hydromorphone, methadone, and oxycodone is somewhat less than oral. Others report bioavailability is significantly higher with some morphine suppositories than with oral morphine (Babul, Darke, Anslow, & Krishnamurthy, 1992). Insertion depth influences the analgesic effects of any suppository and bowel movement after insertion may eliminate the suppository as well as the feces.

TABLE 12.2. OPIOID ANALGESICS FOR MILD TO MODERATE PAIN				
Analgesic	PO dose range (mg)	Duration of action (h)	Maximum 24 h dose (mg)	Comments
Codeine	32–65	3–4		Side and adverse effects similar to stronger opioids. 32 mg is approximately equianalgesic to 650 mg aspirin. Give with caution to patients with impaired ventilation, asthma, increased intracranial pressure, liver failure. Often combined with NSAIDs.
Propoxyphene (Darvon, Darvon-N)	65–130	3–4		May accumulate because of lengthy half-life, especially with regular use. 65 mg is approximately equianalgesic to 650 mg aspirin. Limited usefulness in terminal illness.

Note: Data from American Pain Society, 1992; Foley, 1991; Haviley, et al., 1992; Inturissi, 1990.

Analgesic Tables

To convert from other routes or medications to controlled release morphine, convert to oral immediate release morphine and administer until pain is relieved. After pain relief is achieved, determine the 24-hour dose of immediate release oral morphine, and divide by two or three (depending on whether the controlled release morphine's duration of action is 12 hours or eight hours.

Example: The patient's pain is acceptably managed with morphine 20 mg IM every four hours. This equals 120 mg IM/24 hours, and 360 mg PO/24 hours. The every-12-hour (MS Contin) dose is 180 mg MS Contin (3 MSC 60 mg tablets); and the every-eight-hour (Roxanol) dose is 120 mg.

Tables 12.1 to 12.4 summarize a few salient points—in connection with the above discussion on conversions and dosages—concerning the medications listed there. Readers should also refer to current texts, journals, and other sources for complete information on administering, adjusting, or prescribing these medications.

Only commonly used analgesics are included in these tables. Mixed agonist-antagonists and partial agonists are **not** included because their use in chronic cancer pain is seldom appropriate. It must also be borne in mind that a variety of factors influence drug effects and side effects. These include: patient size, disease status, pain intensity, other medications taken, etc. Discriminative clinical judgement is thus always necessary to effectively administer, adjust, or prescribe these medications.

Psychological Interventions

While many acknowledge the value of non-pharmacological measures to manage pain (Herr & Mobily, 1992), few report using them in

TABLE 12.3.
OPIOID ANALGESICS FOR MODERATE TO SEVERE CANCER PAIN

Analgesic	IM dose (mg)[1]	Oral dose (mg)	Duration of action (h)	Plasma 1/2 life (h)	Comments
Morphine	10	30–60[2]	4–6 IM 4–7 PO	2–3.5	Available in sustained release tablets, rectal suppositories (5, 10, 20, and 30 mg) and suspension.
Hydromorphone (Dilaudid)	1.5	7.5	4–5 IM 4–6 PO	2.3	Available in rectal suppositories (3 mg) and high potency parenteral (Dilaudid HP: 10 mg/mL). Can be given subcutaneously.
Meperidine (Demerol)	75	300	2–3 IM 2–4 PO	2–4	Limited use in terminal illness. Not recommended for long-term use.
Methadone	10	20	4–6	24–36	Tendency to accumulate in tissue and may result in over-sedation. Use with care in older patients.
Levorphanol (Levo-Dromoran)	2	4 (see comments)	4–6 IM 4–7 PO	12–16	See cautions for methadone.
Oxymorphone (Numorphan)	1		4–6	2–3	Not available in oral form. 5 mg rectal suppository = 5 mg morphine IM.
Oxycodone (Percodan, Percocet, Tylox)	15	30	3–4		Dosage limited by combination form (with aspirin or acetaminophen).
Fentanyl (see Table 12.4)					

[1]For single IV bolus use 1/2 the IM dose.
[2]There is disagreement about the IM: oral equivalency. For opioid-naive patients, the recommended **oral** starting dose is 30 mg morphine, or its equivalency.
Note: Data from American Pain Society, 1992; Foley, 1991; Haviley, et al., 1992; Inturissi, 1990.

TABLE 12.4
FENTANYL (DURAGESIC) DOSE PRESCRIPTION BASED UPON DAILY MORPHINE EQUIVALENCE DOSE

Oral 24-hour morphine (mg/day)	IM 24-hour morphine (mg/day)	Duragesic dose (µg/h)
45–134	8–22	25
135–224	23–37	50
225–314	38–52	75
315–404	53–67	100
405–494	68–82	125
495–584	83–97	150
585–674	98–112	175
675–764	113–127	200
765–854	128–142	225
855–944	143–157	250
945–1034	158–172	275
1035–1124	173–187	300

Note: Reprinted with permission from Janssen Pharmaceutica (Manufacturer of Duragesic).

practice (Ferrell, Eberts, McCaffery, & Grant, 1991). The interventions listed below are "rarely a total answer" (Haviley et al., 1992, p. 344). And they are certainly not meant to be used as a kind of "smorgasbord" of suggestions for patients— i.e., "Have you ever tried . . . " Serious effort on the part of nurses to develop expertise in one or more of these interventions is an important goal. Effort, expertise, and confidence in using non-pharmacological methods are necessary before they can be effective, and their implementation is often hampered by the very pain nurses are trying to help patients to deal with (Haviley et al., 1992). To some degree, all of these techniques allow patients to develop an ability to better control themselves and their situation.

Social Support
Social support has a definite but difficult-to-define relationship with morbidity and mortality (Broadhead et al., 1983). Many patients with cancer tend to withdraw socially (Bern-

hard & Ganz, 1991), and thus their suffering increases. Support comes from the patient's significant others and from staff. Increasing the support of others is discussed in chapter 2. The traditional nursing intervention—"giving support" or "lending comfort"—is made up of an important series of actions that develops in the process of building the nurse-patient relationship. Components of this comfort include pity, sympathy, consolation, compassion, commiseration, and reassurance (Morse, Bottorf, Anderson, O'Brien, & Solberg, 1992). Giving consistent and appropriate comfort operationalizes caring, and thus helps the patient through the pain and suffering. (Please see chapters 1, 2, and 3 for a fuller explanation.)

Counseling
Counseling, i.e., intervention to help the patient "integrate the health-illness experience with other life experiences" (Baylor University

School of Nursing, 1991) is clearly indicated in the multidimensional pain experience. Counseling based on the short-term crisis intervention model is appropriate for patients with cancer pain. A key aspect of the crisis intervention model is to apply past coping skills to the current situation—even though the current situation may be perceived as more of a crisis than past events. Goals are limited and applied to the treatment plan (compliance, for example) as well as to dealing with the pain itself. Patient outcomes in relation to practitioners' counseling skills and the ability to "be" with a patient in pain are difficult, if not impossible, to measure in the multidimensional milieu of comprehensive pain treatment.

Distraction

Distraction is considered a cognitive coping technique that encompasses several other techniques, including controlled attention, music therapy, singing, conversation, rhythmic breathing, etc. (Haviley et al., 1992). Children sometimes use play as distraction to deal with pain, and, as previously noted, this sometimes results in their pain being underestimated by others (Hester et al., 1992).

Focusing

Focusing includes learned or acquired mental exercise techniques like: (1) transforming pain into the image of something else that can be controlled by turning it off, and then exercising the control; (2) transforming the context or situation—for example, transforming the self who is sick into the self participating in combat; and (3) dissociating the pain from the body (Fishman, 1990).

Meditation

Meditation is a term meaning to contemplate, or to keep the mind focused, either on itself or on something outside of self. It covers a variety of disciplines, and has been most consistently taught and practiced in Eastern religions, like Buddhism. There are also other conceptions of contemplation, for example, in Catholicism

(Merton, 1953), where meditation may be understood as a form of private devotion or spiritual exercise consisting in deep, continued reflection on some religious theme. The idea of practising meditation is that, through the disciple, the pain may decrease in importance, or be better understood, and thus less distressing (Ram Dass & Gorman, 1985).

Relaxation

Relaxation strategies include guided imagery and progressive muscle relaxation, both of which are helpful in managing pain. This technique is most effective when strategies are combined; it is also similar to the focusing described above.

Hypnosis

Hypnosis has long been used in managing pain, especially for chronic pain. Hypnosis modifies the patient's perception of pain through increasing the ability to concentrate. As is true of all the other interventions in this section, not all patients respond well to any one technique—hypnosis included.

Biofeedback

Biofeedback enables some patients, to some extent, to alter specific body functions, including muscle tension (Haviley et al., 1992), which helps overcome the pain-bracing syndrome.

Other Pain Relief Measures

A number of other techniques exist to reduce pain and to alleviate the symptoms causing pain. These include:

- *Acupuncture and Related Techniques:* Acupuncture, cold laser therapy, and acupressure utilize stimulation of specific peripheral nerves (acupoints) to achieve analgesia.
- *Topical Medications:* Menthol salves are used world-wide for pain. Tiger Balm, Monkey Holding a Peach, and various "sports balms" can all give surprising results for superficial pain, especially for patients with

a tradition of using such medications, e.g., Asian immigrants.

- *Cold or Heat Therapy:* Cold or heat therapy affects some pain by reducing inflammation (cold) or increasing blood flow (heat). Heat therapy also helps relaxation (Haviley et al., 1992).

- *Radiation Therapy:* Radiation therapy reduces tumor size and is useful in several different pain syndromes, or situations (Hellmen, 1990): (1) pressure on nerves from tumor growth responds well to radiation therapy; (2) tumor infiltration of nerves is less responsive; (3) bone pain from isolated metastases responds well to radiation (spinal metastases are commonly treated with radiation, as well as with chemotherapy [MacDonald, 1990]); and (4) obstructive syndromes, such as superior vena cava syndrome, respond to radiation. Depending on several factors, the effects of radiation may be rapid or slow, and, in some cases, include edema and hence temporarily increased symptoms.

- *Chemotherapy:* Chemotherapy can produce analgesia by reducing tumor size (of certain tumors) and possibly by affecting the tumor milieu, which includes tumor secretions and reactive host cells (MacDonald, 1990). Most patients with recurrent breast cancer develop bone metastases accompanied by pain and potential pathological fractures. Some chemotherapeutic agents inhibit the bone metabolism that accompanies bone metastases; others help prevent hypercalcemia and decrease pain and pathologic fractures; and still others inhibit bone formation. Chemotherapy can thus prevent pain, as in the first two situations, or can cause pain, as in the last (MacDonald, 1990). Chemotherapy is also used to slow disease progression and thus decrease pain (Walsh, 1990a). Used skillfully (with due consideration for minimal adverse effects) in this manner, chemotherapy reveals the art of medical oncology.

- *Anesthetic Measures:* Anesthetic measures include trigger point injections and nerve blocks. Blocks may be temporary or permanent. If temporary blocks effectively control pain, then permanent blocks may be used (Foley, 1991).

- *Surgery:* Neurosurgical approaches are most effective for localized, somatic pain (Foley, 1991) and are used when other approaches are unsuccessful (Arbit, 1990). Surgical approaches to cancer pain include:
  1. neurodestructive (neuroablative) surgery, such as cordotomy, which interrupts pain pathways;
  2. neurostimulatory surgery, used to implant an electrode to activate pain inhibitory pathways via transcutaneous, percutaneous, and other electrical nerve stimulation;
  3. orthopedic preemptive surgery, used to repair weight-bearing bones before pathological fracture occurs (Rosier, 1990);
  4. surgical exenteration, indicated in widespread painful pelvic disease (Stillman, 1990); and
  5. other surgical procedures that are, however, less common in pain management.

References

American Pain Society. (1992). *Principles of analgesic use in the treatment of acute pain and cancer pain* (3rd ed.). Skokie, IL: Author.

Arbit, E. (1990). Neurosurgical management of cancer pain. In K.M. Foley, J.J. Bonica, & V. Ventafridda (Eds.). *Proceedings of the Second International Congress on Cancer Pain* (pp. 289–300). New York: Raven Press.

Babul, N., Darke, A.C., Anslow, J.A., & Krishnamurthy, T.N. (1992). Pharmacokinetics of two novel rectal controlled-release morphine formulations. *Journal of Pain and Symptom Management, 7*(7), 400–405.

Baines, M.J. (1990). Management of malignant intestinal obstruction in patients with advanced cancer. In K.M. Foley, J.J. Bonica, & V. Ventafridda (Eds.). *Proceedings of the Second International Congress on Cancer Pain* (pp. 327–335). New York: Raven Press.

Baylor University School of Nursing. (1991). *Self-study report.* Dallas, Texas: Author.

Beaver, W.T. (1990). Nonsteroidal anti-inflammatory analgesics in cancer pain. In K.M. Foley, J.J. Bonica, & V. Ventafridda (Eds.). *Proceedings of the Second International Congress on Cancer Pain* (pp. 109–131).

New York: Raven Press.

Berde, C.B. (1991). The treatment of pain in children. In M.R. Bond, J.E. Charlton, & C.J. Woolf (Eds.). *Proceedings of the VIth World Congress on Pain* (pp. 435–440). Amsterdam: Elsevier.

Bernhard, J. & Ganz, P.A. (1991). Psychosocial issues in lung cancer (part 2). *Chest, 99*(2), 480–485.

Boureau, F., Saudubray, F., d'Arnoux, C., Vedrenne, J., Estève, M., Roquefeuil, B., Kong A Siou, D., Brunet, R., Ranchère, J.Y., Roussel, P., Richard, A., Laugner, B., Muller, A., Doonadieu, S. (1992). A comparative study of controlled-release morphine (CRM) suspension and CRM tablets in chronic cancer pain. *Journal of Pain and Symptom Management, 7*(7), 393–399.

Brescia, F.J., Adler, D., Gray, G., Ryan, M.A., Cimino, J., & Mamtini, R. (1990). Hospitalized advanced cancer patients: A profile. *Journal of Pain and Symptom Management, 5*(4), 221–227.

Broadhead, W.E., Kaplan, B.H., James, S.A., Wagner, E.H., Schoenbach, V.J., Grimson, R., Heyden, S., Tibblin, G., & Gehlbach, S.H. (1983). The epidemiologic evidence for a relationship between social support and health. *American Journal of Epidemiology, 117*(5), 521–537.

Bruera, E., Schoeller, T., & Montejo, G. (1992). Organic hallucinosis in patients receiving high doses of opiates for cancer pain. *Pain, 48*(3), 397–399.

Bruera, E. (1991). Update on adjuvant drugs for cancer pain treatment. In M.R. Bond, J.E. Charlton, & C.J. Woolf (Eds.). *Proceedings of the VIth World Congress on Pain* (pp. 459–465). Amsterdam: Elsevier.

Bruera, E. (1990). Subcutaneous administration of opioids in the management of cancer pain. In K.M. Foley, J.J. Bonica, & V. Ventafridda (Eds.). *Proceedings of the Second International Congress on Cancer Pain* (pp. 210–218). New York: Raven Press.

Coyle, N. (1991). Initial assessment and ongoing evaluation of cancer pain. *American Journal of Hospice and Palliative Care, 8*(6), 27–35.

Cushman, K.E. (1986). Symptom management: A comprehensive approach to increasing nutritional status in the cancer patient. *Seminars in Oncology Nursing, 2*(1), 30–35.

Enck, R.E. (1991). An overview of spinal opioids in pain management. *American Journal of Hospice and Palliative Care, 8*(2), 3–4.

Ferrell, B.R., & McCaffery, M. (1991, November). Maintaining low tech-high touch pain management in hospice. Paper presented at the annual meeting and symposium of the National Hospice Organization, Seattle, WA.

Ferrell, B.R. (1991). Managing pain with long-acting morphine. *Nursing 91, 21*(10), 34–39.

Ferrell, B.R., Eberts, M.T., McCaffery, M., & Grant, M. (1991). Clinical decision-making and pain. *Cancer Nursing, 14*(6), 289–297.

Fishman, B. (1990). The treatment of suffering in patients with cancer pain: Cognitive-behavioral approaches. In K.M. Foley, J.J. Bonica, & V. Ventafridda (Eds.). *Proceedings of the Second International Congress on Cancer Pain* (pp. 301–316). New York: Raven Press.

Fleming, B.M., & Coombs, D.W. (1992). A survey of complications documented in a quality control analysis of patient-controlled analgesia in the postoperative patient. *Journal of Pain and Symptom Management, 78*), 463–469.

Foley, K.M. (1989). Controversies in cancer pain. *Cancer, 63*(11), 2257–2265.

Foley, K.M. (1991). Diagnosis and treatment of cancer pain. In A.I. Holleb, D.J. Fink, & G.P. Murphy (Eds.), *Textbook of clinical oncology* (pp. 555–575). Atlanta: The American Cancer Society.

Gonzales, G.R. (1992). Postherpes simplex type 1 neuralgia simulating postherpatic neuralgia. *Journal of Pain and Symptom Management, 7*(5), 320–323.

Hassenbusch, S.J., Pillay, P., Magdinec, M., Currie, K., Bay, J.W., Covington, E.C., & Tomaszewski, M.Z. (1990). Constant infusion of morphine for intractable cancer pain using an implanted pump. *Journal of Neurosurgery, 73*, 405–409.

Haviley, C., Gagnon, J., MacLean, R., Renz, J., Jones, O., De Witt, W., Nyberg, K., Burns, C., & Pohl, D. (1992). Pharmacological management of cancer pain. *Cancer Nursing, 15*(5), 331–346.

Hellmen, S. (1990). The role of radiation therapy in the management of cancer pain. In K.M. Foley, J.J. Bonica, & V. Ventafridda (Eds.). *Proceedings of the Second International Congress on Cancer Pain* (pp. 41–45). New York: Raven Press.

Herr, K.A., & Mobily, P.R. (1992). Interventions related to pain. *Nursing Clinics of North America, 27*(2), 347–369.

Hester, N.O., Jacox, A., Miaskowski, C. & Ferrell, B. (1992). Excerpts from guidelines for the management of pain in infants, children, and adolescents. *Maternal-Child Nursing, 17*, 146–152.

Inturrisi, C.E. (1990). Opioid analgesic therapy in cancer pain. In K.M. Foley, J.J. Bonica, & V. Ventafridda (Eds.). *Proceedings of the Second International Congress on Cancer Pain* (pp. 133–154). New York: Raven Press.

Kerr, I.G., Sone, M., DeAngelis, C., Iscoe, N., MacKenzie, R., & Schueller, T. (1988). Continuous narcotic infusion with patient-controlled analgesia for chronic cancer pain in outpatients. *Annals of Internal Medicine., 108*(4), 554–557.

Kinzbrunner, B.M., Policzer, J., Miller, B., & Neiber, L. (1990). Non-invasive pain control in the terminally ill patient. *American Journal of Hospice and Palliative Care, 7*(4), 26–29.

Levy, M.H. (1985). Pain management in advanced cancer. *Seminars in Oncology, 12*(4), 394–410.

MacDonald, N. (1990). The role of medical and surgical oncology in the management of cancer pain. In K.M. Foley, J.J. Bonica, & V. Ventafridda (Eds.). *Proceedings of the Second International Congress on Can-*

cer Pain (pp. 27–39). New York: Raven Press.

Mather, L.E. (1991). Novel methods of analgesic drug delivery. In M.R. Bond, J.E. Charlton, & C.J. Woolf (Eds.). *Proceedings of the VIth World Congress on Pain* (pp. 159–173). Amsterdam: Elsevier.

McCaffery, M. & Beebe, A. (1989). *Pain: Clinical manual for nursing practice.* St. Louis: C.V. Mosby.

McCorquodale, S., De Faye, B., & Bruera, E. (1993). Pain control in an alcoholic cancer patient. *Journal of Pain and Symptom Management, 8*(3), 177–180.

McGrath, P.J., Mathews, J.R., & Pigeon, H. (1991). Assessment of pain in children: A systematic psychosocial study. In M.R. Bond, J.E. Charlton, & C.J. Woolf (Eds.). *Proceedings of the VIth World Congress on Pain* (pp. 509–526). Amsterdam: Elsevier.

Mercadante, S., & Maddaloni, S. (1992). Octreotide in the management of inoperable gastrointestinal obstruction in terminal cancer patients. *Journal of Pain and Symptom Management, 7*(8), 496–498.

Merton, T. (1953). *Bread in the wilderness.* New York: New Directions Books.

Monks, R. (1990). Psychotropic drugs. In J.J. Bonica (Ed.), *The management of pain* (pp. 1676–1689). Philadelphia: Lea & Febiger.

Morse, J.M., Bottorf, J., Anderson, G., O'Brien, B., & Solberg, S. (1992). Beyond empathy: Expanding expressions of caring. *Journal of Advanced Nursing, 17,* 809–821.

Murphy, T. (1991). Alternative drug delivery systems. *American Journal of Hospice and Palliative Care, 8*(6), 36–42.

Paice, J.A. (1991). Unraveling the mystery of pain. *Oncology Nursing Forum, 18*(5), 843–849.

Paradis, A. (1992). Patient controlled analgesia. *The Canadian nurse.* August, 1992, 39–41.

Portenoy, R.K. (1989). Cancer pain: Epidemiology and syndromes. *Cancer, 63*(11), 2298–2307.

Portenoy, R.K. (1990). Continuous intravenous infusion of opioid drugs in the management of cancer pain. In K.M. Foley, J.J. Bonica, & V. Ventafridda (Eds.). *Proceedings of the Second International Congress on Cancer Pain* (pp. 219–229). New York: Raven Press.

Porter, J., & Jick, H. (1980). Addiction rare in patients treated with narcotics. *New England Journal of Medicine, 302*(2), 123.

Ram Dass, & Gorman, P. (1985). *How can I help?* New York: Alfred A. Knopf.

Rogers, A.G. (1991). The underutilization of oxycodone. *Journal of Pain and Symptom Management, 6*(7), 452.

Rosier, R. (1990). Bone pain. *American Journal of Hospice and Palliative Care, 7*(6), 25.

Savage, S.R. (1993). Preface: Pain medicine and addiction medicine-controversies and collaboration. *Journal of Pain and Symptom Management, 8*(5), 254–256.

Sawaki, Y., Parker, R.K., & White, P.F. (1992). Patient and nurse evaluation of patient-controlled analgesia delivery systems for postoperative pain management. *Journal of Pain and Symptom Management,*

7(8), 443–453.

Schug, S.A., Zech, D., & Dörr, U. (1990). Cancer pain management according to WHO analgesic guidelines. *Journal of Pain and Symptom Management, 5*(1), 27–32.

Schug, S.A., Zech, D., Grond, S., Jung, H., Meuser, T., & Stobbe, B. (1992). A long-term survey of morphine in cancer pain patients. *Journal of Pain and Symptom Management, 7*(5), 259–266.

Shepard, K.V. (1990). Review of a controlled-release morphine preparation. In K.M. Foley, J.J. Bonica, & V. Ventafridda (Eds.). *Proceedings of the Second International Congress on Cancer Pain* (pp. 191–202). New York: Raven Press.

Stanley, T.H. (1992). The history and development of the fentanyl series. *Journal of Pain and Symptom Management, 7*(3), Supplement, S3–S7.

Stillman, M.J. (1990). Perineal pain: Diagnosis and management, with particular attention to perineal pain of cancer. In K.M. Foley, J.J. Bonica, & V. Ventafridda (Eds.). *Proceedings of the Second International Congress on Cancer Pain* (pp. 359–377). New York: Raven Press.

Twycross, R.G. (1978). Relief of pain. In C.M. Saunders (Ed.). *The management of terminal disease* (pp. 65–98). London: Edward Arnold.

Twycross, R.G. (1990). Management of constipation in the cancer patient with pain. In K.M. Foley, J.J. Bonica, & V. Ventafridda (Eds.). *Proceedings of the Second International Congress on Cancer Pain* (pp. 317–326). New York: Raven Press.

Waldman, S.D., Feldstein, G.S., Donohoe, C.D., & Waldman, K.A. (1988). The relief of body wall pain secondary to malignant hepatic metastases by intercostal nerve block with bipivicaine and methylprednisolone. *Journal of Pain and Symptom Management, 3*(1), 39–43.

Walsh, T.D. (1990a). Symptom control in patients with advanced cancer. *American Journal of Hospice and Palliative Care, 7*(6), 20–29.

Walsh, T.D. (1990b). Prevention of opioid side effects. *Journal of Pain and Symptom Management, 5*(6), 362–367.

Walsh, T.D. (1990c). Adjuvant analgesic therapy in cancer pain. In K.M. Foley, J.J. Bonica, & V. Ventafridda (Eds.). *Proceedings of the Second International Congress on Cancer Pain* (pp. 155–169). New York: Raven Press.

Wesson, D.R., Ling, W., & Smith, D.E. (1993). Prescription of opioids for treatment of pain in patients with addictive disease. *Journal of Pain and Symptom Management, 8*(5), 289–296.

Wilkie, D.J. (1990). Cancer pain management: State of the art nursing care. *Nursing Clinics of North America, 25*(2), 331–343.

World Health Organization (1990). Cancer pain relief and palliative care. Geneva: Author.

III | Physical Care

PROBLEMS AND INTERVENTIONS

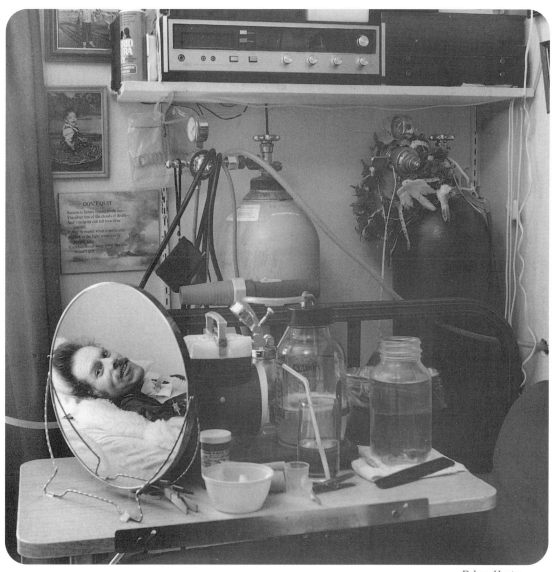

Debora Hunter

Introduction to Patient Care:
The First Encounter

The first encounter with a person who is dying is critically important. This is when the patient and family form their initial (and usually lasting) impression of the practitioner and of his or her abilities. The practitioner and trust in the practitioner are the issues. Trust gained means that the patient and family are far more likely to have hope, to be active participants in the care, and thus to do better overall. Trust or confidence lost means that the patient and family are unlikely to ever have confidence in the practitioner.

The Basic Issue

The basic issue in the first encounter is how the practitioner responds to the (typical) patient and family feelings of being overwhelmed and having no control, as well as to the physical problems of the patient. The most productive response is a quick one, and includes the following considerations.

- Whether it occurs at home or in a facility, the practitioner's first encounter with a patient should never involve delays. This is essential. The practitioner should interview and see to the patient's concerns immediately. From the patient's perspective, reaching the terminal phase of an illness means spending "lifetimes" waiting in offices, clinics, labs, and other places that, for the patient, are full of a great sense of fear. Getting to patients quickly shows in a concrete manner that the practitioner has at least some understanding of their experience. It cannot be expected that patients and their families, at this critical moment, will be able to consider other demands on the practitioner's time, like staff obligations, paperwork, or care of other patients.
- In an initial interview, the practitioner should find out (or better yet, anticipate) what the patient's concerns are, and do something about them right away. It is impossible, of course, to take care of all concerns immediately, but at least doing everything possible to ease the patient's *main* concerns will result in great progress toward building a collabora-

tive relationship. Primary concerns usually center around loss of control and feelings of being overwhelmed. They also usually tend to be involved with: (1) pain and other symptoms; (2) not knowing what to do; (3) not knowing what will happen; (4) not knowing who will help; and (5) physical, emotional, and spiritual exhaustion.

The response to patients' feelings is thus (usually) practical and task-oriented rather than affective or counseling in nature. Of course, patient and family feelings should never be ignored; and at times, counseling may be the primary focus of the first encounter. Nurse behavior perceived by patients with cancer to be the most caring behavior focuses on the practitioner anticipating and acting quickly on the patients' physical needs. Thus, the first issue is whether the patient is hurting, or otherwise in physical distress.

The first encounter also sets the emotional tone for the relationship between patient, family, and practitioner. If practitioners begin by giving direct and honest answers, this is by far the best groundwork.

The First Question

First questions are important. A standard, rhetorical "How are you?" may not be the best beginning. This question asks the patient to tell what may be a terrible truth to a stranger. All too often, the answer given instead will be "okay," or "fine." Then the practitioner is confronted with what to do with a response that is untrue. If there is the slightest indication that the patient might be in pain or have other symptoms, the practitioner should make an immediate determination and response.

Rather than ask "How are you?" practitioners can ask something less threatening but more to the point—for example, "What is going on with you?" The patient can answer this question in a variety of ways and still tell the truth. How he or she really *is*—emotionally, spiritually, and physically—will emerge over time, as the relationship develops between practitioner and patient.

Obligations

Of course, there are always organizational obligations to consider in the first encounter. These include questions to ask, forms to sign, and other issues. Even so, the primary obligation is clear: The patient's well-being is the first consideration. Thus, it is often necessary to find some accommodation between patient needs and organizational obligations. Several initial contacts may be required. How these are structured depends on a variety of factors. If they are planned around patients' needs, the entire course of care may be positively affected.

Although most administrative staff are understanding of patient needs, practitioners may need to educate administrators about their importance. Most will respond well if they feel confident that organizational needs will be met in a timely manner.

Practitioner Expectations in the First Encounter

Experience clearly shows that there is no way to predict what you will find on the first encounter. Practitioners may walk into situations of unimaginable physical, emotional, and/or spiritual suffering. Anger may explode with no discernable provocation. There may be complete denial or complete acceptance. Or the room and the people in it may be filled with spiritual joy. Most often, you will find people who are going through hard times in the best way they can; and much like they have, for most of their lives.

If there are several people present, it is a good idea to clarify who is who, and what each person does in relation to the patient. Be alert to the presence of close, out-of-town relatives because they can sometimes be a source of great difficulty, often based on their feelings of guilt.

The most productive expectation, of course, is no expectation at all. This entails opening oneself to whatever one encounters; never an easy task, but even more necessary in these circumstances than in most others.

Assessing Physical Dimensions of Patients with Cancer

Initial assessments are usually determined, at least in part, by standard forms; often the same forms for every part of the hospital or organization. This means that patients with advanced cancer are assessed in the same way as patients with a broken bone—a classic example of agency demands taking precedence over patient needs.

The initial assessment should be based on the unique situation of each individual patient. Patients with cancer should be assessed in terms of actual and potential problems stemming from their specific tumor and metastatic sites. Other areas to assess include:

- any life-threatening or otherwise serious conditions, including respiratory, cardiac, neurological, bleeding-related, and metabolic conditions;
- pain;
- nausea, vomiting, dysphagia, and other gastrointestinal symptoms;
- infection;
- oral, genitourinary, and skin problems;
- signs of liver, lung, bone, and brain involvement;
- other issues that include fluid intake, elimination patterns, sleep patterns and problems, medications taken (complete information), mobility, and any other issues related to complaints or specific problems of the patient and/or family.

Having made meaningful contact and assessed key issues, the practitioner completes the first encounter by quickly responding to questions or issues arising from it. If, for example, pain is the primary issue, the practitioner does whatever is necessary to control the pain as quickly as possible. When we try to understand dying from the patient and family perspective, we begin to understand the enormity of the situation. The practitioner who responds *quickly* begins the process of making the situation manageable. This is the basis of trust and hope; and thus the basis of effective care.

Neurological Problems and Interventions

Neurological problems, such as delirium, occur to some extent in most patients with terminal illness (Bruera, Fainsinger, Miller, & Kuehn, 1992). Common neurological problems in terminal illness include confusion (delirium, dementia), seizures, motor and/or sensory deficits, decreased consciousness, coma, and/or spinal cord compression. These problems are due to central nervous system (CNS) metastases or primary tumors of the CNS; to non-metastatic processes, such as side effects of treatment, infections, metabolic disorders, neurological paraneoplastic syndromes, and primary neurological disease (Henson & Posner, 1993); and in patients with AIDS, most commonly to AIDS dementia complex, cytomegalovirus infection, cryptococcal meningitis, and toxoplasmic encephalitis (Chaisson & Volberding, 1990). Please see chapter 27 for a discussion of the neurological problems of AIDS and chapter 29 for a discussion of Alzheimer's disease. Increased intracranial pressure is a major factor in some CNS problems, and along with spinal cord compression, is an oncologic emergency.

Confusion: Delirium and Dementia

SYMPTOMS

In general, delirium is an acute "global cognitive disorder" that includes disorientation (most often to time and seldom to person), attention deficits, either agitation or lethargy, and illusions or hallucinations (Martin, 1990, p. 20; Walsh, 1989). There are often changes in mental status from hour to hour and symptoms may worsen at night ("sundowning"). Hallucinations or other troubling psychological events may be manifested only by change in mood, and not voluntarily reported (Bruera, Schoeller, & Montejo, 1992).

Dementia is a chronic gradual decrease in cognition that may begin with slight memory losses or other deficits, either unrecognized or excused by the patient and others. In its early stages, dementia may be mistaken for depression (Walsh, 1989). While dementia predisposes patients to episodes of delirium (Martin, 1990), the "essential diagnostic feature" of

Charles Kemp: TERMINAL ILLNESS: A GUIDE TO NURSING CARE. © 1995 J. B. Lippincott.

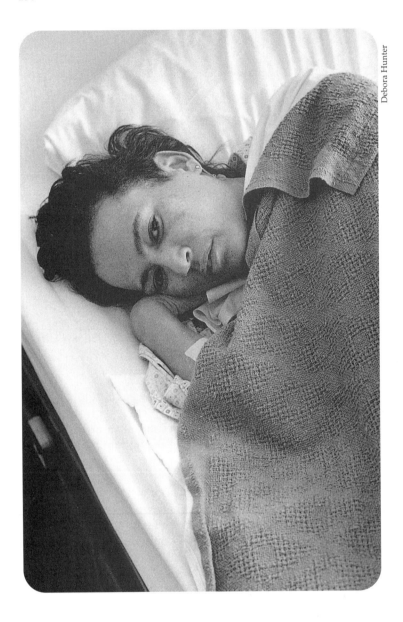

Debora Hunter

delirium (vs. dementia) is "clouding of consciousness" (Walsh, 1989, p. 61). In both delirium and dementia, there may be a decreased control over expression of personality tendencies, with suppressed memories or urges and unconscious material surfacing—to the distress of the patient and family (Walsh, 1989).

ETIOLOGIES

Acute confusion (delirium) may be due to a variety of etiologies, including medications, metabolic disorders, non-malignant CNS disease, pain, infections, fecal impaction/urine retention, sleep deprivation, heart disease,

TABLE 13.1
COMMON CAUSES OF CONFUSION IN PATIENTS WITH CANCER

Treatment	Opioids, steroids, phenothiazines, sedatives, radiation (to brain)
Primary disease	Brain metastases, primary tumor
Distant effects of primary disease	Paraneoplastic syndromes, electrolyte imbalance, e.g. hypercalcemia, hyponatremia, hypoglycemia; and CNS paraneoplastic syndromes (especially with lung, breast, and ovarian cancer) Pain Other symptoms/problems, including anemia, dyspnea, fecal impaction, urine retention Nutritional deficiencies, e.g., cachexia, vitamin B_{12} deficiency
Other causes	Organ failure, including liver, kidney, lung, thyroid, adrenals Infection (and sometimes antibiotics) Non-malignant disease (Alzheimer's disease, atherosclerosis, AIDS dementia) Psychiatric disorder

and/or endocrine disorders. Among the causes of chronic confusion (dementia) are Alzheimer's disease, AIDS dementia, atherosclerosis, intracranial tumors (see discussion of increased intracranial pressure below), drugs, anemia, vitamin B_{12} deficiency, paraneoplastic syndrome, and chronic social isolation (Bruera, Schoeller, & Montejo, 1992; Henson & Posner, 1993; Martin, 1990; Walsh, 1989). Since patients with advanced cancer are at risk for almost all of the above, psychological changes, such as confusion, must be carefully assessed rather than automatically attributed to the disease (see Table 13.1, Common Causes of Confusion in Patients with Cancer). Assessment of a confused patient includes: (1) physical assessment, especially medication review (Walsh, 1989, p. 61) and review of metabolic disorders, including hypercalcemia, hyponatremia, and hypoglycemia (Martin, 1990, p. 22); and (2) a standardized mental status exam, e.g., the Mini-Mental State Examination, shown in Figure 13.1 (Martin, 1990).

INTERVENTIONS

The best option is to modify the etiology, i.e., resolve pain, impaction, insomnia, or hypercalcemia; reduce tumor edema, change medications, etc. In many cases, the etiology cannot be changed, either because the CNS changes are irreversible (e.g., Alzheimer's disease) or because the confusion is part of the dying process (e.g., hypercalcemia in a moribund patient). Symptomatic treatment includes:

- Antipsychotic medications, especially haloperidol (Haldol), which decrease confusion and/or thought disorders and agitation (Billings, 1985). To start, haloperidol 0.5–1.5 mg PO is given twice daily or 0.5–5

Figure 13-1 *Mini-Mental State Examination*

Maximum score 30. Score <20 suggests significant cognitive impairment.

I. Orientation (Maximum score 10)

Ask "What today's date?" Then ask specifically for parts omitted; e.g., "Can you also tell what season it is?"
Ask "Can you tell me the name of this hospital?"
"What floor are we on?"
"What town (or city) are we in?"
"What county are we in?"
What state are we in?"

Date (e.g., January 21)	1 ____
Year	2 ____
Month	3 ____
Day (e.g., Monday)	4 ____
Season	5 ____
Hospital	6 ____
Floor	7 ____
Town/City	8 ____
County	9 ____
State	10 ____

II. Registration (Maximum score 3)

Ask the subject if you may test his/her memory. Then say "Ball," "Flag," "Tree," clearly and slowly, about one second for each. After you have said all 3 words, ask subject to repeat them. This first repetition determines the score (0–3) but keep saying them (up to 6 trials) until the subject can repeat all 3 words. If he/she does not eventually learn all three, recall cannot be meaningfully tested

"Ball"	11 ____
"Flag"	12 ____
"Tree"	13 ____

Record number of trials ____

III. Attention and calculation (Maximum score 5)

Ask the subject to begin at 100 and count backward by 7. Stop after 5 subtractions (93, 86, 79, 72, 65). Score one point for each correct number.
If the subject cannot or will not perform this task, ask him/her to spell the word "world" backwards (D, L, R, O, W). The score is one point for each correctly placed letter, e.g., DLROW = 5, DLORW = 3. Record how the subject spelled "world" backwards:

"93"	14 ____
"86"	15 ____
"79"	16 ____
"72"	17 ____
"65"	18 ____
OR	
Number of correctly placed letters	19 ____

IV. Recall (Maximum score 3)

Ask the subject to recall the three words you previously asked him/her to remember (learned in Registration)

"Ball"	20 ____
"Flag"	21 ____
"Tree"	22 ____

V. Language (Maximum score 9)

Naming: Show the subject a wrist watch and ask "What is this?" Repeat for pencil. Score one point for each item named correctly.
Repetition: Ask the subject to repeat, "No ifs, ands, or buts." Score one point for correct repetition.

Watch	23 ____
Pencil	24 ____
Repetition	25 ____

3-Stage Command: Give the subject a piece of blank paper and say, "Take the paper in your right hand, fold it in half and put it on the floor." Score one point for each action performed correctly.

Takes in right hand	26 ____
Folds in half	27 ____
Puts on floor	28 ____
Closes eyes	29 ____

Reading: On a blank piece of paper, print the sentence, "Close your eyes" in letters large enough for the subject to see clearly. Ask subject to read it and do what it says. Score correctly only if he/she actually closes his/her eyes.

Writing: Give the subject a blank piece of paper and ask him/her to write a sentence. It is to be written spontaneously. It must contain a subject and verb and make sense. Correct grammar and punctuation are not necessary.

Writes sentence   30 ____

Copying: On a clean piece of paper, draw intersecting pentagons, each side about inch, and ask subject to copy it exactly as it is. All 10 angles must be present and two must intersect to score 1 point. Tremor and rotation are ignored
E.g.

Draws pentagons   31 ____

Score: Add number of correct responses. In section III include items 14–18 or item 19, not both. (Maximum total score 30)
Rate subject's level of consciousness: (a) coma, (b) stupor, (c) drowsy, (d) alert

Total score _____

Reprinted with permission from Folstein, M.F., Folstein, F.E., and McHugh, P.R. (1975) Mini-mental state: a practical method for grading the cognitive state of patients for the clinician. *Journal of Psychiatric Research.* 12. 189–198.

mg PO at night for older and physically ill patients and 5 mg PO for stronger patients (Walsh, 1989). Martin (1990) recommends 0.5–1.0 mg PO or IM every 30–60 minutes until agitation decreases, and then on a twice-daily schedule. Chlorpromazine (Thorazine) 10–50 mg PO at night or 10–25 mg PO QID, gives greater sedation and anti-emetic effects (Walsh, 1989). Most experts do not advocate the benzodiazepines, e.g., Valium for confusion. Patients at home, especially those living alone, are the most vulnerable to the possibility of medication mistakes. Medications for such patients should be set up in daily doses with a calendar, and should be carefully monitored.

- The patient's environment should be as familiar as possible and be well-lighted (including a night light). Sensory overload should be avoided, especially at night, and brief, clear, and often repeated explanations given of procedures and other stimulating events. Frequent reminders of person, place, and time may be helpful, including having a clock and a calendar present. Some patients are calmed by television and some are not. Changes in staff should be avoided (Clark, McGee, & Preston, 1992). Regular visits by family and friends should be encouraged and the effects of visits assessed. The patient should be dressed and groomed daily as long as possible. Environmental safety should be assessed. Unsupervised smoking should be discouraged. Structure can be promoted by writing out a schedule or a routine for the patient and others.

- Support to the family is essential. General psychosocial support, teaching, and frequent reassurance are helpful. Counseling or psychotherapy is especially helpful in dealing with anger or "wrong" thoughts, such as wishing the patient would die because he/she is such a terrible burden. See chapter 28 for a further discussion of family issues related to degenerative neurological disorders.

Seizures

Any patient with intracranial tumor(s) or progressive disease is at risk for seizures. Factors that may precipitate seizures in a patient with epilepsy or intracranial tumors include noncompliance with anticonvulsants, sleep deprivation, excess alcohol, stress/anxiety, menses, and medications, including tricyclic antidepressants (Venables, 1989b). Seizures are managed or prevented with phenytoin and/or Phenobarbital, either together or alone (Batzdorf, Black, & Selch, 1990). The dose of corticosteroids should be increased in the presence of these medications (Venables, 1989b).

Motor Sensory Deficits

Motor and sensory deficits in terminal illness are due to a variety of etiologies, including tumor growth, paraneoplastic syndromes, metabolic disorders, treatment, and infections. Motor and sensory complications of AIDS include peripheral neuropathies, autonomic neuropathies, and myopathies. Peripheral neuropathies are common at all stages of HIV infection and AIDS. They may be due to HIV infection or unknown causes, opportunistic infection (especially cytomegalovirus [CMV] or herpes), or medications (Galantino, 1991). Some motor or sensory deficits are cardinal signs of disease progression, and constitute serious complications in cancer and AIDS. Please see the section on neurological complications in chapter 27, and the following section in this chapter.

Increased Intracranial Pressure

Brain metastases are the "most common symptomatic neurological complication of metastatic cancer" (Henson & Posner, 1993) and increased intracranial pressure (ICP) is a major complication. The incidence of brain metastases is increasing because of increased survival of patients with tumors likely to metastasize to the brain (Glover & Glick, 1991).

SYMPTOMS

Headache from increased ICP varies in site and associated symptoms, according to the site of the lesion(s). Typically, the pain is progressive and is usually accompanied by "progressive neurological deficits" (Lipton, Pfeffer, Newman, & Solomon, 1993). Signs and symptoms depend on the nature of the lesion(s), and in addition to, or in the absence of, pain may include decreased level of consciousness, seizures, weakness, nausea and vomiting, bowel and bladder dysfunction, reflex changes, and evidence of cranial nerve involvement (Chernecky & Krech, 1991; Prados & Wilson, 1993). Papilledema (often with visual changes), vomiting, and headache are the "classic triad" of increased ICP (Wegman & Hakius, 1990). Headache may be most severe in early morning, and may awaken the patient (Billings, 1985). Bradycardia simultaneous with increased systolic blood pressure is an "early significant finding" in increased ICP (Chernecky & Krech, 1991). Personality changes and cognitive deficit may occur gradually or, at times, suddenly. Memory and judgement are affected, and agitation or depressed consciousness may be severe. An inability to interpret and/or organize the environment, including other people's facial expressions, may have a negative effect on communications and on other activities (Ragnarsson, 1993).

ETIOLOGIES

Increased intracranial pressure is most often due to tumor (metastatic) and associated edema (Batzdorf, Black, & Selch, 1990) causing pressure, displacement, or obstruction in the brain itself (especially the cortex), but also at the skull and dura or meninges (Wegman & Hakius, 1990).

INTERVENTIONS

Treatment of increased ICP focuses on (1) reducing pressure, and (2) managing associated symptoms (e.g., pain, vomiting, agitation, confusion, and other neurological deficits). Treatment must include explanations and psychosocial support to the family. The idea of cancer in the brain and associated actual or potential symptoms is frightening. Seizures, personality changes, and loss of control are especially feared.

- For reducing ICP, surgery plus radiation result in longer survival rates than does radiation alone, but this combined therapy is not appropriate for patients with disseminated metastases (Prados & Wilson, 1993), which constitutes 40%–60% of cases (Portlock & Goffinet, 1980). Corticosteroids are used along with radiation to treat the increased ICP and cerebral edema of brain tumors (Prados & Wilson, 1993) and may give results as soon as six hours after receiving the medication (Batzdorf, Black, & Selch, 1990)—far more rapidly than does radiation. Corticosteroids alone benefit as many as 75% of patients, but without radiation or surgery, most patients do not survive more than "a few weeks" (Glover & Glick, 1991). Mannitol, an osmotic diuretic, is used if increased ICP does not quickly respond to radiation and corticosteroids. Chemotherapy and other measures, including shunting for hydrocephalus, are used in some cases (Prados & Wilson, 1993).
- Nausea and vomiting are prevented with anti-emetics.
- Activities that increase ICP include suctioning, turning, straining, Valsalva maneuver, hip flexion, lying prone. Activities that are unavoidable should be spaced over time. Valsalva maneuvers can be reduced by preventing constipation. Passive turning for alert patients may help. The patient's head should be elevated or kept in a neutral

position (vs. dependent). Patient safety is a significant consideration. The bed should be kept at its lowest setting (except head elevated). Environmental hazards should be reduced and the patient should not be left alone for long periods of time. Hypertension and fever should be managed and fluids may be restricted (Hunter, 1992; Wegman & Hakius, 1990).

- The treatment of confusional states or deficits is directed to reducing ICP, and failing that, to managing symptoms. The care of patients with confusion is discussed earlier in this chapter. Readers should also refer to the treatment section in chapter 29.

- Associated symptoms may include sensory deficits, visual deficits, aphasia, dysarthria, aprosodia (inability to comprehend or express variations in pitch and other speech patterns), and dysphagia. Adaptive measures, e.g., braces, are sometimes indicated, but when the disease is rapidly progressive, are futile. Range of motion should be maintained up until death, as range of motion loss diminishes quality of life in several respects. Speech or occupational therapy rehabilitation regimes are seldom appropriate in patients with terminal illness; but consultation from these disciplines is indicated in some cases.

- Pain is best managed with steroids and with the treatments discussed above. An opioid plus a phenothiazine can be used if these measures are ineffective (Venables, 1989a).

Spinal Cord Compression

Injury to the spinal cord (usually epidural) results in markedly increased suffering for the patient and significant challenges for all concerned in providing care. Paraplegia, incontinence, constipation, pain, and potential for skin breakdown are the direct sequelae of spinal cord compression (SCC) (Dietz & Flaherty, 1990; Ingham, Beveridge, & Cooney, 1993).

SYMPTOMS

Pain is the most common first symptom of SCC. The pain is generally constant, dull, aching (Henson & Posner, 1993) progressive back pain, usually at or near the lesion, sometimes radicular (Ratanatharathorn & Powers, 1991), commonly exacerbated by movement, coughing, sneezing, or Valsalva maneuver (Miaskowski, 1991), not relieved by lying down and sometimes relieved by sitting up (Glover & Glick, 1991). The painful area is tender to percussion and the pain is exacerbated by "neck flexion or straight leg raising (Arbit, 1990). Pain may exist for months before neurological deficits begin (Zejdlik, 1992). Neurological deficits, the second major manifestation of SCC, usually begin with motor disabilities, most often in the lower extremities. Weakness is the most common neurological deficit (Peterson, 1993). In the early stages, neurological deficits are not necessarily apparent to the patient. (Ratanatharathorn & Powers, 1991). Weakness, ataxia, or occasional stumbling, or even falls, may not appear to be significant to the patient. Evaluation of equilibrium, lower extremity strength, reflexes, gait, including heel-toe walking, should thus be part of the ongoing physical assessment. Bladder dysfunction is a relatively common early sign, consisting of retention manifested by frequent, small voiding (Henson & Posner, 1993). Bowel dysfunction, numbness, paresthesias and sexual impotence may also occur (Hunter, 1992). Impaired genito-urinary sensation, saddle anesthesia, and diminished sensation in the lumbosacral dermatomes is indicative of cauda equina metastases (Glover & Glick, 1991). Diagnostic procedures include plain film of the spine, bone scan, CT scan, myelography, and MRI (Ratanatharathorn & Powers, 1991).

ETIOLOGIES

SCC occurs most often in the thoracic, lumbosacral, and cervical areas at a ratio of approximately 4:2:1 (Henson & Posner, 1993). It is usually due to bone metastasis resulting in bone destruction, or pressure or traction on, or stretching of, nerve structures (Sundaresan, Sachdev, & Krol, 1990). The prognosis is good when diagnosis is early and treatment is appropriate (Dietz & Flaherty, 1990). Delayed diagnosis frequently plays a key role in the development of disabilities (Ratanatharathorn & Powers, 1991) as does rapid onset of symptoms (Dietz & Flaherty, 1990). Tumors commonly associated with cord compression include (but are not limited to) lung, breast, prostate, and lymphoma (Henson & Posner, 1993). Any metastasis to the spine presents the potential for SCC. Primary tumors causing SCC with the poorest response to treatment of SCC are lung and renal cell cancers (Ratanatharathorn & Powers, 1991).

INTERVENTIONS

The importance of early identification of SCC cannot be overstressed in relation to the success of treatment and prevention of devastating complications. Patient and family involvement in detection is important (Peterson, 1993) and should be a standard of care for patients at risk.

- Radiation therapy, combined with steroids (dexamethasone) has been a standard treatment to reduce the compression for more than a decade, even when there is only the suspicion of cord compression (Ratanatharathorn & Powers, 1991).
- Surgery (laminectomy) gives results inferior to radiation and steroids. Laminectomy is indicated because of bone deformity, inability to receive further radiation, high cervical compression, and radio-resistant tumor (Ratanatharathorn & Powers, 1991). Vertebral body resection is effective in relieving the pain of SCC (Arbit, 1990).
- Chemotherapy may be used in a few cases of especially sensitive tumors (Ratanatharathorn & Powers, 1991).

- Disabilities are seldom reversible, so once they occur, adaptive measures should begin. When there is extensive damage to the spine, the patient is maintained as immobile as possible.

Other Neurological Problems

Neurological paraneoplastic syndromes (PNS), while rare (< 1% patients with cancer), can result in a variety of cognitive, sensory, and motor deficits. PNSs are commonly associated with small cell carcinoma of the lung (Henson & Posner, 1993).

References

Arbit, E. (1990). Neurosurgical management of cancer pain. In K.M. Foley, J.J. Bonica, & V. Ventafridda (Eds.), *Proceedings of the Second International Congress on Cancer Pain* (pp. 289–300). New York: Raven Press.

Batzdorf, U., Black, K.L., & Selch, M.T. (1990). Neoplasms of the nervous system: Brain. In C.M. Haskell (Ed.), *Cancer treatment* (3rd ed.) (pp. 436–468). Philadelphia: W.B. Saunders.

Billings, J.A. (1985). *Outpatient management of advanced cancer.* New York: J.B. Lippincott Company.

Bruera, E., Fainsinger, R.L., Miller, M.J., & Kuehn, N. (1992). The assessment of pain intensity in patients with cognitive failure: A preliminary report. *Journal of Pain and Symptom Management, 7*(5), 267–270.

Bruera, E., Schoeller, T., & Montejo, G. (1992). Organic hallucinosis in patients receiving high doses of opiates for cancer pain. *Pain, 48*(3), 397–399.

Chaisson, R.E., & Volberding, P.A. (1990). Clinical manifestations of HIV infection. In G.L. Mandell, R.G. Douglas, & J.E. Bennett (Eds.), *Principles and practices of infectious diseases* (3rd ed.) (pp. 1059–1092). New York: Churchill Livingston.

Chernecky, C., & Krech, R.L. (1991). Complications of advanced disease. In S.B. Baird, R. McCorkle, & M. Grant (Eds.), *Cancer nursing* (pp. 864–874). Philadelphia: W.B. Saunders Company.

Clark, J.C., McGee, R.F., & Preston, R. (1992). Nursing management of responses to the cancer experience. In J.C. Clark & R.F. McGee (Eds.), *Core curriculum for oncology nursing* (2nd ed.) (pp. 67–155). Philadelphia: W.B. Saunders Company.

Dietz, K.A., & Flaherty, A.M. (1990). Oncologic emergencies. In S.L. Groenwald, M.H. Frogge, M. Goodman, & C.H. Yarbro (Eds.), *Cancer nursing: Principles and practice* (pp. 644–668). Boston: Jones and Bartlett.

Folstein, M.F., Folstein, S.E., & McHugh, P.R. (1975). Mini-mental state: A practical method for grading the cognitive state of patients for the clinician. *Journal of Psychiatric Research, 12,* 189–198.

Galantino, M.L. (1991). Pain management and neuromuscular reeducation for the HIV patient. *AIDS Patient Care, 5*(2), 81–85.

Glover, D., & Glick, J.H. (1991). Oncologic emergencies. In A.I. Holleb, D.J. Fink, and G.P. Murphy (Eds.), *Clinical oncology* (pp. 513–533). Atlanta: American Cancer Society.

Henson, J.W. & Posner, J.B. (1993). Neurological complications. In J.F. Holland, E. Frei, R.C. Bast, D.W. Kufe, D.L. Morton, & R.W. Weischselbaum (Eds.), *Cancer medicine* (3rd ed.) (pp. 2268–2286). Philadelphia: Lea & Febiger.

Hunter, J.C. (1992). Nursing care of patients with structural oncological emergencies. In J.C. Clark & R.F. McGee (Eds.), *Core curriculum for oncology nursing* (2nd ed.) (pp. 156–168). Philadelphia: W.B. Saunders Company.

Ingham, J., Beveridge, A., & Cooney, N.J. (1993). The management of spinal cord compression in patients with advanced malignancy. *Journal of Pain and Symptom Management, 8*(1), 1–6.

Lipton, R.B., Pfeffer, D., Newman, L.C., & Solomon, S. (1993). Headaches in the elderly. *Journal of Pain and Symptom Management, 8*(2), 87–97.

Martin, E.W. (1990). Confusion in the terminally ill: Recognition and management. *The American Journal of Hospice and Palliative Care,* May/June 1990, 20–24.

Miaskowski, C. (1991). Oncologic emergencies. In S.B. Baird, R. McCorkle, & M. Grant (Eds.), *Cancer nursing: A comprehensive textbook* (pp. 885–893). Philadelphia: W.B Saunders.

Peterson, R. (1993). A nursing intervention for early detection of spinal cord compressions in patients with cancer. *Cancer Nursing, 16*(2), 113–116.

Portlock, C.S., & Goffinet, D.R. (1980). *Manual of clinical problems in oncology.* Boston: Little, Brown and Company.

Prados, M.D., & Wilson, C.B. (1993). Neoplasms of the central nervous system. In J.F. Holland, E. Frei, R.C. Bast, D.W. Kufe, D.L. Morton, & R.W. Weischselbaum (Eds.), *Cancer medicine* (3rd ed.) (pp. 1080–1119). Philadelphia: Lea & Febiger.

Ragnarsson, K.T. (1993). Principles of cancer rehabilitation medicine. In J.F. Holland, E. Frei, R.C. Bast, D.W. Kufe, D.L. Morton, & R.W. Weischselbaum (Eds.), *Cancer medicine* (3rd ed.) (pp. 1054–1072). Philadelphia: Lea & Febiger.

Ratanatharathorn, V., & Powers, W.E. (1991). Epidural spinal cord compression from metastatic tumor: Diagnosis and guidelines for management. *Cancer Treatment Reviews, 18*(1), 55–71.

Sundaresan, N., Sachdev, V.P., & Krol, G. (1990). Neurosurgical anti-tumor approaches for pain relief. In K.M. Foley, J.J. Bonica, & V. Ventafridda (Eds.). *Proceedings of the Second International Congress on Cancer Pain* (pp. 275–287). New York: Raven Press.

Venables, G. (1989a). Headache. In T.D. Walsh (Ed.), *Symptom control* (pp. 217–227). Oxford: Blackwell Scientific Publications.

Venables, G. (1989b). Seizures. In T.D. Walsh (Ed.), *Symptom control* (pp. 401–410). Oxford: Blackwell Scientific Publications.

Walsh, T.D. (1989). Confusion. In T.D. Walsh (Ed.), *Symptom control* (pp. 57–68). Oxford: Blackwell Scientific Publications.

Wegman, J.A., & Hakius, P. (1990). Central nervous system cancers. In S.L. Groenwald, M.H. Frogge, M. Goodman, & C.H. Yarbro (Eds.), *Cancer nursing: principles and practice* (pp. 751–773). Boston: Jones and Bartlett.

Zejdlik, C.P. (1992). *Management of spinal cord injury.* Boston: Jones and Bartlett.

Respiratory and Cardiovascular Problems and Interventions

Respiratory symptoms are common in patients with advanced cancer. As with many other problems, respiratory problems increase and treatment options decrease as death nears (Coyle, Adelhardt, Foley, & Portenoy, 1990). Infection, most often pneumonia, is the leading cause of death in patients with cancer; and organ failure, most often respiratory, is the second leading cause (Inagaki, Rodriguez, & Bodey, 1974). Respiratory problems of AIDS are most often related to *Pneumocystis carinii* pneumonia, mycobacterial infections, histoplasmosis, and coccidiomycosis (Chaisson & Volberding, 1990). Please see chapter 27 for specific respiratory problems related to patients with AIDS; and chapter 28 for respiratory problems related to degenerative neurological disorders. In addition to dyspnea, respiratory problems of terminal illness include cough and hemoptysis.

Dyspnea and other symptoms increase as death nears, even when there is no lung or pleural involvement (Wachtel, Allen-Masterson, Reuben, Goldberg, & Mor, 1988). Please see chapter 21 for a full discussion of these symptoms when death is imminent.

Dyspnea

Dyspnea is the most common and feared respiratory problem. Depending on the researcher, on when (in what stage of illness) the measurement is taken, on tumor sites, and on other factors, the prevalence of dyspnea among patients with advanced, terminal cancer is as high as 74% (Bruera, Macmillan, Pither, & MacDonald, 1990). Anxiety or fear of suffocation is found in virtually all patients with dyspnea (Cowcher & Hanks, 1990). Anxiety and dyspnea often work in a mutually exacerbating "vicious cycle" (Zerwekh, 1991, p. 881). Thus, treatment of anxiety (in patient and family) is a fundamental part of treatment for dyspnea.

Symptoms and Etiologies/ Assessment

Dyspnea may be present at rest or on exertion, and is influenced by factors such as movement, posture, cough, and environmental conditions.

General assessment includes primary and secondary tumor sites, severity, impact on life, and associated factors that relieve or worsen, such as frequency, duration, and any history of respiratory problems. While no definitive tool yet exists to measure dyspnea, a visual analogue scale can be used to determine progression, treatment efficacy, and other factors (Steele & Shaver, 1992). Specific etiologies/ assessment parameters, other than those for opportunistic infections of AIDS and degenerative neurological disorders (Baines, 1978; Cowcher & Hanks, 1990; Doyle, 1987; Fanta, 1993; Steele & Shaver, 1992), include:

- Obstruction from primary or secondary tumor or enlarged nodes may be characterized by progressive or rapidly increasing dyspnea, hemoptysis, wheezing or stridor, chronic cough, aspiration, and/or pneumonia.
- Loss of function can result from pleural effusion progressing to cardiac tamponade (see section below, and other information in chapter 14), pulmonary edema from cardiac failure, lymphangitis carcinomatosis (see below), paralysis, and/or pneumonia (see below). The increase in bone marrow transplants is chiefly responsible for the increase in bronchiolitis obliterans, a disorder with symptoms that may mimic emphysema and may occur six weeks to two years after treatment (Fanta, 1993).
- Pleural effusion is common with lung or breast cancer and also with lymphoma or leukemia (Portlock & Goffinet, 1980). Symptoms of pleural effusion include trachea displacement toward opposite side with large effusion, decreased breath sounds, possible

pleural rub, and bronchial sounds near top of effusion. Fremitus is absent or decreased but may increase near top of effusion, and the fluid produces soft flat to dull notes to percussion.
- Pneumonia is common and often related to debility and immobility and is characterized by elevated temperature, purulent sputum (although not always present), decreased breath sounds, dullness to percussion at the affected area, and the presence of pleural effusion. Risk factors include debility, immobility, and/or ineffective breathing.
- Pulmonary thromboembolism is often related to debility and immobility. Tumors associated with hypercoagulability are also associated with emboli (Fanta, 1993). These include leukemia, prostate, breast, and colon tumors (Hunter, 1992). Symptoms have sudden onset, are otherwise unexplainable, and include tachypnea, tachycardia, cough, chest pain, and hemoptysis.
- Pericardial effusion may be a precursor to the cardiac emergency of cardiac tamponade. Pericardial effusions are often associated with primary lung tumors or breast cancer, and also with lymphoma, leukemia, and metastatic melanoma (Portlock & Goffinet, 1980). The most common complaints are dyspnea, cough, chest pain, orthopnea, and weakness. Other characteristics are pleural effusion, peripheral edema, jugular vein distension, tachycardia, and tachypnea (Holmes, Livingston, & Turrisi, 1993).
- Lymphangitis carcinomatosis (tumor infiltration of small lymphatic system of lungs) is difficult to diagnose. The primary symptom is dyspnea from tumor edema.
- Ascites is often related to tumors in ovaries, endometrium, breast, colon, stomach, pancreas, and colon; and less often to other tumors (Varricchio, Miller, & Pazdur, 1990). Symptoms include abdominal distension (fluid vs. gas) and tenderness, general dis-

comfort, orthopnea, tachypnea, pleural effusion, and GI symptoms such as early satiation, indigestion, and decreased bowel mobility.

- Anemia is often related to tumors in the liver and colon and to leukemia and multiple myeloma; as well as being secondary to chemotherapy (Boarini, 1990; Cook, 1990; Frogge, 1990; Wujcik, 1990). Manifestations are non-specific and, in addition to dyspnea, include fatigue, weakness, tachycardia, and headache.

- Superior vena cava syndrome (with upper airway edema) is an oncology emergency that is most often associated with mediastinal tumors, especially small cell or squamous cell carcinomas, but also lymphomas (Glover & Glick, 1991). The primary manifestations are engorged neck veins, facial edema, and changes in consciousness. Other symptoms are cough, hoarseness, and stridor.

- Respiratory muscle weakness is often associated with paraneoplastic syndromes, anorexia, and/or cachexia (Fishbein, Kearon, & Killian, 1989). Manifestations include general weakness, anorexia, cachexia, and/or the presence of a paraneoplastic syndrome, such as Eaton-Lambert syndrome.

- Preexisting or other conditions that result in dyspnea may include chronic bronchitis, emphysema, asthma, tuberculosis, or a neuromuscular disorder. Certain treatment sequelae, such as fibrosis secondary to radiation or chemotherapy, may also result in dyspnea.

- And finally, the role of anxiety should be considered.

Interventions

If possible, treatment of dyspnea is directed first to the etiology, and if that is not possible, to palliation of the symptom. One misconception about terminal care is that the latter is the only concern. General and symptomatic treat-

ment of dyspnea centers on supportive measures, administering oxygen and, in many cases, medications (Bruera et al., 1990). The decision for or against aggressive treatment should take into account the expected life span, issues of quality and, of course, the patient's goals.

Independent Interventions

Supportive measures for treating dyspnea (Cowcher & Hanks, 1990; Elpern, 1990; Polomano & McEvoy, 1991; Zerwekh, 1991) include:

- changing the patient's position, which may bring some relief: The head should be elevated, or if dyspnea is due to bronchial obstruction, a position should be found (lying on one side or the other) in which the patient breathes with the most ease;
- limiting activity;
- reducing anxiety, e.g., teaching or encouraging relaxation exercises, prayer, meditation, resolution of conflicts, and exploration of fears. Explaining the situation is helpful to some extent;
- using diet and fluid restrictions for ascites;
- monitoring oral hygiene, which does not reduce dyspnea, but does reduce accompanying problems related to dry mouth and infection; and
- if necessary, modifying the environment, e.g., eliminating irritants, changing humidity, increasing ventilation, etc.

Interdependent Measures

Specific measures (Bruera, et al., 1990; Cowcher & Hanks, 1990; Fanta, 1993; Glover & Glick, 1991) include the following.

- For obstruction in non-moribund patients, chemotherapy or radiation, or, with non-metastatic tracheal tumors, resection may be used. Tracheostomy is necessary in some cases.
- Loss of function is treated according to etiology and supportively. Bronchiolitis oblit-

erans is difficult to treat effectively.

- Pleural effusion is best treated with systemic therapy in patients with small cell lung cancer; and with pleurodesis and sclerodesis if the patient has non-small cell lung cancer (Holmes et al., 1993) or if the effusion is recurrent. Sclerodesis is frequently ineffective and causes pain.
- Pneumonia is treated with antibiotics and risk factors are reduced.
- Pulmonary embolus requires immediate treatment, including oxygen and anticoagulation therapy, except when the patient has a CNS neoplasm.
- Pericardial effusion, especially when rapidly developing, must be treated quickly or tamponade is likely. Pericardiocentesis is the first step, followed, according to tumor sensitivity and other factors, with sclerosing agents, radiation, hormonal therapy, or chemotherapy. Surgery, including pericardiectomy or pleural-pericardial window, may also be used.
- Lymphangitis carcinomatosis is treated primarily with steroids, but usually without great success.
- Ascites, when treatable, may be treated with paracentesis, diuretics, chemotherapy, and/or surgery (shunt).
- Anemia is treated primarily through transfusion, which may result in significant, but often temporary improvement.
- Superior vena cava syndrome requires emergency treatment when there is decreased cardiac output and brain or upper airway edema (Glover & Glick, 1991). Otherwise, treatment is usually high-dose radiation plus corticosteroids or, when the involved tumor is responsive, chemotherapy may also be used.
- Respiratory muscle weakness is treated with glucocorticoids, but any relief is temporary.

The problems inherent in dealing with treatment sequelae bring into focus the complexities of terminal care and the difficulty of balancing issues such as effects of the disease, effects of the treatment, and reasonable hope. Practitioners should keep in mind that some sequelae occur months, and even years, after treatment.

Pre-existing or other conditions are treated according to the problem. Supportive measures for dyspnea include:

- morphine (and perhaps other narcotics), which are essential in relieving dyspnea (Brueraet al., 1990);
- oxygen, which brings temporary relief;
- expectorants, which are sometimes appropriate;
- anxiolytics, especially benzodiazepines, which are useful for calming patients (Cowcher & Hanks, 1990); and
- bronchodilators, which are used primarily when airway obstruction is reversible.

Cough

Opinions about the prevalence of cough as a distressing problem in advanced cancer range from "uncommon" (Hagen, 1991) to "30% of patients" (Cowcher & Hanks, 1990). Cough is most common in bronchogenic cancer (Cowcher & Hanks, 1990). Significant sequelae of pathologic cough include loss of sleep, muscle strain, changes in blood pressure, headache, ruptured blood vessels, and even bone fracture (Hagen, 1991).

SYMPTOMS AND ETIOLOGIES/ ASSESSMENT

Cough may be dry or productive; frequency, severity, and duration are significant; and associated factors include posture and factors that relieve or worsen.

Parameters for etiology and assessment (Baines, 1978; Cowcher & Hanks, 1990; Doyle, 1987; Fanta, 1993; Hagen, 1991) include some of those discussed under dyspnea: obstruction, loss of function, pneumonia, pulmonary embolus, pericardial effusion, and lymphangitis carcinomatosis. Other specific etiologies of cough are:

- aspiration, often associated with extrinsic or intrinsic esophageal obstruction, as well as with tracheo-esophageal fistula;
- vocal cord paralysis, common in primary or secondary tumors of neck or chest, and characterized by bovine cough and hoarseness;
- sputum retention, which may be related to weakness, cachexia, and respiratory infection.
- Congestive heart failure (CHF), which may occur in patients with anemia and a history of cardiac disease. CHF is characterized by fatigue, dyspnea, tachycardia, edema (legs, lungs, dependent), nocturia, chest pain, and cough;
- pre-existing or other conditions, which are similar to those discussed under dyspnea, except that environmental factors—such as dry air, cigarette smoke, or environmental irritants—may play a larger role.

Independent Interventions
supportive measures (Hagen, 1991; Elpern, 1990; Cowcher & Hanks, 1990) in the treatment of cough include:

- Changing position—which may help, especially elevating the head, or if cough is due to bronchial obstruction, finding the position (lying on side) in which the patient breathes with most ease.
- Air should be warmed and humidified.
- Irritants should be removed.
- Teach deep breathing and effective (deep) coughing.

Interdependent Interventions
Occasionally the causative factor can be resolved; more often, the symptom is treated

(Baines, 1978; Cowcher & Hanks, 1990; Hagen, 1991) as follows:

- Expectorants stimulate and increase productivity of the cough.
- Mucolytics decrease secretion viscosity.
- Bronchodilators are used when an airway obstruction is reversible.
- Antihistamines may sometimes help.
- Morphine, or other narcotics are used to suppress cough reflex centrally, and are often given in combination with antihistamines because opioids tend to cause release of histamine.
- Non-opioid centrally acting agents, e.g., dextromethorphan, suppress the cough, and also stimulate the release of histamine.
- Anxiolytics, especially benzodiazepines, may help.
- Other medications and treatments specific to the problem are discussed under dyspnea.

Hemoptysis

SYMPTOMS AND ETIOLOGIES/ ASSESSMENT

The amount of blood is paramount, with massive hemoptysis being a grave sign and small amounts not necessarily ominous; extra-pulmonary origin (nasal, etc.) should be ruled out.

Parameters for etiology and assessment (Cowcher & Hanks, 1990; Portlock & Goffinet, 1980; Rolston & Bodey, 1993) include:

- Tumor, especially bronchogenic, is a common cause of hemoptysis, sometimes massive, with hemorrhage from bronchial arteries. Esophageal tumors may also produce hemoptysis.
- Infection, including pneumonia, candidiasis aspergillosis, and tuberculosis, may result in hemorrhage.
- Pulmonary embolus, and occasionally other cardiac problems may result in hemoptysis.

Independent Interventions

Supportive measures (Cowcher & Hanks, 1990; Elpern, 1990; Portlock & Goffinet, 1980) in the treatment of minor hemoptysis whose origin is understood include:

- Changing position, so that the affected side is dependent, minimizes aspiration.
- Activities should be minimized.
- Reassurance is appropriate in many cases since, in the absence of dysphagia, weight loss, mental deterioration, and/or dyspnea slight hemoptysis is not necessarily an ominous sign (Cowcher & Hanks, 1990).
- Medications that affect bleeding should be reviewed.

Interdependent Interventions

Medications, treatments specific to the problem (Cowcher & Hanks, 1990; Fernandez et al., 1989) include: radiation to identified lesion, chemotherapy, surgery, and medications for infection.

Although surgery may be indicated for massive bleeding, it is necessary to carefully consider quality-of-life issues.

Cardiovascular Problems in Cancer

Cardiovascular problems in cancer are limited primarily to pericardial effusions and cardiac tamponade, metastases to the heart, problems related to secondary problems of cancer (e.g., anemia, hyperthyroidism, SIADH, aldosteronism, amyloidosis), part of multiple systems organ failure, pre-existing problems, effects of treatment, primary pericardial tumors, such as sarcoma or mesothelioma (and principally in the context of AIDS), primary cardiac lymphoma (Chernecky & Krech, 1991; Dietz & Flaherty, 1990; Ewer & Benjamin, 1993; Glover & Glick, 1991; Lang-Kummer, 1990; McFadden & Sartorius, 1992; Moore & Ruccione, 1990; Sarna & Kagan, 1990; Varricchio, Miller, & Pazdur, 1990). Except for pericardial effusion and car-

diac tamponade, most of the above problems that are due to cancer are difficult, or futile, to treat other than palliatively in the context of terminal cancer. Cardiac problems that develop as a result of anemia, SIADH, etc. are sometimes treatable in terminal illness. Except in moribund patients, pre-existing or other cardiac problems, such as dysrhythmias, are treated as they would be in any other patient. See chapter 21 for a discussion of cardiac states as death approaches.

Cardiovascular problems other than those related to cancer are discussed in chapter 30.

PERICARDIAL EFFUSIONS AND CARDIAC TAMPONADE

Cardiac tamponade (pathologic compression) is an oncology emergency resulting from cardiac compression by large pericardial effusion. The rate of effusion is significant, with rapid effusions resulting in more severe tamponade (Glover & Glick, 1991). Small or slow-growing effusions may be non-symptomatic (Varricchio et al., 1990) or, if the heart is encased by tumor or radiation fibrosis, significantly symptomatic (Ewer & Benjamin, 1993). Tumors most likely to metastasize to the heart are lung, breast, melanoma, acute leukemia, lymphoma, and gastrointestinal tumors (Chernecky & Krech, 1991).

The primary symptoms of pericardial effusion are "non-specific" cardiac symptoms (Varricchio et al., 1990). Progression to cardiac tamponade results in more severe symptoms, including dyspnea, retrosternal chest discomfort, or fullness (relieved by bending over) and in cough. Other manifestations of cardiac tamponade include tachycardia, tachypnea, decreased systolic and pulse pressures, changes in consciousness, peripheral cyanosis, neck vein distension, edema, and occasionally nausea, vomiting and abdominal pain.

If the pericardium cannot be drained immediately, treatment may include administrating oxygen (but positive pressure breathing is contraindicated) and medications to improve cardiac contractions and filling. This may result in relief, but symptoms often return within 48 hours (Glover & Glick, 1991). For all but moribund patients, treatment (other than of the tumor) consists of drainage and pericardial sclerosis (Ewer & Benjamin, 1993). Several effective means exist to achieve both, including pericardial catheter drainage and sclerosis via antibiotic, chemotherapy, systemic hormonal therapy, radiation therapy, and pericardiectomy (Glover & Glick, 1991).

References

Baines, M.J. (1978). Control of other symptoms. In C.M. Saunders (Ed.), *The management of terminal disease* (pp. 99–118). London: Edward Arnold.

Boarini, J. (1990). Gastrointestinal cancers: Colon, rectum, and anus. In S.L. Groenwald, M.H. Frogge, M. Goodman, & C.H. Yarbro (Eds.), *Cancer nursing: Principles and practice* (pp. 792–805). Boston: Jones and Bartlett.

Bruera, E., Macmillan, K., Pither, J., & MacDonald, R.N. (1990). Effects of morphine on the dyspnea of terminal cancer patients. *Journal of Pain and Symptom Management, 5*(6), 341–344.

Chaisson, R.E., & Volberding, P.A. (1990). Clinical manifestations of HIV infection. In G.L. Mandell, R.G. Douglas, & J.E. Bennett (Eds.), *Principles and practices of infectious diseases* (3rd ed.) (pp. 1059–1092). New York: Churchill Livingston.

Chernecky, C., & Krech, R.L. (1991). Complications of advanced disease. In S.B. Baird, R. McCorkle, & M. Grant (Eds.), *Cancer nursing: A comprehensive textbook* (pp. 864–874). Philadelphia: W.B Saunders.

Cook, M.B. (1990). Multiple myeloma. In S.L. Groenwald, M.H. Frogge, M. Goodman, & C.H. Yarbro (Eds.), *Cancer nursing: Principles and practice* (pp. 990–998). Boston: Jones and Bartlett.

Cowcher, K., & Hanks, G.W. (1990). Long-term management of respiratory symptoms in advanced cancer. *Journal of Pain and Symptom Management, 5*(5), 320–330.

Coyle, N., Adelhardt, J., Foley, K.M., & Portenoy, R.K. (1990). Character of terminal illness in the advanced cancer patient: Pain and other symptoms during the last four weeks of life. *Journal of Pain and Symptom Management, 5*(2), 83–93.

Dietz, K.A., & Flaherty, A.M. (1990). Oncologic emergencies. In S.L. Groenwald, M.H. Frogge, M. Goodman, & C.H. Yarbro (Eds.), *Cancer nursing: Princi-*

ples and practice (pp. 644–668). Boston: Jones and Bartlett.

Doyle, J.E. (1987). Nursing role in management: vascular disorders. In S.M. Lewis & I.C. Collier (Eds.), *Medical-surgical nursing: Assessment and management of clinical problems* (pp. 893–926). New York: McGraw-Hill.

Elpern, E.H. (1990). Lung cancer. In S.L. Groenwald, M.H. Frogge, M. Goodman, & C.H. Yarbro (Eds.), *Cancer nursing: Principles and practice* (pp. 951–973). Boston: Jones and Bartlett.

Ewer, M.S., & Benjamin, R.S. (1993). Cardiac complications. In J.F. Holland, E. Frei, R.C. Bast, D.W. Kufe, D.L. Morton, & R.W. Weischselbaum (Eds.), *Cancer medicine* (3rd ed.) (pp. 2332–2348). Philadelphia: Lea & Febiger.

Fanta, C.H. (1993), Respiratory complications. In J.F. Holland, E. Frei, R.C. Bast, D.W. Kufe, D.L. Morton, & R.W. Weischselbaum (Eds.), *Cancer medicine* (3rd ed.) (pp. 2349–2358). Philadelphia: Lea & Febiger.

Fernandez, C., Rosell, R., Abad-Esteve, A., Monras, P., Moreno, I., Serichol, M., & Roviralta, M. (1989). Quality of life during chemotherapy in non-small cell cancer patients. *Acta Oncologica, 28*(1), 30.

Fishbein, D., Kearon, C., & Killian, K.J. (1989). An approach to dyspnea in cancer patients. *Journal of Pain and Symptom Management, 4*(2), 76–81.

Frogge, M.H. (1990). Gastrointestinal cancer: Esophagus, stomach, liver, and pancreas. In S.L. Groenwald, M.H. Frogge, M. Goodman, & C.H. Yarbro (Eds.), *Cancer nursing: Principles and practice* (pp. 806–844). Boston: Jones and Bartlett.

Glover, D., & Glick, J.H. (1991). Oncologic emergencies. In A.I. Holleb, D.J. Fink, & G.P. Murphy (Eds.), *Clinical oncology* (pp. 513–533). Atlanta: American Cancer Society.

Hagen, N.A. (1991). An approach to cough in cancer patients. *Journal of Pain and Symptom Management, 6*(4), 257–262.

Holmes, E.C., Livingston, R., & Turrisi, A. (1993). Neoplasms of the thorax. In J.F. Holland, E. Frei, R.C. Bast, D.W. Kufe, D.L. Morton, & R.W. Weischselbaum (Eds.), *Cancer medicine* (3rd ed.) (pp. 1285–1381). Philadelphia: Lea & Febiger.

Hunter, J.C. (1992). Nursing care of patients with structural oncological emergencies. In J.C. Clark & R.F. McGee (Eds.), *Core curriculum for oncology nursing* (2nd ed.) (pp. 156–168). Philadelphia: W.B. Saunders Company.

Inagaki, J., Rodriguez, V., & Bodey, G.P. (1974). Causes of death in cancer patients. *Cancer., 33*(2), 568–573.

Lang-Kummer, J.M. (1990). Hypercalcemia. In S.L. Groenwald, M.H. Frogge, M. Goodman, & C.H. Yarbro (Eds.), *Cancer nursing: Principles and practice* (pp. 520–534). Boston: Jones and Bartlett.

McFadden, M.E., & Sartorius, S.E. (1992). Multiple systems organ failure in the patient with cancer: Nursing implications. *Oncology Nursing Forum, 19*(5), 727–737.

Moore, I.M., & Ruccione, K. (1990). Late effects of cancer treatment. In S.L. Groenwald, M.H. Frogge, M. Goodman, & C.H. Yarbro (Eds.), *Cancer nursing: Principles and practice* (pp. 669–688). Boston: Jones and Bartlett.

Polomano, R., & McEvoy, M.D. (1991). Nursing management of persons with progressive disease: Prototype—lung cancer. In S.B. Baird, R. McCorkle, & M. Grant (Eds.), *Cancer nursing: A comprehensive textbook* (pp. 699–707). Philadelphia: W.B Saunders.

Portlock, C.S., & Goffinet, D.R. (1980). *Manual of clinical problems in oncology*. Boston: Little, Brown and Company.

Rolston, K.V.I., & Bodey, G.P. (1993). Infections in patients with cancer. In J.F. Holland, E. Frei, R.C. Bast, D.W. Kufe, D.L. Morton, & R.W. Weischselbaum (Eds.), *Cancer medicine* (3rd ed.) (pp. 2416–2441). Philadelphia: Lea & Febiger.

Sarna, G.P., & Kagan, A.R. (1990). Non-Hodgkin's lymphomas. In C.M. Haskell (Ed.), *Cancer treatment* (3rd ed.) (pp. 683–718). Philadelphia: W.B. Saunders.

Steele, B., & Shaver, J.S. (1992). The dyspnea experience: Nocioceptive properties and a model for research and practice. *Advances in Nursing Science, 15*(1), 64–76.

Varricchio, C.G., Miller, N., & Pazdur, M. (1990). Edema and effusions. In S.L. Groenwald, M.H. Frogge, M. Goodman, & C.H. Yarbro (Eds.), *Cancer nursing: Principles and practice* (pp. 546–562). Boston: Jones and Bartlett.

Wachtel, T., Allen-Masterson, S., Reuben, D., Goldberg, R., & Mor, V. (1988). The end stage cancer patient: Terminal common pathway. *The Hospice Journal, 4*(4), 43–80.

Wujcik, D. (1990). Leukemia. In S.L. Groenwald, M.H. Frogge, M. Goodman, & C.H. Yarbro (Eds.), *Cancer nursing: Principles and practice* (pp. 930–950). Boston: Jones and Bartlett.

Zerwekh, J. (1991). Supportive care of the dying patient. In S.B. Baird, R. McCorkle, & M. Grant (Eds.), *Cancer nursing: A comprehensive textbook* (pp 875–884). Philadelphia: W.B Saunders.

Skin Problems and Interventions

Skin problems of patients with advanced cancer include decubitus ulcers, malignant ulcers, fistulas, fungating tumors, pruritus, infections, and dermatologic sequelae of treatment (Billings, 1985; De Conno, Ventafridda, & Saita, 1991). Skin problems are universal in persons with AIDS and are discussed in chapter 27. It is important to note that there is a general alteration of skin condition in patients with advanced cancer and other illness, hence problems are more likely. Compromises of the skin may encompass thinning, loss of elasticity, dehydration, deepening of sores and wrinkles, various pigmentation disorders (De Conno et al., 1991), as well as problems related to immuno-suppression, nutrition, and loss of mobility.

Decubitus Ulcers

Decubitus ulcers result from pressure, sometimes exacerbated by trauma (e.g., friction, bruises, multiple, same-site injections), especially at or near bony prominences. The devel-opment of decubitus ulcers is influenced by multiple factors, including immobility and incontinence, hydration, and nutritional, circulatory, and mental status. Patients who are terminally ill are at significant risk of skin breakdown. In one hospice, the prevalence of decubitus ulcers was 13%, with most occurring in the two weeks preceding death (Hanson et al., 1991). The results of decubiti may include pain, infection, protein loss, multiplication of lesions, and increased demands on caregiver effort.

Because of associated morbidity and negative influence on quality of life, decubitus ulcers are best prevented. Preventive measures include attention to frequent assessment, frequent turning, correct positioning, good hygiene, attention to mechanical factors, to hydration and nutrition, to pain status and immobility, to the patient's other physical problems or factors of the patient's disease or treatment, to the bed, to preventive devices, and utilizing the knowledge and abilities of the caregiver(s) to the greatest extent possible. Despite great effort, decubitus ulcers are sometimes "inevitable . . . and do not always indicate bad nursing care" (De Conno et al., 1991).

Charles Kemp: TERMINAL ILLNESS: A GUIDE TO NURSING CARE. © 1995 J. B. Lippincott.

Frequent assessment is mediated by the degree of risk of skin breakdown for a particular patient, the discomfort involved, and life expectancy. During bathing (or better, while massaging), is a good time to carefully inspect the skin. Special attention should be given to the sacrum, ischia, heels, ankles, and trochanters.

Turning the patient every two hours is the standard, since decubitus ulcers can develop in as little as two hours (Billings, 1985). Turning must be done with care to prevent external trauma from shearing force, bruising, and friction.

Patients should be placed at oblique (30-degree) alternating angles on the bed rather than always straight up and down (De Conno et al., 1991).

Skin should be kept clean, dry, and as free as possible from urine, stool, drainage, or perspiration. Frequently cleansed skin is often excessively dry, hence moisturizing lotions can be used judiciously. Powders should be avoided. Soaps used for skin and linens should be non-irritating.

Mechanical and other factors should be avoided or modified. These include wrinkled or rough sheets, crumbs, tape, jewelry, patient's fingernails, vigorous drying with towels, excessive heat, and other external factors that can contribute to the development of decubitus ulcers.

Protein deficiency is strongly linked with decubitus development (Waltman, Bergstrom, Armstrong, Norvell, & Braden, 1991). Hydration and nutrition should be maintained as long as possible, given the patient's desires and capabilities. If eating causes significant distress, however, it should be discontinued if the patient desires.

Since immobility is frequently implicated in decubitus ulcers and pain is a frequent cause of immobility, pain must be controlled. Over-medication with analgesics may result in immobility and not feeling the pain of developing problems. Depending on when death is expected, immobility from weakness or paralysis can be addressed with passive range of motion exercises. However, care should be taken that exercises are not discontinued weeks before death: immobile patients can stiffen quickly and develop subsequent problems. It is essential that pain be controlled before range of motion exercises begin. Ideally, this exercise serves also as a means of positive human contact.

Other physical problems or factors that contribute to skin breakdown include: use of steroids, infection, anemia, and edema (Billings, 1985).

Soft beds are better than hard, and special surfaces, e.g., sheepskin or egg crate foam, are better than the mattress alone. Sheepskin should be brushed daily and kept clean. An alternating pressure mattress, such as the Clinitron bed, is best, especially for high-risk patients or for those with skin breakdown (De Conno et al., 1991). The Clinitron bed is also more comfortable in general, and in particular for patients with pain (Walsh & Brescia, 1990). Preventive devices—including sheepskin pads shaped to fit over heels and sheepskin or blankets between the knees—are helpful for very debilitated patients. Duffield (1989) discourages the use of foam, ring-shaped cushions.

Family caregivers should understand procedures and prevention. Their ability to understand, as well as to provide, good care should be assessed on an ongoing basis.

If decubitus ulcers develop, they should be treated using the above principles of prevention, as well as the following additional principles or techniques:

• *Assessment:* Different organizations have different means of classification and description. It is important that everyone providing care to a particular patient use the same means of classification and description. Regardless of classification scheme, the first stage of a developing decubitus ulcer is intact skin with erythema and, often, pain. Once there is a lesion, classifications begin to differ. For the purposes of describing and recording the patient's condition, at a minimum, the diameter and depth should be measured (not estimated) and the lesion described, e.g., presence of erythema, vesicles, drainage, eschar, or bony involvement. The patient's mobility, mental status, and other relevant factors should be noted. The appearance of the dressing, other skin areas, bed linens, etc. should be described. When appropriate, the family caregiver's mental, socioeconomic, and physical status should also be described.

- *Relief of pressure and other contributing factors:* This is described above. The Clinitron or similar bed is especially helpful. Key issues are relief of pressure and prevention of infection.

- *Treatment of open ulcers:* There are a number of products, theories, and home remedies, many of which are helpful, and new ones are being promoted, even while this book is going to press. Generally accepted measures (De Conno et al., 1991; Billings, 1985; Duffield, 1989) include:

  1. Reestablish blood supply by eliminating pressure. Eliminate other causative factors, e.g., urine, drainage.
  2. Remove any necrotic tissue either surgically, by enzymes, e.g., collagenase, or chemically, e.g., hydrogen peroxide.
  3. Treat infection: Duffield (1989) discourages topical antibiotics and recommends systemic antibiotics, prescribed according to microorganism.
  4. Keep skin area clean with 50% hydrogen peroxide, followed by normal saline, povidone-iodine, or chlorhexidine. Vesicles should not be broken. Topical antiseptics should be discontinued as soon as granulation begins (De Conno et al., 1991).
  5. Dressings should be semi-permeable membrane, or the wound can be left exposed to air. Wet (Ringer's solution) to dry dressing may also be used. Dry

dressings should not be used. Occlusive dressings, including Stomahesive, Duoderm, and others, should not be used on immuno-suppressed patients (Ungvarski, 1992).

Malignant Ulcers, Fistulas, and Fungating Tumors

Malignant ulcers, fistulas, and fungating tumors are visible (and often olfactory) manifestations of advanced disease. Malignant ulceration occurs most frequently in patients with tumors of the head and neck (squamous cell), breast, sarcomas, and recurrent gynecologic tumors (Enck, 1990). Billings (1985, p. 103) notes that "while the disheartening appearance" is seldom amenable to treatment, the associated problems can often be managed. Attendant problems include:

- Bleeding is managed by radiation, cryosurgery, or embolization. Major, irreversible hemorrhage calls for sedation (De Conno et al., 1991). Dark towels can be used to minimize visual effects of bleeding. With lesser bleeding, pressure bandaging may help.
- Odor is due to anaerobic microorganisms (Enck, 1990), and is foul. Frequent cleaning of the area is essential. Povidone iodine, hydrogen peroxide, and chlorhexidine are effective agents. Infection should be treated topically and systemically. Dressings may include packing (charcoal dressings) for absorption of exudates. Good air circulation is helpful to some extent, as are ionizers. Metronidazole 250 mg orally five times day or clindamycin 300 mg orally qid are effective in eliminating odor (Enck, 1990). Both have liabilities and are not effective for long-term use. Metronidazole injection solution incorporated in an 0.8% gel on daily dressings is also effective. The use of

the gel medium is apparently important.

- Drainage to adjacent areas can be distressing psychologically as well as resulting in infection, excoriation, and similar problems. Fistulas that open onto the skin can be managed similarly to an ostomy, both with respect to discharge and protection of surrounding skin. Rectovaginal or rectoperineal fistulas are very distressing to patients. Creative management, using tampons, sanitary pads, and other measures, tax the skills of the practitioner. Unflagging persistence in good treatment and effective management of the conditions has a positive effect on both the patient's physical and psychological well-being.
- Large, malignant ulcers with signs of infection are painful. Treating the infection relieves the pain (Enck, 1990).
- Psychosocial issues are at the fore in the management of these problems. Support and diversion are essential.

Pruritus

Pruritus is common in patients with primary polycythemia, Hodgkin's disease, lymphoma, and leukemia, as well as with other tumor types (De Conno et al., 1991). Pruritus also develops secondarily to systemic processes such as uremia and cholestasis (Billings, 1985), especially when there is obstructive jaundice (Baines, 1978). Itching may also be due to psychological disorder (Amlot, 1989) and other problems indirectly related to terminal illness, e.g., Candida, eczema; and to initial opioid use.

Treating the cause is the best course. When this is not possible, the following measures (Amlot, 1989; DeConno et al., 1991; Billings, 1985; Jenkins, 1988) may reduce pruritus:

- The application of local comfort measures, such as cooling bath with sodium bicarbonate, moisturizing lotions for dry skin, calamine lotion, or medicated lotions (2%

phenol, menthol) and anesthetic gel (0.5–2.0% lidocaine) every two hours. Because of potential development of sensitization phenomena, antihistamine ointments are discouraged by De Conno et al. (1991, p. 253) but Amlot (1989, p. 289) reports that in severe cases, potential benefits outweigh risks.

- Corticosteroids are usually ineffective in systemic disease.
- Other non-pharmacological measures include: keeping the patient's nails trimmed, treating insomnia (pruritus may be worse at night), avoiding coffee and alcohol, and providing distraction. Detergents used for bed linens and clothing should be mild. It may be helpful for some patients to wear gloves at night.
- Medications: systemic and topical therapies should be combined for severe itching. In addition to the aforementioned topical measures, the following are used: antihistamines are more effective for itch due to allergy than for itch due to other problems, and are ineffective for itch due to cholestasis. Diphenhydramine has anxiolytic properties, as does Hydroxyzine (25–50 mg IM or PO every six hours). The latter is effective for both pruritus and anxiety (Amlot, 1989). Promethazine 20–50 mg every 12 hours or Trimeprazine 10 mg every eight hours may also be used (De Conno et al, 1991; Amlot, 1989). Chlorpromazine, up to 200 mg. qid, is effective, but also affects liver function and so is contraindicated for some patients. Aspirin is helpful only to patients with Hodgkin's disease and polycythemia vera. Cimetidine is effective in some patients with polycythemia vera (Amlot, 1989).

Infections

Skin infections in patients with terminal cancer are most commonly bacteriologic, but also viral, fungal, or mixed (De Conno et al., 1991).

Infections are often complicated by some combination of immuno-suppressive medications, neutropenia, debility, and other factors. Some infections are preventable through effective hygiene, wound care, and, to a lesser extent, maintenance of other aspects of health status. Skin infections should be treated on the basis of the microorganism involved. Pain and odor, if any, from the infection should be addressed. Herpes zoster ("shingles") often results in pain and thus anti-inflammatory and opioid drugs may be required. De Conno et al. (p. 254) recommends systemic steroids, and "in selected cases," epidural steroids. (See neuropathic pain in chapters 11 and 12.)

Dermatologic Sequelae of Treatment

Both radiation and chemotherapy can have ill effects on the skin.

The effects of radiation are mediated by dose, skin condition, and other factors, and are most severe in skin folds. Radiation injuries are less common under current treatment modalities than they were previously (Parker, 1991). Late reactions to radiation may be irreversible, and include malfunction of dermal glands.

Patients with advanced cancer may receive radiation for palliation of symptoms, especially for bone pain. Early alterations in skin integrity include erythema, followed sometimes by blisters and desquamation. Other reactions include dryness, pruritus, edema, vesiculation, ulceration, weeping, pain, and alopecia (Mayer, 1988a). Infection may also result. Treatment includes measures to minimize problems, such as avoiding irritants, e.g., harsh soaps, restrictive clothing, trauma. Skin should be cleansed gently with warm water and mild soap. Mild lotions may also be used. Treatment of ulcers and infections is the same as discussed elsewhere.

Skin problems resulting from chemotherapy include necrosis from drug extravasation, alope-

cia, and allergic or hypersensitivity reactions. Other reactions include changes in pigmentation, photosensitivity, nail problems, folliculitis, and radiation recall reactions (Haskell, 1991). In advanced disease, palliative chemotherapy is seldom given in amounts sufficient to cause skin reactions (De Conno et al., p. 249). The possibility of extravasation still exists, however. Most extravasations do not result in more than local irritation (Mayer, 1988b). Treatment includes ice packs for 24 hours after occurrence and wound care, if necessary.

References

Amlot, P. (1989). Itch. In T.D. Walsh (Ed.), *Symptom control* (pp. 285–294). London: Blackwell Scientific Publications.

Baines, M.J. (1978). Control of other symptoms. In C.M. Saunders (Ed.), *The management of terminal disease* (pp. 99–118). London: Edward Arnold.

Billings, J.A. (1985). The management of common symptoms. In J.A. Billings (Ed.). *Outpatient management of advanced cancer* (pp. 40–139). Philadelphia: J.B. Lippincott.

De Conno, F., Ventafridda, V., & Saita, L. (1991). Skin problems in advanced and terminal cancer patients. *Journal of Pain and Symptom Management, 6*(4), 247–256.

Duffield, M. (1989). Bedsores. In T.D. Walsh (Ed.), *Symptom control* (pp. 35–41). London: Blackwell Scientific Publications.

Enck, R.E. (1990). The management of large fungating tumors (malignant ulceration). *American Journal of Hospice and Palliative Care, 7*(3), 11–12.

Hanson, D., Langemo, D.K., Olson, B., Hunter, S., Sauvage, T., Burd, C., & Cathcart-Silberberg, T. (1991). The prevalence and incidence of pressure sores in the hospice setting: Analysis of two methodologies. *American Journal of Hospice and Palliative Care, 8*(5), 18–26.

Haskell, C.M. (1991). Principles and practice of cancer chemotherapy. In C.M. Haskell (Ed.), *Cancer treatment* (pp. 21–43). Philadelphia: W.B. Saunders.

Jenkins, J. (1988) Pruritus. In S.B. Baird (Ed.), *Decision making in oncology nursing* (pp. 80–81). Philadelphia: B.C. Decker.

Mayer, D.K. (1988a). Skin integrity alterations associated with radiation therapy. In S.B. Baird (Ed.), *Decision making in oncology nursing* (pp. 112–113). Philadelphia: B.C. Decker.

Mayer, D.K. (1988b). Skin integrity alterations associated with extravasation. In S.B. Baird (Ed.), *Decision making in oncology nursing* (pp. 118–119). Philadelphia: B.C. Decker.

Parker, R.G. (1991). Principles of radiation oncology. In C.M. Haskell (Ed.), *Cancer treatment* (pp. 15–21). Philadelphia: W.B. Saunders.

Ungvarski, P.J. (1992). Nursing management of the adult client. In J.H. Flaskerud and P.J. Ungvarski (Eds.), *HIV/AIDS: A guide to nursing care* (2nd ed.)

(pp. 146–198). Philadelphia: W.B. Saunders.

Walsh, M., & Brescia, F.J. (1990). Clinitron therapy and pain management in advanced cancer patients. *Journal of pain and symptom management, 5*(1), 46–50.

Waltman, N.L., Bergstrom, N., Armstrong, N. Norvell, K., & Braden, B. (1991). Nutritional status, pressure sores, and mortality in elderly patients with cancer. *Oncology Nursing Forum, 18*(5), 867–873.

Oral Problems and Interventions

Oral problems, ranging from pathological processes to poor hygiene, contribute significantly to decreased quality of life in many patients with advanced cancer, especially those with hematologic malignancies and patients treated for head and neck cancer (Kenny, 1990). As many as 40% of patients in treatment for cancer experience oral problems secondary to treatment (Sonis, 1993). The primary oral complications of cancer are infections, stomatitis, ulcers, dry mouth, and taste alteration (hypogeusia, ageusia, dysgeusia) (De Conno, Ripamonti, Sbanotto, & Ventafridda, 1989). In some cases anorexia, malnutrition, and cachexia result directly from oral complications (De Conno et al., 1989). Patients with AIDS have an extremely high (> 70%) incidence of oral infections and other problems, including candidiasis, oral hairy leukoplakia, herpes simplex, oral warts, recurrent aphthous ulcers, periodontal disease, and lesions due to opportunistic infections and cancer (Boswell & Hirsch, 1992; Greenspan & Greenspan, 1992). Lesions from opportunistic infections (cytomegalovirus and disseminated histoplasmosis) and cancer associated with AIDS are also common. Oral problems of AIDS are discussed in chapter 27.

General Interventions/Prevention

Oral care should be frequent, systematic, and take into consideration the fragility of the oral cavity of patients with advanced disease (Kenny, 1990). Thus, the toothbrush should be a soft one; toothpaste should be mild; mouthwash should be mild and not contain alcohol; and the water-pick device should be operated at a low (power of water jet) setting. Dental flossing should be done with great care, lest the floss cut into the patient's gums. Areas where lesions or pockets of infection exist should be the last areas flossed. Dentures should fit well and be carefully cleaned and removed at night. Oral care for patients who are weak and cachectic may consist primarily of rinsing with salt water. Oral care should be given before sleep. Regular and systematic oral care can help reduce the likelihood of infections, especially bacterial. Oral pain may be partially relieved with popsicles.

Charles Kemp: TERMINAL ILLNESS: A GUIDE TO NURSING CARE. © 1995 J. B. Lippincott.

Infections (of Cancer)

Candidiasis
The most common fungal infection of cancer by far is candidiasis, characterized by oral discomfort, removable white ("cottage cheese") plaques and/or flat red lesions of the mucosa without removable plaques. Candida esophagitis (with or without oral candidiases) causes dysphagia and often retrosternal pain, and nausea and vomiting (Rolston and Bodey, 1993). See also the discussion of candidiasis in chapter 27.

Etiologies/Assessment
Candidiasis is often associated with steroid and/or antibiotic use (Baines, 1978), as well as with other immuno-suppressive treatment. Patients with leukemia are at great risk, followed by those with lymphoma (Rolston & Bodey, 1993). Patients with AIDS are at the greatest risk.

Interventions
An oral care protocol helps, if not in prevention, then certainly in early identification. De Conno et al. (1989) discourage using the commonly prescribed Nystatin, and instead recommend Clotrimazole as having greater efficacy and fewer side effects for both prevention and treatment. Parenteral amphotericin B is very effective and parenteral fluconazole is an alternative (Rolston & Bodey, 1993). Ketoconazole is an alternative, especially in the potentially fatal disseminated candidiasis infection (De Conno et al., 1989).

Aspergillosis
Aspergillosis, primarily pulmonary, is increasingly found in patients who are neutropenic or receiving chronic steroid therapy. Symptoms are non-specific. Treatment is with amphotericin B. Patients who recover from aspergillosis are at risk for pulmonary hemorrhage (Rolston & Bodey, 1993).

Cryptococcosis
Cryptococcosis infections may be disseminated, including to the central nervous system, and are challenging to diagnose. Treatment is with amphotericin B alone or with 5-Fluorocytosine (Rolston & Bodey, 1993).

Viral Infections
Viral infections are primarily from herpes simplex virus (HSV). HSV infections are characterized by removable painful yellowish membranes on mucosa and vesicular eruptions on or adjacent to lips.

Viral infections are less common than candidiasis (De Conno et al., 1989), but may increase over time because of the increase in sexually transmitted herpes zoster in the 1980s.

Currently the most effective treatment is IV acyclovir (De Conno et al., 1989).

Bacterial Infections
Bacterial infections are characterized by small oral hemorrhages, periodontal pain, fever, signs of periapical abscess, and signs of secondary infection in adjacent structures; other signs of inflammation may be missing (De Conno et al., 1989).

Bacterial infections result from a variety of pathogens and are common during and after chemotherapy.

Interventions call for treatment including antibiotic therapy and dental care.

Stomatitis

Symptoms of stomatitis are inflammation and denudation of the oral mucosa, ulcers (sometimes infected with Candida), and bleeding (Kenny, 1990).

Stomatitis is commonly drug-induced (Kenny, 1990) or may also be related to infection, poor dental hygiene, denture problems, vitamin deficiency, radiation therapy, or blood dyscrasias (Billings, 1985).

Interventions take into consideration the

fact that radiation and chemotherapy complications are reduced or prevented through frequent, systematic oral care. Treatment includes regular oral care before and after meals and before bedtime. Oral care for a patient with stomatitis typically consists of (De Conno et al., 1989; Kenny, 1990):

- lip lubricant is used if indicated;
- cleansing rinses, such as sodium chloride solution, 0.9%; bicarbonate of soda; hydrogen peroxide, 3%–6%; or povidone iodine, 1%, which can be used several times each day;
- analgesic rinses, which include Xylocaine viscous 2% 5–15 mL every 4 hours; dyclonine hydrochloride 0.5% 5–10 mL every 2 hours; equal parts up to 30 ml of diphenhydramine hydrochloride elixir 12.5 mg/5 mL and aluminum hydroxide, which can be used every two hours. Benzydamine hydrochloride is effective, but not yet available in the United States. (Sonis, 1993).

Ulcers

Recurrent aphthous ulcers are the most common oral ulceration in persons with AIDS. They are less common in patients with cancer. Ulcers are found in and out of the mouth.

Ulcers are a result of: (1) the neutropenia found most often in patients with hematologic malignancies; (2) local factors, such as trauma, infection, drug toxicity; or (3) from unknown causes (De Conno et al., 1989).

Intervention consists of treatment that is the same as for stomatitis.

Dry Mouth (Xerostomia)

Xerostomia is characterized by thirst and discomfort. In addition, radiation-induced dental caries is common in patients with xerostomia (Sonis, 1993).

Xerostomia is very common in advanced

disease and is due to a variety, and often a combination of factors. Among these are decrease in saliva caused by radiation, medications, infection, and other factors; erosion of buccal mucosa caused by disease, treatment, infection, and other factors; and dehydration caused by anorexia, vomiting, diarrhea, mouth breathing, O2 therapy, difficulty swallowing, and other factors (Baines, 1978; De Conno et al., 1989).

Interventions call for treatment that includes addressing specific etiologies when possible, e.g., changing medications or reducing the dosage, treating the infection, or increasing fluids by mouth. Medications to palliate xerostomia include Pilocarpine, dihydroergotamine, and 2% citric acid solution (De Conno et al., 1989). Sugarless gum, hard candy, popsicles or other means of hydration are suggested by Billings (1985, p. 78). "Artificial saliva" may be used to reduce problems of dry mouth (Baines, 1978). De Conno et al. offer the following suggestions for artificial saliva:

- glycerin, Cologel, normal saline (1:1:8);
- methylcellulose, lemon essence, water; and
- hydrophilic chewing gum.

Xerostomia may be associated with dehydration and imminent death.

Taste Changes (Hypogeusia, Ageusia, Dysgeusia)

Common taste changes are decreased tolerance of bitter and increased tolerance of sweet tastes (Grant, 1986), De Conno et al. (1989) report "an increased threshold of detection for all four basic tastes" in some patients (p. 27). A common food aversion is for meat.

Taste disorders may be caused by cancer treatment, medications, or protein, vitamin, and zinc deficiencies.

Interventions call for offering only foods that do not taste or smell unpleasant to the patient. If the problem is increased threshold to tastes, then hot, strong-smelling foods may be helpful. Maximum nutrition with minimum intake is the general goal when taste disorders influence dietary intake. Alternative intake, such as nasogastric feeding or hyperalimentation, are seldom appropriate.

References

Baines, M.J. (1978). Control of other symptoms. In C.M. Saunders (Ed.), *The management of terminal disease* (pp. 99–118). London: Edward Arnold.

Billings, J.A. (1985). The management of common symptoms. In J.A. Billings (Ed.). *Outpatient management of advanced cancer* (pp. 40–139). Philadelphia: J.B. Lippincott.

Boswell, S.L., & Hirsch, M.S. (1992). Therapeutic approaches to the HIV-seropositive patient. In V.T. DeVita, S. Hellman, & S.A. Rosenberg (Eds.), *AIDS: Etiology, diagnosis, treatment, and prevention* (3rd ed.) (pp. 417–433). Philadelphia: J.B. Lippincott Company.

De Conno, F., Ripamonti, C., Sbanotto, A., & Ventafridda, V. (1989). Oral complications in patients with advanced cancer. *Journal of Pain and Symptom Management, 4*(1), 20–29.

Grant, M. (1986). Nutritional interventions: Increasing oral intake. *Seminars in Oncology Nursing, 2*(1), 36–43.

Greenspan, J.S., & Greenspan, D. (1992). Oral lesions associated with HIV infection. In G.P. Wormser (Ed.), *AIDS and other manifestations of HIV infection* (2nd ed.) (pp. 489–498). New York: Raven Press.

Kenny, S.A. (1990). Effect of two oral care protocols on the incidence of stomatitis in hematology patients. *Cancer Nursing, 13*(6), 345–353.

Rolston, K.V.I., & Bodey, G.P. (1993). Infections in patients with cancer. In J.F. Holland, E. Frei, R.C. Bast, D.W. Kufe, D.L. Morton, & R.W. Weischselbaum (Eds.), *Cancer medicine* (3rd ed.) (pp. 2416–2441). Philadelphia: Lea & Febiger.

Sonis, S.T. (1993). Oral complications. In J.F. Holland, E. Frei, R.C. Bast, D.W. Kufe, D.L. Morton, & R.W. Weischselbaum (Eds.), *Cancer medicine* (3rd ed.) (pp. 2381–2388). Philadelphia: Lea & Febiger.

Gastrointestinal Problems and Interventions

Common gastrointestinal (GI) problems include dysphagia, nausea, vomiting, anorexia, cachexia, constipation, diarrhea, incontinence, and bowel obstruction. While there is conflicting information on the prevalence of specific GI problems in end-stage disease, the most common and troublesome are anorexia, and nausea and vomiting.

Dysphagia

SYMPTOMS AND ETIOLOGIES/ ASSESSMENT

Dysphagia may include difficulty swallowing solids only, or solids and liquids. Dysphagia may be manifested by difficulty swallowing, frequent choking, or odynophagia (pain when swallowing). Some liquids may be harder to swallow than others. Water, for example, is difficult for some patients to swallow, while thicker fluids may be easier. Other patients may experience difficulty with the mucus associat-

Charles Kemp: TERMINAL ILLNESS: A GUIDE TO NURSING CARE. © 1995 J. B. Lippincott.

ed with milk products. When present with cognitive failure and weight loss of 10 kilograms or more, dysphagia with solids or liquids is an accurate indicator that death is likely to occur in less than four weeks (Bruera, Miller, Kuehn, MacEachern, & Hanson, 1992).

Dysphagia may be due to dysfunction of the tongue, or stricture or lesions of the esophagus (Grant & Ropka, 1991). Dysphagia from tumor extension "requires at least 90% . . . of the circumference of the esophagus be involved with tumor" (Skinner & Skinner, 1993, p. 1391). Dysphagia accompanied by odynophagia and chest pain may indicate esophagitis from fungal, bacterial, or viral infection (Roubein & Levin, 1993). In patients with AIDS, dysphagia is most commonly due to esophageal candidiasis or cytomegalovirus infection (Polis & Kovacs, 1992).

INDEPENDENT INTERVENTIONS

When dysphagia is not due to infection, and is not total:

- Only soft foods should be eaten, and liquids taken in small amounts at frequent intervals through the day.

- When dysphagia is due to infection, avoid spicy, acidic, salty, sticky, and excessively hot or cold foods. Popsicles may, however, help with pain (Ungvarski, 1992).
- Alcohol and tobacco exacerbate dysphagia.
- The patient's head should be kept elevated during and for 30 minutes after meals.
- Having a suction machine available may help if choking is a problem.
- Walsh (1990a, p. 22) warns against the use of tetracyclines or aspirin in the presence of dysphagia.

INTERDEPENDENT INTERVENTIONS

When dysphagia is due to infection, interventions are directed to resolving the infection. As dysphagia worsens and/or the patient deteriorates, palliative radiation may give symptomatic relief. Palliative surgery—including esophagectomy and surgical bypass, and endoprosthetic intubation—do not prolong life, but often bring symptomatic relief (Frogge, 1990; Skinner & Skinner, 1993). The care of patients with endoprosthesis is focused on preventing complications. The most troublesome complication is reflux of gastric contents, leading to pneumonia. Frogge (1990, p. 817) gives these directions:

- The head of the bed is kept elevated at all times and meals must be taken in an upright position.
- Take small swallows.
- To clear the tube, drink at least one half glass of water or carbonated beverage at the end of each meal.
- "Aggressive pulmonary hygiene" is required.

Gastrostomy and jejunostomy allow nutritional support, but do not relieve symptoms. The clinician should begin, with the patient and family, to explore the positive meanings of giving and receiving food in relation to the liabil-ities of attempting to eat in some situations in advanced disease.

Nausea and Vomiting

Probably the most distressing GI problem is nausea, which is frequent and constitutes the "second most common problem" in cancer (Fainsinger, Miller, Bruera, Hanson, & MacEachern, 1991, p. 9) and a very common problem in AIDS (Dworkin, 1992). More than 60% of patients with terminal cancer experience nausea and vomiting sometime in the last six weeks of life (Wachtel, Allen-Masterson, Reuben, Goldberg, & Mor, 1988).

SYMPTOMS AND ETIOLOGIES/ ASSESSMENT

With or without retching or vomiting, nausea is distressing to patients. While usually a well-defined sensation, nausea may also be experienced as vague abdominal discomfort. The incidence of nausea in terminal illness is high enough that all patients should be periodically assessed for the problem. Patterns may exist, and their determination may provide insight about the etiology.

While specific causes of nausea and vomiting are often difficult to determine, conditions and considerations concerning the common and sometimes interrelated causes of nausea and vomiting in cancer (Baines, 1978; Glover & Glick, 1991; Grant, 1987; Hogan, 1990; Morrow, Lindke, & Black, 1991) include the following:

- Medications, including opioids, steroids, and digoxin, should be reviewed, including length of time taken.
- Cancer treatment, especially brain and total body radiation, as well as chemotherapy, should be reviewed.
- Hypercalcemia occurs in 10%–20% of all patients with cancer (Lowitz, 1990) and thus

is a significant cause of nausea and vomiting. While hypercalcemia is discussed in greater detail in chapter 20, several points should be made here. Hypercalcemia is most common in cancer of breast and lung with bony metastasis, but is not limited to these. The primary manifestations of the disorder are anorexia, nausea, constipation, polydipsia, and polyuria.

- Bowel obstruction is relatively common in patients with abdominal tumors, especially colorectal and ovarian. In early stages, nausea and vomiting are accompanied or preceded by colicky abdominal pain, increased bowel sounds, abdominal distension, and diarrhea. In later stages the pain and distension increase and the patient also experiences constipation. Bowel obstruction is more completely covered at the end of this chapter.
- Increased intracranial pressure is usually due to primary or secondary brain tumor(s) and/or to related cerebral edema. The primary manifestations of increased intracranial pressure are headache (especially in the morning), blurred vision, nausea and vomiting, lethargy, changes in mentation, and neurological signs (sensory, motor, autonomic). Increased intracranial pressure is discussed in greater detail in chapter 13.
- Uremia is often due to primary or secondary bladder, breast, or kidney tumor(s). Manifestations include decreased urine output, cardiac changes (< BP early, > BP later, congestive heart failure), nausea, vomiting, anorexia, stomatitis, GI bleeding, diarrhea, constipation, and lethargy and changes in mentation.
- Pancreatic disease may be due to primary or secondary pancreatic tumor. Manifestations include nausea and vomiting, anorexia and weight loss, and phlebitis.
- Gastric irritation from carcinoma of stomach may cause nausea and vomiting.
- Psychological distress may be a precipitating factor, triggered by a variety of inter-personal problems, treatment (past or present) stimuli, and other psychosocial issues.
- Other etiologies include: uncontrolled pain or other symptoms, acute GI infection unrelated to the disease, and unexplained nausea and anorexia (Bruera, Catz, Hooper, Lentle, & McDonald, 1987).

INDEPENDENT INTERVENTIONS

While etiologies may be difficult to determine, one characteristic of nausea and vomiting to keep in mind is that the problem, regardless of etiology, is often self-perpetuating and/or self-exacerbating. Independent interventions (Billings, 1985; Grant, 1987; Grant & Ropka, 1991; Ouwekerk & Keizer, 1990; Pervan, 1990) include:

- Determining and acting upon (i.e., by providing information and encouragement through teaching) any misconceptions on the part of the patient and the family—e.g., that nausea from opioids will be a long-lasting problem (Walsh, 1990b).
- Modifying diet (in the absence of a prescribed diet), according to the following guidelines:
  1. Increase soft drinks, soda crackers, salty foods, fresh fruits, non-acidic juices, chicken soup or broth, jello, bland and/or soft foods, non-gas- forming foods, cold foods, and foods that the patient thinks will be tolerated.
  2. Decrease fatty, fried, strong-smelling foods.
  3. Avoid smells, sights of cooking; bathrooms smells may also contribute to the problem, and should be minimized.
  4. Institute smaller, more frequent meals, taken when nausea and vomiting are least problematic; fasting may be necessary.
  5. Insure adequate hydration, except that liquids should be minimized before, during, and immediately after meals.

- Teaching and supporting the patient and their family in using imagery, progressive muscle relaxation, music therapy, or distraction techniques (see Psychological Interventions in chapter 11); providing psychological support to patient and family; resting and elevating the patient's head; and keeping the patient's room cool are all techniques that may help alleviate nausea.

INTERDEPENDENT INTERVENTIONS

Baines (1978), Billings (1985), Grant & Ropka (1991), and Pervan (1990) all suggest measures centering on resolving the underlying causes of nausea, and on the use of antiemetics to control symptoms. As with other aspects of symptom management, the key is to prevent the problem. The widely studied problem of anticipatory nausea and vomiting (ANV) has been shown to be non-responsive to medication—except that studies have not adequately addressed preventive medications (Redd, 1990). In patients who have a problem with nausea and vomiting, antiemetics are given on a regular schedule so that the patient does not experience the problem. In patients who have not had a problem with nausea and vomiting, antiemetics are given at the first sign of nausea. To be most effective, antiemetics are given:

- in therapeutic dosages, so that nausea is eliminated;
- at proper (preventive) intervals, so that the patient does not reexperience nausea, e.g., 30 minutes before taking opioids; and
- by an effective route, so that the patient does not loose medication through vomiting or through ineffective absorption.

Oral is the preferred route. If necessary, maintenance antiemetics may be given rectally. Initially, in cases of severe vomiting, medications may be given parenterally. If a particular medication is not effective, a medication with a different site of action is a logical next step. Antiemetics commonly used, singly or in combination, for patients with advanced disease (Grant & Ropka, 1991; Kris & Gralla, 1990; Pervan, 1990) include:

- metoclopramide 1–3 mg/kg IV;
- haloperidol 0.5–5.0 mg PO;
- dexamethasone 4–10 mg PO;
- droperidol 2.5–10 mg IM;
- prochlorperazine 10 mg PO; 25 mg PR (can also be given IM or IV); and
- diazepam 5 mg PO.

Side effects may be more pronounced in older patients. These medications (other than dexamethasone) may be given in conjunction with corticosteroids. Metoclopramide is known to be more effective when given together with dexamethasone. Combinations, including as many as five drugs given intravenously and orally, is even more effective (Atoner et al., 1993). Pervan (1990) also reports encouraging research on a 5-HT_3 antagonist, granisetron.

INTERVENTIONS FOR SPECIFIC PROBLEMS

For the specific problems noted above, interventions include the following:

- Nausea due to medications is most often opioid-induced nausea. Such nausea usually results "only with initial narcotic doses" (Lindley, Dalton, & Fields, 1990), with a change from short-acting to long-acting morphine (Ferrell, 1991), or may simply be a part of opioid therapy in some patients (Campora et al., 1991). Whatever the case, the previously noted independent actions and antiemetics are usually effective. It is best if antiemetics can eventually be decreased or discontinued (Levy, 1985), but this is not possible for some patients. Some clinicians attempt to relieve the problem by changing the route of administration, e.g., from oral to parenteral (Campora et al., 1991). McCaffery and Ferrell (1991) report that this measure is futile since narcotics ultimately have the same actions, differing only in degree, regardless of route.

- Nausea due to cancer treatment is treated with independent measures and with the antiemetic medications noted above.
- In hypercalcemia, the cause is treated as symptoms are managed. Please see chapter 20.
- Bowel obstruction is discussed in the last section of this chapter.
- Nausea and vomiting from increased intracranial pressure is an oncologic emergency and the underlying problem must be palliated quickly, lest the patient die within a "short period of time" (Wachtel et al., 1988). Corticosteroids are the mainstay. Diuretics are also sometimes used (Billings, 1985). The patient's head should be elevated. Please refer to chapter 13.
- Nausea and vomiting from uremia is treated by addressing kidney function when possible, and palliatively when kidney failure is advanced.
- Nausea and vomiting from pancreatic disease is most often palliated.
- Nausea and vomiting from gastric irritation is palliated. Antacids may occasionally be effective.
- Nausea and vomiting from psychological distress is addressed through uncovering and dealing with precipitating factors. If the problem occurs in conjunction with a treatment, the patient can be given increased medication prior to the treatment. "Anticipatory" vomiting is often difficult to manage (Ouwekerk & Keizer, 1990) and is thus best prevented through action well in advance of expected precipitating factors.
- Interventions for treating nausea and vomiting from other etiologies include the following:
  1. When related to pain or to other symptoms, the nausea and vomiting is treated palliatively as the other problems are resolved or palliated.
  2. When related to stimuli such as smells, sights, tastes, etc., the stimulus or the patient is removed; or if either of these alternatives is impossible, the patient's response is modified by increasing the dose of antiemetic.
  3. Any acute GI infection unrelated to the disease is treated and/or palliated.
  4. Unexplained nausea and anorexia (Bruera et al., 1987) should be treated palliatively.

Anorexia and Weight Loss

With a prevalence of 90%, anorexia is a significant contributing factor to the weight loss found in 84% of patients with terminal cancer (Wachtel et al., 1988). Anorexia and weight loss are "the most common symptoms in terminal cancer patients," and occur, to some extent, in all cancers (p. 73). Anorexia and weight loss are universal in patients with advanced AIDS. If weight loss is due to poor appetite alone, nutritional support or other measures may stabilize or even increase the patient's weight in earlier stages of disease. In later stages, anorexia can be considered an "adaptive process" within the process of dying (Miller & Albright, 1989, p. 36). If weight loss is due to the more complex cachexia, nutritional support will not reverse the process (Lindsey, 1986). While there is disagreement on exactly what constitutes cachexia, Lindsey (1986, p. 19) gives a functional definition that serves our purposes here: "systemic derangement of host metabolism which results in progressive wasting."

ETIOLOGIES/ASSESSMENT

With anorexia and weight loss common, and in most cases inevitable, among patients with terminal illness, identifying specific causes is an

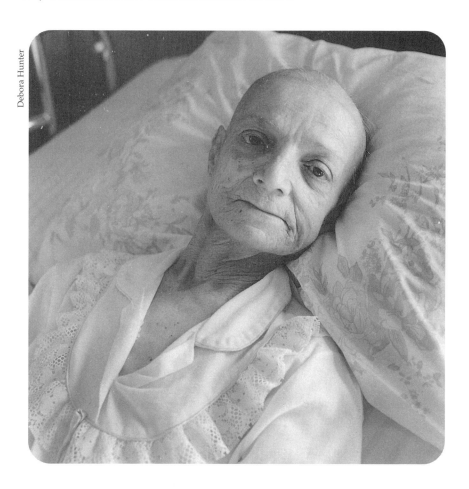

Debora Hunter

extremely challenging, and perhaps ultimately unproductive, task. A general assessment includes intake patterns, food likes and dislikes, and determining the meaning of food or eating to the patient and family. Common causes of anorexia include the following.

- A number of physical symptoms often contribute to, or cause anorexia, such as pain, nausea, vomiting, diarrhea, constipation, dysphagia, dyspnea, various infections, stomatitis, etc. Each of these, and other symptoms, are discussed elsewhere in this book. In general, most people who are seriously ill and/or suffering distressing symptoms have poor appetites.

- Fatigue: although discussed in greater depth elsewhere in this book, significant factors leading to fatigue (Cushman, 1986) include anemia, dsypnea, complications of treatment (accumulation of waste products), and cycles of poor nutritional status exacerbated by fatigue from poor nutritional status. Paraneoplastic syndromes may also cause fatigue (Holmes, Livingston, & Turrisi, 1993). Note that fatigue and weakness are not the same things (see chapter19).

- Psychological or spiritual distress is another cause, and may include anxiety and/or depression, or feelings of hopelessness or uselessness, all of which may result in little enthusiasm or energy for preparing or eating food.

- Causes stemming from other problems also exist. Taste disorders, for example, are discussed in chapter16. Early satiety, feelings of fullness shortly after beginning to eat, is another example. These feelings may be absent at breakfast, and become more pronounced at later meals. Poorly-fitting dentures and other causes of dental or oral pain may also play a role in anorexia.

INDEPENDENT INTERVENTIONS

Interventions for treating the problems noted above include the following (Billings, 1985; Grant & Ropka, 1991.):

- If anorexia is due to an identifiable problem—such as particular symptoms, early satiety, taste disorders, or poorly fitting dentures—then act on those problems. Early satiety, for example, can be partially managed by increasing nutritional value and size of morning meals. Taste disorders are discussed in chapter 16.
- Altering diet is usually helpful—at least to some extent. Small meals, on the patient's schedule, and according to the taste and whims of the patient, are the most helpful measure (Miller & Albright, 1989). Time taken to determine what appeals to the patient is time well spent. Giving and taking food often have profound (and sometimes unrecognized) meaning to patients and their families. Helping the family become proficient in preparing food appropriate to the terminal situation can have a tremendous positive effect on patient and family. Homemade milkshakes or Carnation Instant Breakfast are better tolerated by some patients than are dietary supplements, hence may have greater value (Miller & Albright, 1989). General guidelines for altering diet include the following:
  1. Determine the meaning to the patient and family of giving and taking food.

Indirect questions may be necessary, including asking both the patient and family how it feels when the patient doesn't want to eat, rejects food, or continues to lose weight. It is possible, with some families, to encourage and instruct them in trying to redirect their food-related personal values from symbolic nurturing to symbolic sharing. Partaking of half-a-bite of food by sharing it in "sacred meals" eaten with loved ones constitutes a kind of victory over the disease (R. Bowie, personal communication, April, 1992) eaten with loved ones constitutes a kind of victory. More often, however, strong and perhaps unconscious beliefs about food cannot be modified. Families may require frequent support in their helplessness and frustration related to diminished intake.

  2. Experiment by trying foods with different tastes, textures, temperatures, seasonings, degrees of spiciness, degrees of moisture, colors, etc.
  3. Experiment with different liquids. Nutritional supplements, such as Ensure, etc. are difficult for some patients to tolerate; water is difficult for some to drink. Cold, clear liquids are usually well tolerated, and even enjoyed. Try soft drinks, non-acidic fruit juices or seltzers, flavored jello (liquid or congealed), popsicles, tea (warm or iced), and any other drinks that sound good to the patient.
  4. Evaluate the nutritional quality of intake and, if possible and appropriate, modify to improve the quality. Patients who are not moribund may benefit from supplementary sources of protein and calories.
- Insure a minimum of procedures, treatments, psychological upsets (negative *or* positive), or other stressors or activities prior to meals. At the same time, if a dear friend arrives before a meal, it may be better to forgo the meal.

- Depression as the primary etiology of anorexia requires comprehensive interventions, discussed in the section on depression in chapter 1. For patients living at home, making food as easy as possible to prepare or eat may increase consumption. Frozen foods, meals on wheels, and similar measures may thus help.

INTERDEPENDENT INTERVENTIONS

Options to address the problem of anorexia are limited (Baines, 1978: Billings, 1985) and include the following:

- Steroids have a striking effect on anorexia, giving weeks or even months of improved quality of life. Over-use, however, creates significant problems.
- Antidepressant are used when depression is an etiology in the anorexia.
- If the problem is due to medication, that particular medication may be decreased, or another substituted.
- Oral nutritional supplements may be of little or no value in extending life; and total parenteral nutrition (TPN) actually shortens the survival of some patients with advanced cancer (Miller & Albright, 1989).

Constipation

SYMPTOMS AND ETIOLOGIES/ ASSESSMENT

About 50% of patients with terminal cancer are constipated (Wachtel, et al., 1988). In addition to the decreased frequency of bowel movements, problems of constipation include the accompanying discomfort, fecal impaction with diarrhea and incontinence, anorexia, nausea and vomiting, urinary retention and incontinence, and confusion. Severe constipation influences the absorption of oral medications, thus sometimes markedly increasing pain.

Undiagnosed fecal impaction is a key factor in significant numbers of patients whose pain becomes unmanageable (Glare & Lickiss, 1992).

The patient's bowel history is significant. Constipation may be a lifelong pattern, or may have a more recent etiology. Note however that in patients with far-advanced cancer, constipation may be an unalterable consequence of diminished intake, and thus not necessarily a problem. In the earlier stages of disease, a "reasonable goal" is a bowel movement every two-three days (Levy, 1985). Specific etiologies include:

- Medications are a common cause of constipation. Opioids inevitably cause constipation (Levy, 1985). Other medications that contribute to constipation—often in concert with immobility, depression, and inadequate fluids and fiber (Cushman, 1986; Twycross, 1990)—include NSAIDs, drugs with anticholinergic properties, and diuretics.
- Cancer treatment, especially Vinca alkaloids, may cause constipation.
- Diet, especially one low in fiber and fluid intake, contributes to constipation.
- Decreased activity level contributes to constipation.
- Depression has psychological and physical effects on elimination.
- Changes in bowel habits may be indirectly related to illness, e.g., decreased privacy.

INDEPENDENT INTERVENTIONS

Independent interventions for treating constipation include the following (Levy, 1985; Grant & Ropka, 1991):

- When possible, modify intake to increase fiber and fluids, and avoid constipating foods, e.g., dairy products and fried foods. Please note, however, that "dietary modifications and bulk laxatives alone are seldom tolerable or adequate" (Levy, 1985, p. 403) for patients with advanced cancer who are taking opioids. As death nears, all intake inevitably decreases.

- When possible, increase activity (note that good pain control is necessary to do so).
- Assist patients and family to resolve the anger or hopelessness that may lie behind depression. Please see section on depression in chapter 1.
- Offer privacy and bathroom assistive devices.

INTERDEPENDENT INTERVENTIONS

Interdependent interventions for treating constipation are noted below (Baines, 1978; Billings, 1985; Grant & Ropka, 1991; Levy, 1985). It should be noted that treatment for constipation in tied to: (1) resolution of the problem; and (2) changes in risk factors; specifically, use of opioids (if opioids are increased, then the prevention/treatment of constipation should escalate).

- When the patient is at risk for constipation (i.e., taking opioids, with a decreased activity level, or with a decreased fluid intake), give a prophylactic stool softener, e.g., diocytyl sodium sulfosuccinate *and* a laxative, e.g., Doxidan or Senokot S.
- When the patient is constipated (no bowel movement in 48 hours of treatment, as above), give (continued) stool softener *and* a laxative, such as Senokot, Dulcolax, or Milk of Magnesia.
- If constipation continues, check for impaction. If there is no impaction, give (continued) stool softener *and* a laxative such as Dulcolax suppository, magnesium citrate *or* Fleets enema.

Diarrhea

Diarrhea occurs most often in patients with stomach/esophageal cancers (50%), followed by those with pancreatic or cervical/uterine cancers. Patients with primary brain tumors are least likely to experience diarrhea (Wachtel et al., 1988). Patients with AIDS have a very high incidence of diarrhea refractory to treatment (Pomerantz & Harrison, 1990).

SYMPTOMS AND ETIOLOGIES/ ASSESSMENT

Diarrhea may be profuse, or there may be a pattern of expelling small amounts of watery stool. Incontinence is a confounding factor.

A number of potential etiologies are listed below. General assessment of diarrhea includes usual patterns of elimination and, with respect to the diarrhea, determination of the onset, amount, appearance, associated symptoms, dietary patterns, *and* perirectal or stomal skin condition. Specific etiologies (Billings, 1985; Cushman, 1986; Grant & Ropka, 1991) include the following situations.

- Cancer treatment, including radiation or chemotherapy, may result in increased peristalsis, inflammation, and overproduction of mucous. Surgery may sometimes contribute to diarrhea.
- Pancreatic insufficiency is characterized by steatorrhea, i.e., pale, bulky, greasy stools, and gas (Baines, 1978).
- GI infection can cause acute diarrhea, especially in immuno-suppressed patients, but in others as well. Sudden-onset diarrhea may be due to infection from food poisoning, often resulting, when patients live at home, from food kept over-long or poorly stored. Infection may also be due to poor hygiene on the part of the patient and/or the caregiver. This is especially a problem with confused patients who tend to scratch or otherwise put their fingers in their anus.
- Fecal impaction may cause small amounts of watery stool to be expelled around the impaction.
- Diarrhea may be a sign of partial intestinal

obstruction. Please see the section on obstruction at the end of this chapter.

- Chronic diarrhea may also be due to diverticulitis, ulcerative colitis, colon tumor, hyperthyroidism, or diabetes (Hamdy, 1989).
- Drug toxicity from laxatives, antacids, or antibiotics sometimes causes diarrhea.
- Stress can be a precipitating or contributing factor.
- Supplemental feedings of high osmolality can result in diarrhea.
- Common etiologies in patients with AIDS include *Microsporidia*, *Cryptosporidium*, and salmonella infections (Ungvarski, 1992).

INDEPENDENT INTERVENTIONS

Independent interventions for treating diarrhea include the following (see Grant & Ropka, 1991; Ungvarski, 1992):

- Diet can be modified, e.g., increasing low-residue foods that are high in protein and calories, giving small and frequent meals, eliminating high-lactose foods, avoiding spicy, greasy, or (GI) irritating foods, such as caffeine, and avoiding extremely cold or hot foods.
- Fluid should be increased to prevent fluid and electrolyte loss, especially in very old or young patients. Patients should take two-to-three quarts of noncarbonated fluids per day.
- Comfort measures include protective ointments or anesthetics applied to perirectal area, e.g., A&D Ointment, hydrocortisone, or Tucks. Since skin problems almost invariably accompany chronic diarrhea, these comfort measures should begin *before* problems develop. After several days of diarrhea, even the softest toilet paper is painful. Squeeze bottles, one with warm soapy water to cleanse and the other with clear water to rinse are far superior to toilet paper. When the diarrhea pattern is one of small amounts of stool, adult diapers can be worn at home and "panty liners" used if

the patient is able to go out.
- Food storage, caregiver, or patient hygiene, or other habits related to infection may need to be modified.

INTERDEPENDENT INTERVENTIONS

Interdependent interventions for treating diarrhea include the following (see Billings, 1985; Grant & Ropka, 1991; Cushman, 1986):

- The primary antidiarrheal medications include: (1) opioids, if the patient is not already taking them—e.g., codeine, tincture of opium; and (2) Lomotil or Lomodium. Octreotide has been used with some success in patients with AIDS (Manfredi et al., 1993).
- If diarrhea is due to pancreatic insufficiency, pancreatic replacements are given, along with antidiarrheal medications. Diet modification includes high protein, high carbohydrates, and vitamin replacement (Billings, 1985).
- GI infections are diagnosed and treated medically. The opportunistic infections of AIDS, e.g., cryptosporidiosis, are extremely difficult to manage. Behavioral etiologies are addressed if necessary.
- Fecal impactions are removed and preventive measures instituted. Note that digital removal of an impaction is contraindicated in persons with neutropenia or thrombocytopenia (Donoghue, 1988).
- Interventions for obstructions are addressed below.
- Diverticulitis, colitis, hyperthyroidism, and tumors are treated medically and supportively. Not all treatment options may be open, e.g., withholding fluids.
- Drug toxicity (especially laxatives, antacids, or antibiotics) is treated by changing the medication, if possible.
- The temporary use of antianxiety medications for patients with diarrhea may also be indicated (Hamdy, 1989).

Fecal Incontinence

SYMPTOMS AND ETIOLOGIES/ ASSESSMENT

Fecal incontinence is most often due to diarrhea, whether from impaction, infection, or other causes. Temporary fecal incontinence is common. Many patients will deny and hide incontinence. Combined incontinence of urine and feces is more resistant to treatment, especially when it occurs with slow onset (Hamdy, 1989).

For etiologies and assessment, see also preceding section on diarrhea. Note also the following points:

- Anxiety may play a role in some cases.
- Fecal incontinence is commonly associated with dementia, especially when incontinence is manifested with formed stools several times per day (Hamdy, 1989).
- Incontinence is occasionally related to the nature of the toilet the patient is using (for example, is the patient able to get to a sitting position?) or its location, or the patient's inability to remove clothing.

INTERVENTIONS

- Diarrhea and/or anxiety are treated according to the methods described above. Other interventions are represented by the circumstances described below.
- Dementia presents a major management problem. When death is not imminent, developing a bowel routine should be considered. If possible, placing the patient on the toilet shortly after breakfast and coffee is probably the easiest routine. Glycerine suppositories after breakfast also help, but may not always work for patients with dementia. Constipation can be induced with (for example) codeine given every 4 hours with laxative suppos-

itories, or Fleets enemas every two or three days to force evacuation (Hamdy, 1989). Codeine or other opioids may also help with agitation.
- Rearranging furniture may help, including placing a portable toilet next to the bed if the patient cannot get to the toilet, or installing rails in the bathroom toilet. Modifying clothing may also help.

Bowel Obstruction

Bowel obstruction presents difficult decisions. Practitioners skilled in palliative care may be comfortable with treating the problem palliatively, while those used to acute care tend to treat obstruction aggressively, except when the patient is obtunded.

SYMPTOMS AND ETIOLOGIES/ ASSESSMENT

In the early stages of obstruction, there is usually colicky abdominal pain, increased bowel sounds, abdominal distension, and diarrhea. Few patients complain of constipation. In later stages, the pain and distension increase and the patient experiences nausea and vomiting and constipation. The most prevalent symptoms (> 75%) are nausea and vomiting, intestinal colic, and other abdominal pain (Baines, 1990).

Bowel obstruction is relatively common in patients with abdominal tumors, especially colorectal and ovarian (Baines, 1990).

INTERDEPENDENT INTERVENTIONS

In the early or partial stages, patients with bowel obstruction can be treated with liquid or soft diet, stool softeners, and antiemetics, especially metoclopramide (Zerwekh, 1991). The conventional or "conservative" treatment of intravenous fluids, antiemetics, and nasogastric suction may resolve obstruction, or obstruction may spontaneously resolve in some cases (Baines, 1990). Prolonged conservative treatment unfortunately is uncomfortable and a "barrier" between the patient and family (Baines, 1990). Surgery to resolve intestinal obstruction in patients with advanced intra-abdominal cancer results in a high level of complications, mortality, and reobstruction (Chan & Woodruff, 1992). The problem of complete bowel obstruction illustrates the challenging decisions necessary in oncology. If death is imminent, then symptoms of obstruction should be treated and the obstruction left unresolved. The difficulties in the decision lie in predicting when someone will die. Although "three simple determinations (cognitive failure, dysphagia, and weight loss) . . . can predict survival of more or less than four weeks" (Bruera et al., 1992, p. 341) the uncertainty of predicting life expectancy and of making the best decision remains a major challenge. Surgical relief of the obstruction, i.e., gastrostomy or colostomy, is "only . . . justified in someone with a few months to live" (Baines 1978, p. 102). The abdominal pain and vomiting can be palliated, although the patient may vomit once or twice a day, for as long as three months (Storey, 1991). Liquid diets are helpful, although patients may choose an occasional favorite meal—inevitably vomited later. The St. Christopher's Hospice regimen for symptom-oriented management of obstruction (Baines, 1990) includes:

- For intestinal colic: discontinue stimulative laxatives, metoclopramide, domperidone, and any other agent likely to increase peristalsis. Analgesics, usually along with an antispasmodic, are given.
- For vomiting: use prochlorperazine suppositories 25 mg every eight hours; chlorpromazine suppositories 50–100 mg every eight hours; haloperidol 5–15 mg/24 hours IV; or methotrimeprazine 50–150 mg/24 hours, which are also effective. Baines (1990) notes that methotrimeprazine is the "most effective antiemetic in obstructive vomiting" (p. 333). Hyoscine hydrobromide (e.g., Donnatal) and somatostatin are also effective (Mercadante & Maddaloni, 1992).
- For abdominal pain: medications are given orally if there is minimal vomiting; or continuously subcutaneously if vomiting is a problem.
- For diarrhea: treat as discussed above.

References

Atoner, A., Onat, H., Ozturk, N., Aykan, F., Inanc, S., Topuz, E., & Dincol, K. (1993). The efficacy of a five-drug antiemetic combination during chemotherapy regimens containing cisplatin or cyclophosphamide-doxorubin. *Journal of Pain and Symptom Management*, 8(3), 126–131.

Baines, M.J. (1990). Management of malignant intestinal obstruction in patients with advanced cancer. In K.M. Foley, J.J. Bonica, & V. Ventafridda (Eds.), *Advances in pain research and therapy, Volume 16: Proceedings of the Second International Congress on Cancer Pain.* (pp. 327–335). New York: Raven Press.

Baines, M.J. (1978). Control of other symptoms. In C.M. Saunders (Ed.), *The management of terminal disease* (pp. 99–118). London: Edward Arnold.

Billings, J.A. (1985). The management of common symptoms. In J.A. Billings (Ed.). *Outpatient management of advanced cancer* (pp. 40–139). Philadelphia: J.B. Lippincott.

Bruera, E., Catz, Z., Hooper, R., Lentle, B., & McDonald, N. (1987). Chronic nausea and anorexia in advanced cancer patients: A possible role for autonomic dysfunction. *Journal of Pain and Symptom Management*, 2(1), 19–21.

Bruera, E., Miller, M.J., Kuehn, N., MacEachern, T., & Hanson, J. (1992). Estimate of survival of patients admitted to a palliative care unit: A prospective study. *Journal of Pain and Symptom Management*, 7(2), 82–86.

Campora, E., Merlini, L., Pace, M., Bruzzone, M., Luzzani, M., Gottlieb, A., & Rosso, R. (1991). The incidence of narcotic-induced emesis. *Journal of Pain and Symptom Management*, 6(7), 428–430.

Chan, A., & Woodruff, R.K. (1992). Intestinal obstruction in patients with widespread intraabdominal malignancy. *Journal of Pain and Symptom Management*, 7(6), 339–342.

Coyle, N., Adelhardt, J., Foley, K.M., & Portenoy, R.K. (1990). Character of terminal illness in the advanced cancer patient: Pain and other symptoms during the last four weeks of life. *Journal of Pain and Symptom Management*, 5(2), 88.

Cushman, K.E. (1986). Symptom management: A comprehensive approach to increasing nutritional status in the cancer patient. *Seminars in Oncology Nursing, 2*(1), 30–35.

Donoghue, M.M. (1988). Impaction. In S.B. Baird (Ed.), *Decision making in oncology nursing* (pp. 140–141), Philadelphia: B.C. Decker.

Dworkin, B.M. (1992). Gastrointestinal manifestations of AIDS. In G.P. Wormser (Ed.), *AIDS and other manifestations of HIV infection* (2nd ed.) (pp. 419–432). New York: Raven Press.

Fainsinger, R., Miller, M.J., Bruera, E., Hanson, J., & Maceachern, T. (1991). Symptom control during the last week of life on a palliative care unit. *Journal of Palliative Care, 7*(1), 5–11.

Ferrell, B.R. (1991). Managing pain with long-acting morphine. *Nursing 91, 21*(10), 34–39.

Frogge, M.H. (1990). Gastrointestinal cancer: Esophagus, stomach, liver, and pancreas. In S.L. Groenwald, M.H. Frogge, M. Goodman, & C.H. Yarbro (Eds.), *Cancer nursing: Principles and practice* (3rd ed.) (pp. 806–844). Boston: Jones and Bartlett Publishers.

Glare, P., & Lickiss, J.N. (1992). Unrecognized constipation in patients with advanced cancer: A recipe for disaster. *Journal of Pain and Symptom Management, 7*(6), 369–371.

Glover, D., & Glick, J.H. (1991). Oncologic emergencies. In A.I. Holleb, D.J. Fink, and G.P. Murphy (Eds.), *Clinical oncology* (pp. 513–533). Atlanta: American Cancer Society.

Grant, M. (1987). Nausea, vomiting, and anorexia. *Seminars in Oncology Nursing, 3*(4), 277–286.

Grant, M., & Ropka, M.E. (1991). Alterations in nutrition. In S.B. Baird, R. McCorkle, & M. Grant (Eds.), *Cancer nursing: A comprehensive textbook* (pp. 717–741). Philadelphia: W.B Saunders.

Hamdy, R. (1989). Fecal incontinence. In T.D. Walsh (Ed.), *Symptom control* (pp. 259–263). Oxford: Blackwell Scientific Publications.

Hogan, C.M. (1990). Advances in the management of nausea and vomiting. *Nursing Clinics of North America, 25*(2), 475–497.

Holmes, E.C., Livingston, R., & Turrisi, A. (1993). Neoplasms of the thorax. In J.F. Holland, E. Frei, R.C. Bast, D.W. Kufe, D.L. Morton, & R.W. Weischselbaum (Eds.), *Cancer medicine* (3rd ed.) (pp. 1285–1337). Philadelphia: Lea & Febiger.

Kenny, S.A. (1990). Effect of two oral care protocols on the incidence of stomatitis in hematology patients. *Cancer Nursing, 13*(6), pp 345–353.

Kris, M.G., & Gralla, R.J. (1990). Management of vomiting caused by anticancer drugs. In K.M. Foley, J.J. Bonica, & V. Ventafridda (Eds.), *Advances in pain research and therapy, Volume 16: Proceedings of the Second International Congress on Cancer Pain.* (pp. 337–343). New York: Raven Press.

Levy, M.H. (1985). Pain management in advanced cancer. *Seminars in Oncology, 12*(4), 394–410.

Lindley, C.M., Dalton, J.A., & Fields, S.M. (1990). Narcotic analgesics: Clinical pharmacology and therapeutics. *Cancer Nursing, 13*(1), 28–38.

Lindsey, A.M. (1986). Cancer cachexia. *Seminars in Oncology Nursing, 2*(1). pp 19–29.

Lowitz, B.B. (1990). Paraneoplastic syndromes. In C.M. Haskell (Ed.), *Cancer treatment* (3rd ed.) (pp. 841–849). Philadelphia: W.B. Saunders.

Manfredi, R., Vezzadini, P., Costigliola, P., Ricchi, E., Pia Fanti, M., & Chiodo, F. (1993). Elevated plasma levels of vasoactive intestinal peptide in AIDS patients with refractory idiopathic diarrhoea. Effects of treatment with octreotide. *AIDS, 7*(20), 223–226.

McCaffery, M., & Ferrell, B.R. (1991, November). *High-tech pain control.* Paper presented at the meeting of the National Hospice Organization. Seattle, Washington.

Mercadante, S., & Maddaloni, S. (1992). Octreotide in the management of inoperable gastrointestinal obstruction in terminal cancer patients. *Journal of Pain and Symptom Management, 7*(8), 496–498.

Miller, R.J., & Albright, P.G. (1989). What is the role of nutritional support and hydration in terminal cancer patients. *American Journal of Hospice Care, 6*(6), 33–38.

Morrow, G.R., Lindke, J.L., & Black, P.M. (1991). Predicting development of anticipatory nausea in cancer patients: Prospective examination of eight clinical characteristics. *Journal of Pain and Symptom Management, 6*(4), 215–223.

Ouwekerk, J., & Keizer, H.J. (1990). Psychologic aspects of the treatment of emesis in cancer nursing. *Seminars in Oncology Nursing, 6*(4), Supplement 1 (November), 6–9.

Pervan, V. (1990). Practical aspects of dealing with cancer therapy-induced nausea and vomiting. *Seminars in Oncology Nursing, 6*(4), Supplement 1 (November), 3–5.

Polis, M.A., & Kovacs, J.A. (1992). Fungal infections in patients with acquired immunodeficiency. In V.T. DeVita, S. Hellman, & S.A. Rosenberg (Eds.), *AIDS: Etiology, diagnosis, treatment, and prevention* (3rd ed.) (pp. 167–180). Philadelphia: J.B. Lippincott Company.

Pomerantz, S., & Harrison, E. (1990). End-stage symptom management. *AIDS Patient Care, 4*(1), 18–20.

Redd, W.H. (1990). Management of anticipatory nausea and vomiting with cancer chemotherapy. In K.M. Foley, J.J. Bonica, & V. Ventafridda (Eds.), *Advances in pain research and therapy, Volume 16: Proceedings of the Second International Congress on Cancer Pain.* (pp. 345–357). New York: Raven Press.

Roubein, L.D., & Levin, B. (1993). Gastrointestinal complications. In J.F. Holland, E. Frei, R.C. Bast, D.W. Kufe, D.L. Morton, & R.W. Weischselbaum (Eds.), *Cancer medicine* (3rd ed.) (pp. 2370–2380). Philadelphia: Lea & Febiger.

Skinner, D.B., & Skinner, K.A. (1993). Neoplasms of the esophagus. In J.F. Holland, E. Frei, R.C. Bast, D.W. Kufe, D.L. Morton, & R.W. Weischselbaum (Eds.), *Cancer medicine* (3rd ed.) (pp. 1382–1394). Philadelphia: Lea & Febiger.

Storey, P.S. (1991). Obstruction of the GI tract. *American Journal of Hospice and Palliative Care, 8*(3), 5.

Twycross, R.G. (1990). Management of constipation in the cancer patient with pain. In K.M. Foley, J.J. Bonica, & V. Ventafridda (Eds.), *Advances in pain research and therapy, Volume 16: Proceedings of the Second International Congress on Cancer Pain.* (pp. 317–326). New York: Raven Press.

Ungvarski, P.J. (1992). Nursing management of the adult client. In J.H. Flaskerud & P.J. Ungvarski (Eds.), *HIV/AIDS: A guide to nursing care* (2nd ed.) (pp. 146–198). Philadelphia: W.B. Saunders Company.

Wachtel, T., Allen-Masterson, S., Reuben, D., Goldberg, R., & Mor, V. (1988). The end stage cancer patient: Terminal common pathway. *The Hospice Journal, 4*(4), 43–80.

Walsh, T.D. (1990a). Symptom control in patients with advanced cancer. *American Journal of Hospice and Palliative Care, 7*(60), 20–29.

Walsh, T.D. (1990b). Prevention of opioid side effects. *Journal of Pain and Symptom Management, 5*(6), 362–367.

Zerwekh, J. (1991). Supportive care of the dying patient. In S.B. Baird, R. McCorkle, & M. Grant (Eds.), *Cancer nursing: A comprehensive textbook* (pp. 881–882). Philadelphia: W.B Saunders.

Genitourinary Problems and Interventions

The primary genitourinary (GU) problems are incontinence, obstruction, and sexual dysfunction. GU dysfunction also occurs as a sign of spinal cord compression (see chapter 13). Problems sometimes classified as genitourinary, such as candidiasis, fistulas, malignant ulcers, and pruritus, are outlined in chapter 15.

Urinary Incontinence

Urinary incontinence is a troublesome problem for patients and caregivers. It is embarrassing and shameful to many people, and is often taken, fearfully, as a sign of deterioration. For significant numbers of patients, incontinence is the deciding factor in submitting to extended care placement.

SYMPTOMS AND ETIOLOGIES/ ASSESSMENT

The symptoms of urinary incontinence vary according to etiology. Specific etiologies and

Charles Kemp: TERMINAL ILLNESS: A GUIDE TO NURSING CARE. © 1995 J. B. Lippincott.

related symptoms include the following situations:

- Incontinence only at night may be the result of over-sedation, or related to polyuria from heart failure (Hamdy, 1989).
- Incontinence primarily in the morning may be associated with diuretics given in the morning.
- Incontinence accompanied by dysuria may be related to infection.
- Incontinence that results from movement, lifting, coughing, laughing, etc. is considered stress incontinence.
- Incontinence in which there is no awareness of full bladder or urgency may result from retention or atonic bladder. Causes include diabetic neuropathy, spinal cord injury, and other neurological dysfunction. This form of incontinence is common with pelvic lesions (Enck, 1989).
- Incontinence as the result of urgency coupled with inability to reach the toilet in time is the most common form, and may be due to problems of access, complicated by a variety of physical problems. This form of incontinence may be benign with respect to mortality, or it may also be due to primary

brain tumors or metastasis (Enck, 1989). Some patients are simply unable to manage zippers, buttons, reaching a sitting position, or other mechanical impediments.

- The possibility of polyuria from hypercalcemia should be considered.
- Incontinence may result from mechanical problems such as bladder or other obstruction from tumor, fecal impaction, prostrate enlargement, fistula, etc.
- The effects of pelvic radiation and/or surgery may include incontinence.

INDEPENDENT INTERVENTIONS

Caregiver and patient attitudes are of primary importance in this condition. Some people are able to operate with the attitude that incontinence is just another problem to manage; more often, incontinence is viewed as a major problem and, in fact, may thus *become* a major problem. The practitioner who approaches the problem with a positive, matter-of-fact attitude can help promote more functional attitudes in caregivers and patients alike. Note, however, that behavioral programs, such as those used for bladder training, are seldom appropriate for patients who are terminally ill.

Independent interventions for treatment by caregivers (Clark, McGee, & Preston, 1992; Hamdy, 1989) include the following:

- Identify any specific etiologies noted above and act on those if possible.
- Modify some aspect of the situation, e.g.:
  1. Rearrange environment, including (perhaps) obtaining portable commode.
  2. Modify the patient's clothing.
  3. Teach patient to void as soon as the urge is felt.
  4. Limit fluids in the evening and decrease sedatives to limit night incontinence.
- Minimize the effects of incontinence with the following measures.

1. Use urinals and towels to catch and soak up the urine. Although such measures are thought by some to be unsuitable for long-term use (Enck, 1989), many caregivers use these measures for years with a family member who is chronically ill. Frequent changes are necessary, but in some cases this situation is not as difficult to manage as is an indwelling catheter; and it does not have as many inherent liabilities as a catheter.
2. Frequent skin care is also necessary. Vaseline is helpful in protecting the skin.
3. Using Attends or other products that allow patients to go out for limited periods of time.

INTERDEPENDENT INTERVENTIONS

Interdependent interventions for treatment by caregivers (Enck, 1989; Fainsinger, MacEachern, Hanson, & Bruera, 1992; Hamdy, 1989) include:

- Anticholinergic medications, which may help, but often also interact with other medications commonly taken by patients with terminal illness; they may also be difficult for debilitated persons to tolerate.
- A catheter, either condom or indwelling, is sometimes necessary for some patients, especially for those with discomfort from retention, and a slow physical deterioration (Fainsinger et al., 1992). Hamdy (1989, p. 254) makes three key points about the use of indwelling catheters.
  1. Because bladder capacity is often reduced, especially with pelvic disease, a 30 mL balloon should not be filled to capacity; 5–10 mL is adequate. The smaller balloon size causes less discomfort.
  2. Leakage of urine around the catheter

may be due to stimulation of the detrusor muscle, hence bladder relaxants, such as emepronium bromide or flavoxate hydrochloride, may be helpful.

3. Regular bladder flushing with normal saline or antiseptics, e.g., chlorhexidine 1:5000 or neomycin 0.2% solution, helps prevent infection. Fluid intake should be high.

The primary complication of urinary catheters is (sometimes asymptomatic) bacteriuria, which markedly increases in prevalence over time, until almost all patients catheterized for a month or more have bacteria in their urine. Encrustation and bladder spasms may also occur (Fainsinger et al., 1992).

Obstructive Uropathy

SYMPTOMS AND ETIOLOGIES

The possibility of gradual—usually bladder neck—obstruction is indicated by changes in urinary habits, especially retention (manifested by hesitancy, urgency, nocturia, frequency, and decreased force of stream), flank pain, hematuria, or intractable urinary tract infections (Garnick, 1993; Glover & Glick, 1991). Rapid obstruction of the ureter often results in severe pain (Garnick, 1993). Alternating polyuria and oliguria suggest the possibility of partial kidney obstruction (Glover & Glick, 1991). Infection, calculi, and decreased renal function may occur. Regional mass (or masses) will sometimes be found on examination.

Primary or metastatic retroperitoneal tumors or regional lymph involvement can result in obstruction (Garnick, 1993).

INTERVENTIONS

While a lower urinary tract obstruction can sometimes be relieved with an indwelling catheter, surgery is often necessary (Glover & Glick, 1991). The presence of tumor or other obstructive processes in or at the urethra or bladder results in difficulties and complications in catheter insertion, hence catheterization should be undertaken with care. Ureteral obstruction in non-moribund patients requires surgery.

Sexual Dysfunction

This section is concerned only with physical etiologies of sexual dysfunction. A more complete discussion of the subject can be found in chapter 1.

SYMPTOMS AND ETIOLOGIES/ ASSESSMENT

Sexual dysfunction in patients with advanced cancer often encompasses all phases of the sexual response cycle—desire, excitement, orgasm, and resolution (Anderson & Schmuch, 1991).

Pain (general, or sexual-functioning-related), stress, depression, and fatigue play significant roles in decreasing sexual activity, even when desire exists. In general, tumors and treatments most associated with sexual functioning, especially physically but also psychologically, are also most associated with sexual dysfunction (Anderson & Schmuch, 1991). Thus primary and metastatic GU and regional (colon, rectum, lumbosacral) tumors, as well as breast tumors, produce significant dysfunction. CNS tumors, especially those resulting in spinal cord compression, can cause sexual dysfunction. Many cancer treatments, including chemotherapy, hormone therapy, regional radiation, or surgery, can affect one or more sexual response(s). Other common factors influencing sexual response(s) in patients with advanced disease include opioids, alcohol, and a variety of other medications and substances, as well as preexisting conditions, such as diabetes, hypertension, and arthritis (Anderson & Schmuch, 1991; Clark, McGee, & Preston, 1992).

INTERVENTIONS

By the time the disease has progressed to terminal, not much can be done to improve physiologic sexual functioning. Pain, stress, depression, and other extrinsic factors may be relieved to some extent, but their "cure"—e.g., opioids, tranquilizers, antidepressants—may also diminish sexual function. The reader is referred to chapter 1 for a discussion of loss of sexual intimacy.

References

Anderson, B.L., & Schmuch, G. (1991). Sexuality and cancer. In A.I. Holleb, D.J. Fink, & G.P. Murphy (Eds.), *Clinical oncology* (pp. 606–616). Atlanta: American Cancer Society.

Clark, J.C., McGee, R.F. & Preston, R. (1992). Nursing management of response to the cancer experience. In J.C. Clark & R.F. McGee (Eds.), *Core curriculum for oncology nursing* (pp. 67–155), Philadelphia: W.B. Saunders.

Enck, R.E. (1989). The management of urinary incontinence. *American Journal of Hospice Care, 6*(6), 9–10.

Fainsinger, R., MacEachern, T., Hanson, J., & Bruera, E. (1992). The use of urinary catheters in terminally ill cancer patients. *Journal of Pain and Symptom Management, 7*(6), 333–338.

Garnick, M.B. (1993). Urologic complications. In J.F. Holland, E. Frei, R.C. Bast, D.W. Kufe, D.L. Morton, & R.W. Weischselbaum (Eds.), *Cancer medicine* (3rd ed.) (pp. 2323–2331). Philadelphia: Lea & Febiger.

Glover, D., & Glick, J.H. (1991). Oncologic emergencies. In A.I. Holleb, D.J. Fink, & G.P. Murphy (Eds.), *Clinical oncology* (pp. 513–533). Atlanta: American Cancer Society.

Hamdy, R. (1989). Urinary incontinence. In T.D. Walsh (Ed.), *Symptom control* (pp. 247–257). Oxford: Blackwell Scientific Publications.

19

Dehydration and Fatigue

Prior to the inception of hospice care for the terminally ill, and the development of expertise in palliative care for this patient category, it was generally assumed that decreased fluid intake indicated a need for fluid replacement via intravenous infusion or nasogastric tube (Collaud & Rapin, 1991). With greater attention paid to the patient's quality of life, however, realization grew that "alterations in nutrition, fluid balance, and elimination are predictable" (Zerwekh, 1991, p. 880) and are not necessarily calls to attempt to reverse the condition. In patients who are cachectic and dying, attempting to reverse or maintain hydration and nutrition is not only futile, but may also be harmful (Brescia, 1991). As in all other aspects of terminal care, the central issue of dehydration is the well-being of the patient: If death is imminent, nothing is gained by rehydration; if time and/or quality of life can be extended, rehydration is indicated.

Charles Kemp: TERMINAL ILLNESS: A GUIDE TO NURSING CARE. © 1995 J. B. Lippincott.

Problems of Dehydration

The two principal physical problems of dehydration in persons who are terminally ill are: (1) dry mouth (xerostomia); and (2) thirst (Collaud & Rapin, 1991). These problems may be complicated by dysphagia (Wachtel, Allen-Masterson, Reuben, Goldberg, & Mor, 1988). Contrary to the problems of dehydration found in others, persons who are terminally ill do not usually experience headaches, nausea, vomiting, or cramps (Musgrave, 1990)—perhaps because of medications they are already taking. Moreover, dehydration in patients with terminal illness may not necessarily result in electrolyte imbalances, such as hypercalcemia (Brown & Chekryn, 1989).

A third problem of dehydration is the emotional issues surrounding the fundamental need for living beings to take in fluids. Although there may be no gain for the patient in taking in fluids, still, for the family and other caregivers, there may be a very strong desire to *give* fluids. Even though patients close to death often lose the desire for fluids, the issue for family and others remains a potent one.

OTHER EFFECTS OF DEHYDRATION

Several authors (Zerwekh, 1991; Musgrave, 1990) note effects of dehydration that should be considered in decisions about means of hydration. Musgrave (1990, p. 63) specifically notes that some effects of dehydration are "beneficial." Among these are the following.

- Decrease in urine output: Incontinence and its attendant psychological, cosmetic, care, and physical issues become less problematic. Decreased urine may obviate the need for catheterization, or the effort associated with frequent cleaning, and changing sheets and bedpans.
- Decrease in gastric secretions: A decrease in vomiting may be noted, especially when there is an intestinal obstruction.
- Decrease in pulmonary secretions and edema: In this respect, hydration may actually decrease quantity as well as quality of life. The futile trauma of suctioning pharyngeal secretions may also be avoided.
- Decrease in other fluid accumulations, such as ascites and peripheral edema: Decreased edema at any site, or in general, promotes comfort. Decreased edema at tumors may decrease pain from nerve compression.

TREATMENT OF DEHYDRATION

Assuming that neither quantity nor quality of life can be increased through rehydration, the issue in treatment is comfort related primarily to xerostomia and thirst. For patients with sufficient strength, and who are able to swallow, oral fluids are helpful for both these problems, as well as for the emotional well-being of caregivers. Giving and receiving drink is more than a physiological issue (Collaud & Rapin, 1991). When a patient is unable to swallow, just a few drops of water or other fluid, lovingly and gently offered from a favorite cup or glass, can be significant and even, in some respects, healing for all concerned.

Xerostomia and thirst are further treated by regular oral care, e.g., every two hours, regardless of mental status. Depending on the patient's ability to swallow, oral care consists of:

- small, frequent sips of fluids, including ice chips, or chips of popsicle;
- very fine spray from an (e.g., perfume) atomizer—these are available at minimal cost from drug or variety stores;
- swabbing with glycerin, Cologel, normal saline (1:1:8) or methylcellulose, or lemon essence and water (De Conno, Ripamonti, Sbanotto, & Ventafridda, 1989); and
- gentle cleansing of the mouth with a soft, moist brush, and a trace of toothpaste.

Fatigue

Fatigue is common in virtually all patients with advanced disease (Irvine, Vincent, Bubela, Thompson, & Graydon, 1991). Although weakness may accompany fatigue, the two are *not* the same, nor are they always associated. Fatigue is "characterized by subjective feelings of discomfort and decreased functional status related to decreased energy" (Pickard-Holley, 1991, p. 14). Weakness is more accurately thought of as a symptom resulting from neurological dysfunction, and having no voluntary aspect. Common etiologies of fatigue include the disease itself, secondary infections, effects of treatment, insomnia, anemia, malnutrition, prolonged immobility, depression, and/or emotional exhaustion (Hubsky & Sears, 1992; Irvine et al., 1991; Ungvarski, 1992). Extreme fatigue often results in, or contributes to, sadness or depression; this, in turn, exacerbates the fatigue.

In persons without disease, fatigue is usually resolved with increased rest or sleep. For persons whose fatigue is a sequela of illness, the condition is not easily overcome by rest (Pickard-Holley, 1991). Nevertheless, while fatigue may be a given in advanced disease, there are interventions to help patients live as fully as possible within the constraints of fatigue.

The primary intervention is, if possible, to resolve the problem that causes the fatigue. Many of the etiologies above are subject to resolution or modification. In some other situations, e.g., "multiple sclerosis fatigue" or chronic HIV infection, fatigue is a given and there is little, if anything, that will change it. Change must then occur in the patient and environment.

Planned and paced activities help minimize the effects of fatigue (Ungvarski, 1992). There seems to be a universal tendency among patients of all sorts to over-extend themselves when they are feeling better than usual. This is followed inevitably by hours, or even days, of recovery time. In helping plan activities, the nurse should assist the patient to identify activities that are: (1) essential; *and* (2) pleasant or uplifting. These are then prioritized, with the top priorities including some essentials and some pleasant or uplifting activities. This means that some activities that are important may have to be assigned to someone else. While giving up activities is difficult for many people, efforts to assure them about who will accomplish the needed tasks, and when they will be accomplished, often eases the reluctance.

Many people find it difficult to reorder any aspect of their lives, especially in the context of illness. But reordering is necessary. For example, eating breakfast, resting, and then bathing—rather than the reverse order—may help some patients accomplish the top priority (nutritional intake) more often, despite their tendency to stick to old habits and to bathe first.

Most people have difficulty resting when they feel well, or at least well enough to continue an activity. Thus, every planned activity should be either of short duration or divided into several stages, each one accompanied by *planned* rest. Finally, other modifications may be possible in the manner in which activities are conducted. For ambulatory patients, activities that can be accomplished while sitting rather than while standing might include

showering, shaving, brushing teeth, putting on makeup, preparing food, etc. Furniture might need rearranging to increase sitting time. These measures may seem, on the face of it, simple and easy to accomplish. However, few people are able to initiate such changes themselves.

Modifying the environment helps in many cases. Placement of phone, medications, drinking water, toilet chair, and other essentials decreases energy expenditure. Attention should be paid to the presence, for instance, of low-slung chairs, beds, and other furniture that require excessive effort to get in and out of. As patients' energy is decreased, the environment available to them should also decrease in size. Since the situation in terminal illness means that everyone is eventually limited to using only several rooms, and finally to one room only, the room(s) chosen might as well be the best ones available. The quality of life for those who are dying seems to depend to a great extent on the ability to adapt well to the circumstances. A classic manifestation of adaptability in dying is having the patient's bed in the living room or den. Assistive devices can be installed to help the patient get in and out of the bath, go to the toilet, etc.

Fatigue and weakness, or further disability, can be mutually reinforcing: the greater the fatigue, the less exercise the patient can get, and the more weakness will result. Therefore, some kind of exercise is necessary for most patients, whether it be in order to accomplish a task or simply for its own sake (Ungvarski, 1992). This may entail as little (or as much) as getting out of bed daily or passive range of motion exercises. Patients who do not require any exercise include those with end-stage heart disease and those who are moribund.

Heat plays a role in increasing fatigue. Baths or showers should be warm, not hot. The patient's room temperature should be cool (Hubsky & Sears, 1992). Finally, the patient's (and often also the family's) psychological state may play a role in fatigue. Depression plays a role in many cases. Fatigue can even function as a sort of defense mechanism, which facilitates avoidance of unpleasant interactions. Addressing fatigue always includes a psychosocial component, sometimes with respect to the response to fatigue and sometimes with respect to fatigue as a behavior in response to other factors.

References

Brescia, F.J. (1991). Killing the known dying: Notes for a death watcher. *Journal of Pain and Symptom Management, 6*(5), 337–339.

Brown, P., & Chekryn, J. (1989). The dying patient and dehydration. *Canadian Nurse, 85*(5), 14–16.

Collaud, T., & Rapin, C-R. (1991). Dehydration in dying patients: Study with physicians in French-speaking Switzerland. *Journal of Pain and Symptom Management, 6*(4), 230–240.

De Conno, F., Ripamonti, C., Sbanotto, A., & Ventafridda, V. (1989). Oral complications in patients with advanced cancer. *Journal of Pain and Symptom Management, 4*(1), 20–29.

Hubsky, E.P., & Sears, J.H. (1992). Fatigue in multiple sclerosis: Guidelines for nursing care. *Rehabilitation Nursing, 17*(4), 176–180.

Irvine, D.M., Vincent, L., Bubela, N., Thompson, L., & Graydon, J., (1991). A critical appraisal of the research literature investigating fatigue in the individual with cancer. *Cancer Nursing, 14*(4), 188–199.

Musgrave, C.F. (1990). Terminal dehydration: To give or not to give intravenous fluids. *Cancer Nursing, 13*(1), 62–66.

Pickard-Holley, S. (1991). Fatigue in cancer patients. *Cancer Nursing, 14*(1), 13–19.

Ungvarski, P.J. (1992). Nursing management of the adult client. In J.H. Flaskerud & P.J. Ungvarski (Eds.), *HIV/AIDS: A guide to nursing care* (2nd ed.) (pp. 146–198). Philadelphia: W.B. Saunders Company.

Wachtel, T., Allen-Masterson, S., Reuben, D., Goldberg, R., & Mor, V. (1988). The end stage cancer patient: Terminal common pathway. *The Hospice Journal, 4*(4), pp 43–80.

Zerwekh, J. (1991). Supportive care of the dying patient. In S.B. Baird, R. McCorkle, & M. Grant (Eds.), *Cancer nursing: A comprehensive textbook* (pp. 881–882). Philadelphia: W.B Saunders.

Oncology Emergencies and Paraneoplastic Syndromes

Most of the oncology emergencies found in terminal illness are covered in other chapters of this book, as follows: increased intracranial pressure and spinal cord compression are discussed in chapter 13; superior vena cava syndrome and airway obstruction, and cardiac tamponade are discussed in chapter 14; and obstructive uropathy is discussed in chapter 18. Other disorders sometimes termed oncology emergencies may also be classified as paraneoplastic syndromes (Lowitz, 1990).

Paraneoplastic syndromes are problems that occur at a distance from the primary, or metastatic, tumors. Mechanisms of action may occur as ectopic hormone production, as auto-immune or immune responses, or as other, unknown responses (Holmes, Livingston, & Turrisi, 1993). Syndromes usually considered oncologic emergencies are discussed below, and include hypercalcemia and syndrome of inappropriate antidiuretic hormone. Other paraneoplastic syndromes are also discussed below.

Any of these oncology emergencies and/or paraneoplastic syndromes may occur as part of the final stage of disease. In some cases, there is ultimately no reasonable treatment. In other cases, however, treatment may result in palliation of symptoms.

Hypercalcemia

Hypercalcemia is the most common metabolic oncology emergency, and occurs in 10%–20% of patients with cancer (Lang-Kummer, 1990). The tumors most commonly associated with hypercalcemia are breast and lung (both > 25%), followed by renal, ovarian, multiple myeloma, pancreatic, esophageal, and head and neck cancers (Finley, 1992; Glover & Glick, 1991; Lowitz, 1990). Despite the association of hypercalcemia with bony metastases and hyperparathyroidism, two tumors that frequently involve bone—prostate cancer and small cell carcinoma of the lung—rarely result in hypercalcemia (Pritchard & Burch, 1993).

In addition to the above, two key factors that increase the risk of hypercalcemia are

Charles Kemp: TERMINAL ILLNESS: A GUIDE TO NURSING CARE. © 1995 J. B. Lippincott.

immobility and dehydration (Dietz & Flaherty, 1990). Anorexia, nausea, vomiting, and pain contribute directly or indirectly to these. The use of thiazide diuretics, vitamin A and D, and some hormones increases the risk of hypercalcemia (Lang-Kummer, 1990).

Clinical characteristics of hypercalcemia are similar in many respects to those of the underlying disease. Neuromuscular symptoms include malaise, apathy, muscle weakness, fatigue, and hyporeflexia. These may progress to mental changes, seizures, and coma. Gastrointestinal characteristics include nausea, vomiting, anorexia, constipation, and abdominal pain. Renal changes include polyuria and polydipsia and, ultimately, renal failure. A sudden increase in serum calcium levels may result in cardiac arrhythmias and death (Dietz & Flaherty, 1990; Glover & Glick, 1991; and Miaskowski, 1991).

Clearly, prevention is important in the consideration of hypercalcemia. The patient whose physical, psychological, and spiritual pain are well-managed is more likely to be mobile and take adequate fluids, and is thus less likely to develop hypercalcemia (or a host of other problems).

Mild hypercalcemia is treated with an increase in oral fluids, supplemented with sodium phosphate (Lowitz, 1990). Treatment of more severe hypercalcemia begins with intravenous rehydration. Calcium supplements and vitamin A and D should be discontinued. Dietary calcium intake, except perhaps with lymphomas, can be continued. Medications that decrease bone resorption of calcium include intravenous mithramycin and a newer class of medication, the bisphosphonates; the latter includes etidronate, given intravenously to lower serum calcium levels and orally to maintain the lower level. Calcitonin provides a prompt, but shortlived decrease in serum levels and symptoms. Corticosteroids are sometimes effective in patients with multiple myeloma, lymphoma, or breast cancer (Glover & Glick, 1991; Lowitz, 1990; Pritchard & Burch, 1993).

Syndrome of Inappropriate Anti-Diuretic Hormone (SIADH)

SIADH occurs in almost 10% of patients with small cell carcinoma of the lung (SCLC) and is the most common paraneoplastic syndrome associated with SCLC (Holmes et al., 1993). SIADH is found less frequently in patients with cancer of the pancreas, prostate, esophagus, duodenum, and brain; with Hodgkin's disease; and in patients with pulmonary or central nervous system metastases. Morphine use and withdrawal of steroids may also contribute to SIADH (Finley, 1991; Glover & Glick, 1991). The result of SIADH is hyponatremia.

Characteristics of mild hyponatremia include anorexia, nausea, myalgias, and slight neurological changes, such as irritability, lethargy, or headache. These can progress to hyporeflexia, increasing weakness, confusion, somnolence, and coma. Nausea and vomiting, anorexia, thirst, decreased urine output, and weight gain may also occur (Finley, 1991; Glover & Glick, 1991; Holmes et al., 1993).

Treatment for SIADH ideally is treatment of the underlying cause—the tumor. Failing that, fluids are restricted to 500–1,000 mL/24 hours and demeclocycline, 800 mg–1000 mg/24 hours, is given (Lowitz, 1990). Patients will benefit from a (decreased) fluid intake schedule and hourly mouth rinsing to compensate for decreased fluids (Finley, 1991).

Paraneoplastic Syndromes Not Usually Considered Emergencies

Ectopic Adrenocorticotropic Hormone Syndrome (Ectopic ACTH)

Ectopic ACTH is most commonly found in patients with SCLC, pancreatic cancer, bronchial carcinoid tumors, and neural tumors (Lowitz, 1990; Volker, 1991). Because of rapid onset of the disorder and characteristics of advanced disease, patients with ectopic ACTH related to advanced cancer lack the typical moon facies, obesity of the trunk and other stigmata of Cushing's syndrome. Characteristics include generalized weakness, weight loss, hypertension, and hypokalemia. Treatment may be limited to blood pressure control and potassium replacement (Holmes et al., 1993).

Hypoglycemia
In terminally ill patients, hypoglycemia is found most often in patients with mesenchymal tumors, and hepatic, adrenal, and gastrointestinal carcinomas (Odell, 1993). Symptoms include extreme fatigue, weakness, dizziness, tremors, and, if untreated, seizures (Glover & Glick, 1991; Szeluga, Groenwald, & Sullivan, 1990). Treatment is intravenous dextrose (Glover & Glick, 1991).

Hypocalcemia
Hypocalcemia is relatively uncommon, and occurs most often in: patients with advanced liver or breast cancer, especially with widespread bony metastases in the latter case; and in patients with visceral or mesenchymal tumors. Tetany is the primary characteristic of hypocalcemia. Related symptoms include paraesthesias and muscle cramps. Neurological symptoms include laryngospasm, lethargy, and changes in mentation. Seizures may also occur. Treatment is usually via intravenous calcium (Lowitz, 1990).

Carcinoid Syndrome
Carcinoid syndrome results most frequently from neoplasm of the gastrointestinal tract, usually accompanied by liver metastases, and also from bronchogenic carcinomas and intracranial neoplasm (Donehower, 1991; Volker, 1992). Carcinoid syndrome is characterized by flushing of the skin, especially facial; and diarrhea, bronchoconstriction, and cardiac anomalies. Wheezing and abdominal pain often accompany the flushing attacks. Flushing may be tran-

sient and mild, or in the case of tumors arising in the foregut (bronchus, stomach, first portion of the duodenum, and pancreas) severe and, ultimately, disfiguring (Vinik, Thompson, & Averbuch, 1993). Treatment is directed to the tumor. Failing that, flushing and other problems respond well to octreotide (Somatostatin) therapy (Vinik et al., 1993). Symptomatic treatment, including niacin supplements, phenothiazines, and corticosteroids, is sometimes effective (Haskell & Giuliano, 1990).

Central Nervous System (CNS) Paraneoplastic Syndromes
A number of CNS paraneoplastic syndromes exist. Many are associated with lung, breast, or ovarian cancer, as well as with other tumors. These syndromes include: peripheral, sensory, and autonomic neuropathies; motor system disorders; several degenerative syndromes of the CNS; CVA from several etiologies; necrotic myelopathy; and blindness. All are challenging to treat (Lowitz, 1990).

Other
Paraneoplastic Syndromes Associated with lung cancer and hepatic cell carcinoma are discussed in Part IV of this book. Syndromes associated with lung cancer include:

- Eaton-Lambert syndrome (pseudomyasthenia);
- hypertrophic osteoarthropathy;
- digital clubbing;
- polyarthritis;
- hematologic disorders (thrombocytosis, hypercoagulation, thrombocytopenia, and anemia);
- neurological disorders (these are rare, but may occur); and
- nephrotic syndrome.

Paraneoplastic syndromes in hepatic cell carcinoma may include:
- hypercalcemia;
- hypoglycemia;

- Cushing's syndrome;
- osteoporosis;
- excessive gonadotropin production;
- feminization;
- hyperlipidemia; and
- a variety of bleeding disorders, including disseminated intravascular coagulation.

References

Dietz, K.A., & Flaherty, A.M. (1990). Oncologic emergencies. In S.L. Groenwald, M.H. Frogge, M. Goodman, & C.H. Yarbro (Eds.), *Cancer nursing: Principles and practice* (pp. 644–668). Boston: Jones and Bartlett.

Donehower, M.G. (1991). Endocrine cancers. In S.B. Baird, R. McCorkle, & M. Grant (Eds.), *Cancer nursing: A comprehensive textbook* (pp. 584–596). Philadelphia: W.B Saunders.

Finley, J.P. (1992). Nursing care of patients with metabolic and physiological oncological emergencies. In J.C. Clark & R.F. McGee (Eds.), *Core curriculum for oncology nursing* (2nd ed.) (pp. 169–192). Philadelphia: W.B. Saunders Company.

Glover, D., & Glick, J.H. (1991). Oncologic emergencies. In A.I. Holleb, D.J. Fink, & G.P. Murphy (Eds.), *Clinical oncology* (pp. 513–533). Atlanta: American Cancer Society.

Haskell, C.M., & Giuliano, A.E. (1990). Carcinoid tumors. In C.M. Haskell (Ed.), *Cancer treatment* (3rd ed.) (pp. 418–426). Philadelphia: W.B. Saunders.

Holmes, E.C., Livingston, R., & Turrisi, A. (1993). Neoplasms of the thorax. In J.F. Holland, E. Frei, R.C. Bast, D.W. Kufe, D.L. Morton, & R.W. Weischselbaum (Eds.), *Cancer medicine* (3rd ed.) (pp. 1285–1337). Philadelphia: Lea & Feiberger.

Lang-Kummer, J.M. (1990). Hypercalcemia. In S.L. Groenwald, M.H. Frogge, M. Goodman, & C.H. Yarbro (Eds.), *Cancer nursing: Principles and practice* (pp. 520–534). Boston: Jones and Bartlett.

Lowitz, B.B. (1990). Paraneoplastic syndromes. In C.M. Haskell (Ed.), *Cancer treatment* (3rd ed.) (pp. 841–849). Philadelphia: W.B. Saunders.

Miaskowski, C. (1991). Oncologic emergencies. In S.B. Baird, R. McCorkle, & M. Grant (Eds.), *Cancer nursing.* (pp. 885–893). Philadelphia: W.B Saunders.

Odell, W.D. (1993). Ectopic hormones and humoral syndromes of cancer. In J.F. Holland, E. Frei, R.C. Bast, D.W. Kufe, D.L. Morton, & R.W. Weischselbaum (Eds.), *Cancer medicine* (3rd ed.) (pp. 896–904). Philadelphia: Lea & Feiberger.

Pritchard, D.J., & Burch, P.A. (1993). Orthopedic complications. In J.F. Holland, E. Frei, R.C. Bast, D.W. Kufe, D.L. Morton, & R.W. Weischselbaum (Eds.), *Cancer medicine* (3rd ed.) (pp. 2290–2293). Philadelphia: Lea & Feiberger.

Szeluga, D.J., Groenwald, S.L., & Sullivan, D.K. (1990). Nutritional disturbances. In S.L. Groenwald, M.H. Frogge, M. Goodman, & C.H. Yarbro (Eds.), *Cancer nursing: Principles and practice* (pp. 495–519). Boston: Jones and Bartlett.

Vinik, A.I., Thompson, N.W., & Averbuch, S.D. (1993). Neoplasms of the gastroenteropancreatic endocrine system. In J.F. Holland, E. Frei, R.C. Bast, D.W. Kufe, D.L. Morton, & R.W. Weischselbaum (Eds.), *Cancer medicine* (3rd ed.) (pp. 1180–1209). Philadelphia: Lea & Feiberger.

Volker, D.L. (1992). Pathophysiology of cancer. In J.C. Clark & R.F. McGee (Eds.), *Core curriculum for oncology nursing* (2nd ed.) (pp. 265–285). Philadelphia: W.B. Saunders Company.

Imminent Death and Interventions

Causes of Death

The most frequent causes of death in patients with cancer (Inagaki, Rodriguez, & Bodey, 1974) are:

- Infection (47%) comes primarily from pneumonia and septicemia. Patients with tumors of the lung, head, and neck, and with melanoma, are most likely to die from pneumonia; and patients with gastrointestinal and genitourinary tumors are more likely to develop septicemia, but may also die from pneumonia. Obstructive tumors and neutropenia are often associated with death from infection.
- Organ failure (25%) is most frequently (in decreasing order) respiratory, cardiac, hepatic, central nervous system (CNS), and renal. Respiratory and CNS failure are caused by tumor; hepatic and renal failure are usually caused by tumor; and cardiac failure is caused in approximately equal numbers by heart disease or tumor.

Charles Kemp: TERMINAL ILLNESS: A GUIDE TO NURSING CARE. © 1995 J. B. Lippincott.

- Infarction (11%) is most often of the lungs or heart. Lung infarction is a result of either tumor in the lung or distal thrombosis, causing embolization. Arteriosclerosis is the primary cause of myocardial infarction.
- Carcinomatosis or carcinosis (10%) is widespread metastatic disease and occurs most often in patients with melanoma or breast cancer. Cachexia and/or electrolyte imbalances are commonly associated with carcinomatosis.
- Hemorrhage (7%) occurs most frequently in the gastrointestinal tract and brain, and is usually caused by GI tumor or melanoma.

Ultimately, death from any of these, or other, causes is a result of a lack of oxygen to the brain (Nuland, 1994).

The abnormalities that, together, are most predictive of impending death (survival of less than four weeks) in patients with cancer are cognitive failure, dysphagia, and significant weight loss (Bruera, Miller, Kuehn, MacEachern, & Hanson, 1992). Advanced cancer and a major infection (pneumonia or septicemia) are predictive of imminent death (survival of less than one week).

In patients with AIDS, The greatest risk of death occurs with significantly decreased CD4 cell count, diagnosis of wasting syndrome, *Mycobacterium avium-intracellulare* complex infection (MAI), or lymphoma (Hanson, Horsburgh, Fann, Havlik, & Thompson, 1993). Other conditions indicating reduced survival time, but not imminent death, include *Pneumocystis carinii* pneumonia, Kaposi's sarcoma, toxoplasmosis, cryptococcosis, cryptosporidiosis, or esophageal candidiasis (Hanson et al., 1993).

Symptoms that have been a problem previously often continue to cause difficulties, and may increase in severity in the last weeks of life. Contrary to some reports, there is seldom a "crescendo of pain" during that time and, in fact, for some patients, pain and nausea may decrease (Fainsinger, Miller, Bruera, Hanson, & MacEachern, 1991). Changes in consciousness are common and include, in the final week or weeks, confusion and/or agitation. Social withdrawal is also common, and does not necessarily mean distress or deterioration: There usually is little to say in the face of eternity. Drowsiness or unresponsiveness frequently occur in the final days.

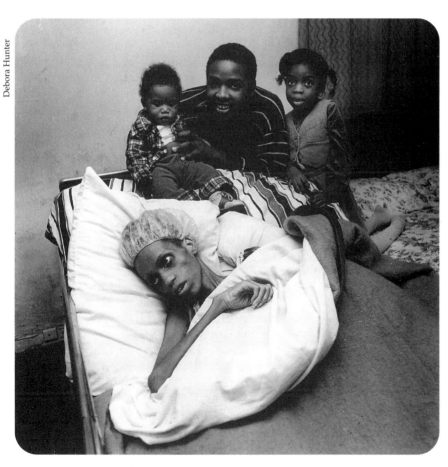

Debora Hunter

Providing Care to Moribund Patients

The first intervention in caring for moribund (dying) patients is to teach the family what to do and what to expect. Family members and others involved with the patient often imagine that death is a catastrophic event, filled with terrible physical agony. Understanding that this is seldom the case is immensely comforting. Now, more than ever, the family will benefit from involvement in giving care. Providing care keeps people busy with giving out their love, vs. sitting or pacing and feeling helpless.

This is truly the last chance to say what needs saying and to do what needs doing. The nurse may need to be very directive with a patient or family member, to help one or the other—or both—say healing words of forgiveness or acceptance.

This is also the last chance to tell the truth, to say good-bye, and to do whatever else is necessary to end a life well. Some words can be a lovely, final gift; some people need help saying them.

Dying at home presents challenging decisions and often a need for great support to the family. There is almost always the question: Is there anything more we should be doing, or that would be done if she or he was in the hospital? The presence or availability of the nurse when death occurs at home is extremely helpful.

Different political areas (cities, counties, etc.) have different procedures for what happens after a person dies at home. Knowing what will happen when authorities are informed of the death can prevent difficult crises. Resuscitation, for example, will be attempted by many emergency services—regardless of cause of death or of what the family says. It is thus necessary to learn about local procedures and to make alternative plans if possible. When death is due to advanced incurable disease and resuscitation is not desired by the patient, waiting for at least an hour or more

after death to contact authorities is probably the simplest measure to prevent resuscitation attempts. A physician or, in some areas, hospice nurses can come to the home and pronounce death and thus prevent problems. With enough lead time, some medical examiner offices issue "do not resuscitate" bracelets or documents prior to death.

While it is not possible to predict the exact course of a person's death, certain events are common in the final few days or hours of life. These are given below, along with a discussion of care.

- Anorexia occurs in about 90% of patients within the last two weeks of life (Wachtel, Allen-Masterson, Reuben, Goldberg, & Mor, 1988) and in even more in the last days. Many people have an intense desire to give food to even the most cachectic moribund patients. This may be an unconscious means of nurturing and showing love (Zerwekh, 1991). However, in so far as feeding a loved one can be considered a sign of love and nurturing, it is in any case a secondary and indirect sign; both patient and family will benefit from primary, or more direct expressions of love. Forcing food on patients who are clearly dying may also be a form of denial, or a manifestation of helplessness. Whatever the cause of the desire to give food, it is, at best, a burden for the patient. When dysphagia is the cause of anorexia, forcing food can result in choking. The nurse can: (1) help the family clarify their feelings and goals in wanting the patient to eat; and (2) teach them alternative means of expressing their love and care.
- Some patients also refuse fluids in their final days or hours. This is discussed more fully in chapter 19. Suffice it to say here that forcing fluids or initiating intravenous infusions for hydration is nearly always contraindicated in persons who are imminently terminal. Nothing is gained by these attempts and, more to the point, depending on tumor

involvement and other factors, such measures can actually increase pulmonary edema, peripheral edema, urine output, secretions, vomiting, and ascites (Zerwekh, 1991). Xerostomia and thirst are the primary problems resulting from decreased fluids in patients who are close to death. Treatment consists of oral care (preferably given by the family) at least every two hours; occasional sips, even of one-two drops, of fluid; and/or fine spray from an atomizer. This is discussed in greater detail in chapter 19.

- Dreams and visions of persons who died previously tend to increase in frequency in terminal patients during their final weeks and days. These are usually comforting to the person who is dying. Family members sometimes reject or devalue such occurrences. Powerful themes and symbols appear in these dreams and visions. Among these are a bridge or a river to cross, a door through which lies the "other side," a tunnel leading to the light, traveling, angels, religious figures, and deceased loved ones. Early on in the dying process, it is very helpful (to patient, family, and nurse) for the person who is dying to describe these experiences and to talk about what they mean. Later, when the person is able perhaps only to mumble, one simply listens to whatever is intelligible.

- Many patients withdraw, not in despair, but in acceptance of death (or life). These people speak very little, even to loved ones or to favorite caregivers. This a natural part of the process, and it is very helpful to family members to understand that it is not depression or rejection of others in a negative sense. We can probably say that the person who withdraws in this way is looking toward eternity rather than to finite life. Once family members understand the process, it is usually well-accepted.

- Symptoms such as pain, nausea, and vomiting are treated with the same vigor as at any point in the illness. The oral route for medications becomes less available, and the rectal and subcutaneous routes assume more importance. While there is disagreement about the degree of pain experienced during the final days of life (Fainsinger et al., 1991), it is clear that some patients experience a decrease in pain, some experience an increase in pain, and for some patients, pain does not change.

- Respiratory symptoms are often a significant problem in imminently terminal patients. The character of agonal respirations (near the end of life) is generally increasingly shallow and/or labored as death nears. Periods of apnea increase in frequency and/or respirations slow. Problems include pulmonary secretions increasing and the patient having increasing difficulty managing them, i.e., difficulty coughing, clearing, and swallowing effectively. Dyspnea often increases as death nears, even when there is no lung or pleural involvement (Wachtel et al., 1988). The specific cause(s) of dyspnea should be sought, and the interventions chosen should be based on etiology, if possible. In general, intervention options for dyspnea (Bruera, Macmillan, Pither, & MacDonald, 1990; Fainsinger et al., 1991; Zerwekh, 1991) include oxygen, opioids, tranquilizers, steroids, atropine to decrease secretions, and independent comfort measures, as described in chapter 19. Increased dyspnea and secretions, sometimes referred to as the "death rattle," leads to great anxiety in the family (Lindley-Davis, 1991). There is sometimes what is or seems to be a final struggle for breathe. While suctioning may not extend either the length or quality of life, it may be comforting to the family, especially if they do not themselves carry out the procedure. Atropine is probably a better choice than suctioning. Neither, however, slows the process. Zerwekh (1991) states that suctioning is used primarily when there is an artificial airway.

- The pulse rate increases and there is a corresponding decrease in cardiac efficiency, i.e., the pulse (usually) is weak and irregular. Blood pressure decreases.
- Changes in consciousness include drowsiness or unresponsiveness, and in some patients, confusion and/or agitation. The latter is treated according to etiology, e.g., with opioids for pain, and oxygen and/or opioids for dyspnea as described elsewhere in this text. Confusion or agitation of unknown etiology may be treated with tranquilizers or with low-dose, anti-psychotics.
- Patients who become unresponsive or comatose receive basic and non-intrusive care as follows. Use artificial tears when the patient does not blink. Provide very gentle mouth care. Give minimal skin care, primarily to keep the skin clean and dry (bowel movements are unusual and urine output is generally minimal). If the patient is incontinent, Attends or heavy towels may be effective enough to avoid catheterization. Vital signs are seldom necessary. If the patient is not incontinent, monitor for retention. The question of how much of what medications to give is difficult to answer definitively. Pain and antiemetic medications should generally be continued as before.
- The nurse should reassure the family about the normalcy of events and help them continue to provide as much care as possible. Knowing that the patient is likely to be able to hear is very helpful to family members, and motivates them to talk to the patient. The importance of family involvement in care at this point cannot be too highly stressed.
- Cyanosis, beginning distally and progressing, results from cardiac and respiratory deficiencies. The skin is usually cool and mottled. The patient may perspire and edema may develop.
- Some patients briefly "rally" for a few

moments or even hours, and perhaps make a memorable statement or two. Many patients do not.

Depending on room temperature, a light blanket or sheet should be used. Lighting should be whatever the patient is used to. Other than loved ones who heretofore have been able to come, visitors should generally be only those (usually) few that have been with the patient in his or her final weeks. Conversation should not be hushed and children should not be kept out. The brief presence of an infant grandchild is very appropriate.

Finally, the duty to those who are dying comes down to this: "Watch with me." This is what we do and what we teach others to do in this time of truth.

After Death

Whether at home or in the hospital, there is a tendency to hurry through whatever happens after a person dies. In hospitals, for example, nurses often ask the family to leave a few minutes after the death while they "wrap" or otherwise prepare the body for transport to (of course) the basement. At home, the ambulance service may be called to transport the body a few minutes after the death. Why? This rush is probably related to the family's pain and the staff's discomfort. There is also the fact that there may be *no* particular reason; that this is just the way it's done.

It should be understood by all, after some consideration of the facts, that there is, in reality, no reason to hurry. In fact, there usually is reason not to hurry. Slowing the after-death events means that the family has more time to begin understanding the reality of what has happened, and to begin the process of saying good-bye. Spending time with the body before it is made up (as if going to a party) by the funeral home helps the family see that the person is truly gone, physically. Some families want to wash the face or otherwise tend to the body. Some want to sit with the body, and some want to stay awhile, then go away, and then come back. Some want to keep the body at home until the next day. Whatever the case, the only reason not to encourage families to take as much time as they like have to do with public health rules—and these rules apply only to a few patients; even then, they are usually relevant only after the patient has been dead for at least 24 hours.

References

Bruera, E., Macmillan, K., Pither, J., & MacDonald, R.N. (1990). Effects of morphine on the dyspnea of terminal cancer patients. *Journal of Pain and Symptom Management, 5*(6), 341–344.

Bruera, E., Miller, M.J., Kuehn, N., MacEachern, T., & Hanson, J. (1992). Estimate of survival of patients admitted to a palliative care unit: A prospective study. *Journal of Pain and Symptom Management, 7*(2), 82–86.

Fainsinger, R., Miller, M.J., Bruera, E., Hanson, J., & MacEachern, T. (1991). Symptom control during the last week of life on a palliative care unit. *Journal of Palliative Care, 7*(1), 5–11.

Hanson, D.L., Horsburgh, C.R., Fann, S.A., Havlik, J.A., & Thompson, S.E. (1993). Survival prognosis of HIV-infected patients. *Journal of Acquired Immune Deficiency Syndrome, 6*(6), 624–629.

Inagaki, J., Rodriguez, V., & Bodey, G.P. (1974). Causes of death in cancer patients. *Cancer, 33*(2), 568–573.

Lindley-Davis, B. (1991). Process of dying: Defining characteristics. *Cancer Nursing, 14*(6), 328–333.

Nuland, S.B. (1994). *How we die.* New York: Alfred A. Knopf.

Wachtel, T., Allen-Masterson, S., Reuben, D., Goldberg, R., & Mor, V. (1988). The end stage cancer patient: Terminal common pathway. *The Hospice Journal, 4*(4), pp 43–80.

Zerwekh, J. (1991). Supportive care of the dying patient. In S.B. Baird, R. McCorkle, & M. Grant (Eds.), *Cancer nursing: A comprehensive textbook* (pp. 875–884). Philadelphia: W.B Saunders.

IV | Metastatic Spread

IMPLICATIONS FOR PATIENT CARE

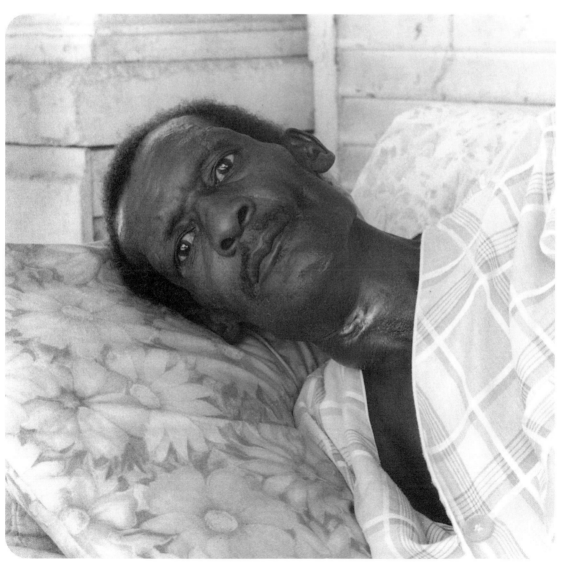

Debora Hunter

Introduction to Metastatic Spread: Common Symptoms

Ninety-seven percent of patients with terminal cancer have metastatic disease, and this is the primary cause of mortality in patients with cancer (Dudjak, 1992; Shure, 1991). Patterns of spread are "one of the oldest problems in oncology" (Weiss, 1992, p. 91). While no tumor is completely predictable, there is a likely pattern of spread for many tumors (Hubbard & Loitta, 1991). Spread is by direct invasion of the tumor into local areas, direct "seeding" to other organs, and lymphatic and hematogenous spread (Fidler & Hart, 1985).

This section applies current clinical knowledge of metastases and resultant problems to help practitioners anticipate problems and thus *minimize or prevent* their ill effects. It is essential to remember that the listing of metastatic sites is not inclusive of all patients. Some have fewer sites and problems; some have other sites and problems; and in many there may only be "tentative evidence of metastatic disease" (Kupchella, 1990, p. 68). Although many cancers metastasize to the adrenals (Weiss, 1992), clinical significance of such metastasis is rare (Faig & Hoffman, 1993), hence adrenal metastasis is not discussed in the following material. As always, the focus, strengthened but not blinded by knowledge, is on what is happening *with the individual patient*.

This section is divided into five chapters, according to major organs and systems.

Chapter 22. Major Organs: Lung Cancer, Pancreatic Cancer, Liver Cancer, Brain Cancer

Chapter 23. Female Reproductive: Breast Cancer, Ovarian Cancer, Uterine Cancer

Chapter 24. Gastrointestinal: Colorectal Cancer, Stomach Cancer, Esophageal Cancer, Oral Cancer

Chapter 25. Urinary Tract: Renal Cancer, Other Urinary Cancer (except bladder), Bladder Cancer, Prostate Cancer

Chapter 26. Blood/Lymph and Skin: Non-Hodgkin's Lymphoma, Leukemia, Multiple Myeloma, Melanoma

These categories take in the 18 primary tumor sites (Table IV.1) that each cause more than 5,000 deaths per year in the United States. The chapters in this section include brief discussions of metastatic sites, symptoms, and oncologic emergencies common to tumors for each primary site. Tables in each of the chapters provide a quick reference for identifying the *Problems* and *Assessment Parameters* associated with sites of *Metastatic Spread*. Under *Problems* in the tables, and in the text of the chapters themselves, oncologic emergencies are presented in **boldface**. There is some inevitable repetition in this section. For example, many tumors typically spread to bone and, rather than refer readers to problems of bony metastases, bone tumor problems instead are listed for each tumor, for easy reference.

TABLE IV.1
ESTIMATED 1990/1992 DEATHS BY TUMOR SITE

Rank	Site	Estimated deaths, 1990	Estimated deaths, 1992
1	Lung	142,000	146,000
2	Colon-rectum	60,900	58,300
3	Breast	44,300	46,300
4	Prostate	30,000	34,000
5	Pancreas	25,000	25,000
6	Non-Hodgkin's lymphoma	18,200	19,400
7	Leukemia	18,100	18,200
8	Stomach	13,700	13,300
9	Ovary	12,400	13,000
10	Liver, biliary	11,900	12,300
11	Brain, CNS	11,100	11,800
12	Kidney, other urinary	10,300	10,700
13	Uterus	10,000	10,000
14	Esophagus	9,500	10,000
15	Bladder	9,700	9,500
16	Multiple myeloma	8,900	9,200
17	Oral	8,350	7,950
18	Melanoma	6,300	6,700

Note. American Cancer Society, 1992.

References

American Cancer Society. (1992). *Cancer Facts and Figures—1992.* Atlanta: Author.

Dudjak, L.A. (1992). Cancer metastasis. *Seminars in Oncology Nursing, 8*(1), 40–49.

Faig, J.C., & Hoffman, A.R. (1993). Endocrine complications. In J.F. Holland, E. Frei, R.C. Bast, D.W. Kufe, D.L. Morton, & R.W. Weischselbaum (Eds.), *Cancer medicine* (3rd ed.) (pp. 2398–2402). Philadelphia: Lea & Febiger.

Fidler, I.J., & Hart, I.R. (1985). Principles of cancer biology: Cancer metastasis. In V.T. DeVita, S. Hellman, and S.A. Rosenberg (Eds.), *Cancer: Principles and practice of oncology.* Philadelphia: J.B. Lippincott.

Hubbard, S.M., and Loitta, L.A. (1991). The biology of metastases. In S.B. Baird, R. McCorkle, and M. Grant (Eds.), *Cancer nursing* (pp. 130–142). Philadelphia: W.B Saunders.

Kupchella, C.E. (1990). The spread of cancer: Invasion and metastasis. In S.I. Groenwald, M.H. Frogge, M. Goodman, and C.H. Yarbro (Eds.), *Cancer nursing: Principles and practice* (pp. 58–71). Boston: Jones and Bartlett.

Shure, D. (1991). Extrathoracic and endocrine manifestations of lung cancer. In R.A. Bordow & K.M. Moser (Eds.), *Manual of clinical problems in pulmonary medicine* (pp. 463–465). Boston: Little, Brown and Company.

Weiss, L. (1992). Comments on hematogenous metastatic patterns in humans as revealed by autopsy. *Clinical and Experimental Metastasis, 10*(3), 191–199.

Major Organs
(Lung, Pancreas, Liver, Brain):
Metastatic Spread/
Common Symptoms

Lung Cancer

Lung cancer is the leading cause of cancer death for both women and men, with total estimated 1992 deaths of 146,000. About 53,000 women will die from lung cancer in 1992 (vs. 46,000 from breast cancer) and about 93,000 men will die from lung cancer in the same time period (American Cancer society [ACS], 1992).

The most common lung cancers (according to World Health Organization classification) are squamous cell (epidermoid), small cell (SCLC), adenocarcinoma, and large cell (Minna, Pass, Glatstein, & Ihde, 1989). The following is a list of the significant characteristics of the different tumor types.

- Squamous cell carcinomas tend to spread by local invasion, and hence have fewer distant sites of metastases. The extremely painful superior sulcus or Pancoast tumors most often result from squamous cell carcinomas (Johnson, Hainsworth, & Greco, 1982). Common sites of metastases are con-

tralateral thorax, bone, marrow, lymph, and liver (Piemme, 1988; Portlock & Goffinet, 1980). Common problems of squamous cell carcinomas include deep chest pain, atelectasis, bronchial obstruction with pneumonitis, hilar adenopathy, and a tendency to cavitate (Minna et al., 1989).

- Small cell carcinomas are the most aggressive of the lung cancers and the most likely to result in distant metastases (Figlin, Holmes, Petrovich, & Sarna, 1990). Small cell carcinomas are also more likely than other lung cancers to spread to bone marrow (Portlock & Goffinet, 1980). Small cell carcinomas may be endocrinologically active (Figlin et al., 1990), hence patients may be more likely to develop the paraneoplastic syndromes discussed on the following page and noted in Table 22.1 (Volker, 1992). Common sites of metastases are con-

Charles Kemp: TERMINAL ILLNESS: A GUIDE TO NURSING CARE. © 1995 J. B. Lippincott.

tralateral thorax, bone, marrow, liver, lymph, meninges, and brain (Piemme, 1988). Common problems of small cell carcinomas include deep chest pain, atelectasis, pneumonitis, and hilar and mediastinal adenopathy (Minna et al., 1989).

- Adenocarcinomas are associated with multiple pulmonary nodules, as well as with metastases to pleura and scalene (chest) nodes (Figlin et al., 1990). Common sites of metastases are contralateral thorax, bone, liver, lymph, and brain (Piemme, 1988). Common problems include pain, pleural and chest wall involvement, and a tendency for pleural effusion (Minna et al., 1989).
- Large cell carcinomas are often large grossly as well as microscopically. Large cell carcinomas are the least common of the four major types. Metastatic patterns are similar to the other forms of lung cancer. Pleural effusions and cavitation are not uncommon (Minna et al., 1989). Lung cancer also metastasizes to the heart (Chernecky & Krech, 1991). In general, metastases to adrenals, and kidneys are asymptomatic (Shure, 1991).

The tendency for widespread metastases and the intrinsic pulmonary symptoms in lung cancer present a complicated clinical challenge. Common selected symptoms of lung cancer include: dyspnea and a combination of other pulmonary symptoms; persistent and often severe pain; fever (sometimes of unknown origin); nausea and/or vomiting; constipation, diarrhea, and anorexia; and weight loss. Other significant symptoms are cough, hepatomegaly, lymphadenopathy, neurologic sequelae of brain metastases, and paraneoplastic syndromes (Faber, 1991; Figlin et al., 1990; Wachtel, Allen-Masterson, Reuben, Goldberg, & Mor, 1988; Walsh, 1990).

Lung cancer is also associated with a number of other paraneoplastic syndromes (Holmes, Livingston, and Turrisi, 1993). Among these are:

- Eaton-Lambert syndrome (Pseudomyas-

thenia), characterized by severe muscle weakness and fatigue;
- hypertrophic osteoarthropathy, characterized by inflammation of the joints of the fingers and toes, and sometimes also of the distal ends of long bones;
- digital clubbing, which may accompany hypertrophic osteoarthropathy or may occur independently (polyarthritis, similar to rheumatoid arthritis, may also occur);
- hematologic disorders, which include thrombocytosis, hypercoagulation, thrombocytopenia, and anemia;
- neurological disorders, which are rare, but clinically significant; and
- nephrotic syndrome, which is usually a paraneoplastic syndrome rather than a result of tumor invasion or metastases.

The *oncologic emergencies* most often associated with lung cancer are **pericardial effusion and cardiac tamponade, superior vena cava syndrome, tracheal obstruction, spinal cord compression, increased intracranial pressure** (from metastasis to the brain and/or carcinomatosis meningitis), **hypercalcemia,** and **syndrome of inappropriate antidiuretic hormone secretion (SIADH, hyponatremia)** (Glover & Glick, 1991; Miaskowski, 1991).

The spread, problems, and assessments associated with lung cancer are illustrated in Table 22.1.

Pancreatic Cancer

Cancer of the pancreas is the fifth leading cause of cancer death for women and men, and occurs about equally in both populations (ACS, 1992).

Almost all tumors of the pancreas are adenocarcinomas and are usually diagnosed at an advanced stage (Haskell, Selch, & Ramming, 1990; Frogge, 1990). Common sites of metastases are bone, lung, liver, bowel, and regional and distal lymph nodes. (Piemme, 1988; Weiss, 1992).

TABLE 22.1 LUNG CANCER: SPREAD, PROBLEMS, AND ASSESSMENT *		
Metastatic spread	**Problems**	**Assessment parameters**
Thorax, bilaterally, including lymph	Dyspnea (also see chapter 14)	*Pleural effusion:* cough; trachea displaced; fremitus absent, decreased—may increase near top of effusion; percussion dull to flat; absent, decreased breath sounds; possible pleural rub
		Pneumonia: > temperature; purulent sputum (not always); percussion dull; < breath sounds; pleural effusion
		Lymphangitis carcinomatosis: dyspnea from pulmonary edema
		Pulmonary embolus: chest pain; hemoptysis; tachypnea; cough; tachycardia
		Cardiac tamponade: retrosternal chest pain relieved by sitting forward; orthopnea; cough; tachypnea; tachycardia; < cardiac output (< cerebral blood, peripheral cyanosis, < systolic and pulse pressures, and pulsus paradoxus); occasional nausea and vomiting and abdominal pain
		Superior vena cava syndrome: dilated neck or thoracic veins; facial edema, plethora; tachypnea; cyanosis; cough, hoarseness, upper extremity edema
		Obstruction: rapidly progressive dyspnea; hemoptysis; chronic cough; wheezing; stridor; aspiration; pneumonia; respiratory muscle weakness
		Anemia: weakness, fatigue, anorexia, headache, tachycardia
		Cachexia
		Preexisting conditions: COPD; TB; fibrosis secondary to treatment
		Ascites may contribute to dyspnea
	Pain	Pain may be mixed somatic and neuropathic, with chest wall involvement (see discussion of pain from different tumor types)
	Cough	May be associated with **obstruction;** pleural effusion; pulmonary edema from lymphangitis carcinomatosis; pneumonia; **pulmonary embolus;** pericardial effusion or **tamponade;** vocal cord paralysis; respiratory muscle weakness; congestive heart failure; other preexisting conditions
	Hemoptysis	Bronchogenic tumor is a common cause; other causes include pneumonia; **pulmonary embolus;** non-malignant disease; pulmonary
		Irreversible hemorrhage possible with end-stage cancer
	Lymphadenopathy	Lymphedema: enlarged lymph, edema (area or lower extremities); pain; cellulitis, lymphangitis.

(cont'd.)

Note: It is essential to read the description of the patient's tumor type.

	TABLE 22.1 (CONT'D.)	
Metastatic spread	**Problems**	**Assessment parameters**
Liver	Pain	Pain typically upper right abdominal or non-specific, characteristic of visceral pain; pain may radiate to right scapula
	Ascites	Abdominal distension, bulging flanks, fluid wave, weight gain, and discomfort; anorexia, early satiety, indigestion, < bowel mobility; dyspnea, orthopnea, tachypnea; weakness, fatigue; changes in color of urine, stool; pruritus.
Bone	Pain	Pain is usually localized to some extent, especially with metastases to bony thorax; back pain may indicate **spinal cord compression** (see chapter 13); pathologic fractures other than spine are possible; pain may be associated with other processes
	Metabolic changes	**Hypercalcemia:** (Often non-specific) symptoms include fatigue, weakness, anorexia, nausea, polyuria, polydipsia, and constipation; progressing to changes in mentation, seizures, coma
Brain	CNS symptoms	**Increased intracranial pressure:** Pain usually present, more severe in the morning; progressive neurological deficits (motor, sensory, cognitive); nausea, vomiting (see chapter 13)
		Confusion, seizures: See chapter 13
Marrow	Bleeding disorders	Thrombocytopenia: purpura, ecchymosis, petechiae; > bleeding after injection
Kidney	Weakness	Anemia: weakness, anorexia, headache, tachycardia
Other	Various problems	Problems of therapy, e.g., opioids, corticosteroids, antidepressants, radiation, chemotherapy
		Fever of unknown origin (common with liver involvement)
		Dysphagia
		Cardiac disorders
	Metabolic changes	**Syndrome of inappropriate antidiuretic hormone secretion (SIADH, hyponatremia):** Anorexia, nausea, myalgia (including abdominal wall), slight neurological changes; progression to > neurological changes: confusion, lethargy, seizures
		Also see paraneoplastic syndromes below
	Paraneoplastic syndromes	Eaton-Lambert syndrome, hypertrophic osteoarthropathy, digital clubbing (may accompany hypertrophic osteoarthropathy or may occur independently), polyarthritis, hematologic disorders (thrombocytosis, hypercoagulation, thrombocytopenia, and anemia), neurological disorders

Common symptoms include pain, especially abdominal (> 80%), anorexia (> 60%), early satiety (> 60%), xerostomia (> 50%), sleep disturbances (> 50%), weight loss (> 50%), fatigue (> 40%), weakness (> 40%), nausea (> 40%), constipation (> 40%), depression (> 40%), and dyspepsia (> 30%) (Krech & Walsh, 1991). Pain is often dull, boring, and worse at night; or pain may be in the back and relieved by sitting up, bending forward, or lying in a curled up position; and finally, pain is "frequently vague and ill-defined, and thus confusing (Beazley & Cohn, 1991a, p. 220). Ascites may develop late in the course of the disease (Frogge, 1990) and jaundice is common (Beazley & Cohn, 1991a). A variety of other problems, primarily gastrointestinal, are also common. Diarrhea is especially troublesome in later stages (Wachtel et al., 1988). Dyspnea is also common, even without evidence of pulmonary disease or anemia (Walsh, 1990).

The *oncologic emergency* most often associated with pancreatic cancer is **syndrome of inappropriate antidiuretic hormone secretion [SIADH]** (Miaskowski, 1991). Chronic subclinical disseminated intravascular coagulation is "frequently documented" in patients with cancer of the pancreas (Portlock & Goffinet, 1980).

The spread, problems, and assessments associated with pancreatic cancer are illustrated in Table 22.2.

Liver Cancer (Including Liver Metastases)

Primary liver and biliary passages cancer is the tenth leading cause of cancer death overall, with total estimated 1992 deaths of 12,300, about equally divided between women and men (ACS, 1992). Because of the recent immigration of large numbers of people, including many refugees, from areas such as Africa and Southeast Asia where liver cancer is far more common than it is in the United States, we may begin to see an increase in the number of patients with primary liver tumors (Beazley & Cohn, 1991b).

Most primary liver tumors are fast-growing, hepatocellular carcinomas with a high mortality rate (Frogge, 1990). Metastases do not always occur; when they do, they are usually to lung(s), portal vein, and lymph (Haskell et al., 1990).

Most cancers metastasize to the liver by the time of death (Ensminger & Knol, 1993). Symptoms are sometimes ill-defined, and include epigastric pressure, fullness, and discomfort. An abdominal mass or distension may be seen. Intravascular growth may include cardiac vessels, and esophageal varices are common. Fever and ascites are typical (Haskell et al., 1990).

Pain from liver involvement is commonly upper right abdominal, sometimes radiating to the right scapula. In the later stages of the disease, pain worsens, and is often more severe at night. Ascites is common and the abdomen is frequently distended; there may be anorexia or early satiety and weight loss. "Profound, progressive weakness and fatigue are characteristic of liver cancer" (Frogge, 1990). Muscle wasting, fever, and progressive jaundice also are common (Engstrom, McGlynn, & Weese, 1993; Frogge, 1990).

Paraneoplastic syndromes are common in hepatic cell carcinoma, and may include: hypercalcemia, hypoglycemia, Cushing's syndrome, osteoporosis, excessive gonadotropin production, feminization, hyperlipidemia, polycythemia, microangiopathic hemolytic anemia, leucocytosis, erythrocytosis, disseminated intravascular coagulation, dysfibrinogenemia, and cryofibrinogenemia (Beazley & Cohn, 1991b; Engstrom et al., 1993; Haskell et al., 1990).

Death from a primary hepatic neoplasm may be from liver failure or hemorrhage (Haskell et al., 1990); or related to the wasting and weakness of the disease (Frogge, 1990). In the latter case, patients may develop rapidly progressive pulmonary congestion and pneumonia.

TABLE 22.2
Pancreatic Cancer: Spread, Problems, and Assessment

Metastatic spread	Problems	Assessment parameters
Regional extension (see liver and bowel below)	Pain	Pain is often dull, boring, worse at night, sometimes in back, and relieved by sitting, bending forward, lying curled up; abdominal pain may be vague, ill-defined; see liver
	GI	Early satiety, anorexia, weight loss, dyspepsia, jaundice
Liver	Pain	Pain may be upper right abdominal or non-specific and characteristic of visceral pain; Pain may radiate to the right scapula and worsen at night
	Ascites	Abdominal distension, bulging flanks, fluid wave, weight gain, and discomfort; early satiety, indigestion, decreased bowel mobility (potential for obstruction); dyspnea, orthopnea, and tachypnea; weakness and fatigue; anorexia
Bowel	GI disturbances	Diarrhea, constipation, abdominal pain, intestinal obstruction
Bone	Pain	Pain is usually localized to site(s) of lesion to at least some extent
Regional lymph, other structures	Lymphadeno-pathy	Lymphedema: Enlarged lymph, edema (area or lower extremities) pain; cellulitis, lymphangitis
Lungs	Dyspnea, cough, hemoptysis	(See Table 22.1): pleural effusion, pneumonia, embolus, preexisting conditions, ascites may contribute to dyspnea; lymph metastases may be involved; dyspnea may occur without pulmonary involvement (also see chapter 14)
Other	Various problems	Problems of therapy, e.g., opioids, corticosteroids, tricyclic antidepressants, radiation, chemotherapy
		Fever of unknown origin is common with liver metastases
		Syndrome of Inappropriate Antidiuretic Hormone Secretion (SIADH): Personality changes, weight gain, weakness, anorexia, nausea, vomiting, lethargy, seizures, coma
		Fever of unknown origin (common with liver involvement)

Oncologic emergencies associated with hepatic cancer include **hypercalcemia** and **hypoglycemia** (Beazley & Cohn, 1991b).

The spread, problems, and assessments associated with liver cancer are illustrated in Table 22.3.

Brain Cancer

Primary brain and central nervous system cancer is the eleventh leading cause of cancer death overall, with total estimated 1992 deaths of 11,800, about equally divided between women

	TABLE 22.3	
	LIVER CANCER: SPREAD, PROBLEMS, AND ASSESSMENT	
Metastatic spread	**Problems**	**Assessment parameters**
Liver, regional	Pain	Pain may be upper right abdominal or non-specific and characteristic of visceral pain; pain may radiate to the right scapula and worsen at night
	Ascites	Abdominal distension, bulging flanks, fluid wave, weight gain, and discomfort; anorexia, early satiety, indigestion, decreased bowel mobility (potential for obstruction); dyspnea, orthopnea, and tachypnea; weakness and fatigue; changes in color of urine and stool; pruritus Progressive jaundice
	Bleeding	From esophageal varices: May be massive hemorrhage
	General abdominal symptoms	Epigastric fullness, pressure, discomfort; early satiety, constipation, diarrhea; anorexia, cachexia.
Lung(s)	Dyspnea, other pulmonary symptoms	(See Table 22.1): Pleural effusion, pneumonia, embolus, obstruction, preexisting conditions; ascites may be cause of dyspnea. (Also see chapter 14.)
Other	Various problems	Problems of therapy, e.g., opioids, corticosteroids, tricyclic antidepressants, radiation, chemotherapy Fever of unknown origin is common with liver cancer Weakness, fatigue; muscle wasting
Paraneoplastic syndromes	Metabolic changes	**Hypercalcemia:** (Often non-specific) symptoms include fatigue, weakness, anorexia, nausea, polyuria, polydipsia, and constipation; progressing to changes in mentation, seizures, and coma **Hypoglycemia:** Extreme fatigue, weakness, dizziness, and confusion Cushing's syndrome; osteoporosis; excessive gonadotropin production; feminization; hyperlipidemia; polycythemia; microangiopathic hemolytic anemia; leucocytosis; disseminated intravascular coagulation; dysfibrinogenemia; cryofibrinogenemia

and men (ACS, 1992). CNS tumors are the second leading cause of death from childhood cancer (Ranshoff, Koslow, & Cooper, 1991).

Most (malignant) primary brain tumors are glioblastomas and astrocytomas (Prados & Wilson, 1993). These tumors are characterized by local invasiveness and rarely metastasize beyond the CNS (Ranshoff et al., 1991; Wegmmann & Hakius, 1990).

CNS metastases are common with several systemic cancers, notably lung, breast, colon, kidney, testis, and melanoma, but also with others (Piemme, 1988; Weiss, 1992).

While differences exist among the various

TABLE 22.4		
BRAIN CANCER: SPREAD, PROBLEMS, AND ASSESSMENT		
Metastatic spread	**Problems**	**Assessment parameters**
Local extension	CNS symptoms	**Increased intracranial pressure:** Pain usually present, may be more severe in the morning; progressive neurological deficits (motor, sensory, cognitive); nausea, vomiting (see more complete discussion in chapter 13)
		Confusion: See chapter 13
		Seizures: See chapter 13
		Spinal cord compression: Back pain may be local (somatic: Constant, dull, aching) or radicular or both; exacerbated by movement, neck flexion, straight leg raising; decreased by sitting up; tender to percussion. Neurological deficits begin subtly and may not be apparent to the patient: weakness, ataxia, stumbling; urine retention (frequent, small voiding); bowel dysfunction; impotence; numbness
Other	Metabolic changes	Problems of therapy, especially corticosteroids; also other medications, procedures

brain tumors, depending on the location of tumor, problems are generally similar (Robinson, Roy, & Seager, 1991). A more complete discussion of problems of primary and metastatic brain tumors is found in chapter 13.

Oncologic emergencies associated with brain tumors are **increased intracranial pressure** and **spinal cord compression.**

The spread, problems, and assessments associated with brain cancer are illustrated in Table 22.4.

References

American Cancer Society. (1992). Cancer facts and figures—1992. Atlanta: Author.

Beazley, R.M., & Cohn, I. (1991a). Tumors of the pancreas, gallbladder, and extrahepatic ducts. In A.I. Holleb, D.J. Fink, & G.P. Murphy (Eds.), *Clinical oncology* (pp. 219–236). Atlanta: American Cancer Society.

Beazley, R.M., & Cohn, I. (1991b). Tumors of the liver. In A.I. Holleb, D.J. Fink, & G.P. Murphy (Eds.), *Clinical oncology* (pp. 237–244). Atlanta: American Cancer Society.

Chernecky, C., & Krech, R. L. (1991). Complications of advanced disease. In S.B. Baird, R. McCorkle, & M. Grant (Eds.), *Cancer nursing: A comprehensive textbook* (pp 885–893). Philadelphia: W.B Saunders.

Engstrom, P.F., McGlynn, K., & Weese, J.L. (1993). Primary neoplasms of the liver. In J.F. Holland, E. Frei, R.C. Bast, D.W. Kufe, D.L. Morton, & R.W. Weischselbaum (Eds.), *Cancer medicine* (3rd ed.) (pp. 1430–1441). Philadelphia: Lea & Febiger.

Ensminger, W.D., & Knol, J.A. (1993). Metastatic neoplasms of the liver. In J.F. Holland, E. Frei, R.C. Bast, D.W. Kufe, D.L. Morton, & R.W. Weischselbaum (Eds.), *Cancer medicine* (3rd ed.) (pp. 1441–1447). Philadelphia: Lea & Febiger.

Faber, L.P. (1991). Lung Cancer. In A.I. Holleb, D.J. Fink, & G.P. Murphy (Eds.), *Clinical oncology* (pp. 194–212). Atlanta: American Cancer Society.

Figlin, R.A., Holmes, E.C., Petrovich, Z., & Sarna, G.P. (1990). Thoracic Neoplasms. In C.M. Haskell (Ed.), *Cancer treatment* (pp. 165–191). Philadelphia: W.B. Saunders.

Frogge, M.H. (1990). Gastrointestinal cancer: Esophagus, stomach, liver, and pancreas. In S.L. Groenwald, M.H. Frogge, M. Goodman, & C.H. Yarbro (Eds.), *Cancer nursing: Principles and Practice* (3rd ed.) (pp. 806–844). Boston: Jones and Bartlett Publishers.

Glover, D., & Glick, J.H. (1991). Oncologic emergencies. In A.I. Holleb, D.J. Fink, & G.P. Murphy (Eds.), *Clinical oncology* (pp. 513–533). Atlanta: American Cancer Society.

Haskell, C.M., Selch, M.T., & Ramming, K.P. (1990). Gastrointestinal neoplasms: Stomach. In C.M. Haskell (Ed.), *Cancer treatment* (3rd ed.) (pp. 217–229). Philadelphia: W.B. Saunders Company.

Holmes, E.C., Livingston, R., & Turrisi, A. (1993). Neoplasms of the thorax. In J.F. Holland, E. Frei, R.C. Bast, D.W. Kufe, D.L. Morton, & R.W. Weischselbaum (Eds.), *Cancer medicine* (3rd ed.) (pp. 1285–1337). Philadelphia: Lea & Febiger.

Johnson, D.H., Hainsworth, J.D., & Greco, F.A. (1982). Pancoast's syndrome and small cell lung cancer. *Chest: The Cardiopulmonary Journal, 82*(5), 602–606.

Krech, R.L., & Walsh, T.D. (1991). Symptoms of pancreatic Cancer. *Journal of Pain and Symptom Management, 6*(6), 360–367.

Miaskowski, C. (1991). Oncologic emergencies. In S.B. Baird, R. McCorkle, & M. Grant (Eds.), *Cancer nursing* (pp. 885–893). Philadelphia: W.B Saunders.

Minna, J.D., Pass, H., Glatstein, E., & Ihde, D.C. (1989). Cancer of the lung. In V.T. DeVita, S. Hellman, & S.A. Rosenberg (Eds.), *Cancer: Principles and practice of oncology* (pp. 591–622). Philadelphia: J.B. Lippincott.

Piemme, J.A. (1988). Secondary primary or metastatic cancer. In S.B. Baird (Ed.) *Decision making in oncology nursing* (pp. 20–23). Philadelphia: B.C. Decker.

Portlock C.S., & Goffinet, D.R. (1980). *Manual of clinical problems in oncology.* Boston: Little, Brown and Company.

Prados, M.D., & Wilson, C.B. (1993). Neoplasms of the central nervous system. In J.F. Holland, E. Frei, R.C. Bast, D.W. Kufe, D.L. Morton, & R.W. Weischselbaum (Eds.), *Cancer medicine* (3rd ed.) (pp. 1080–1119). Philadelphia: Lea & Febiger.

Ranshoff, J., Koslow, M., & Cooper, P.R. (1991). Cancer of the central nervous system and pituitary. In A.I. Holleb, D.J. Fink, & G.P. Murphy (Eds.), *Clinical oncology* (pp. 329–337). Atlanta: American Cancer Society.

Robinson, C.R., Roy, C., & Seager, M.L. (1991). Central nervous system tumors. In S.B. Baird, R. McCorkle, & M. Grant (Eds.), *Cancer nursing* (pp. 608–636) Philadelphia: W.B. Saunders.

Shure, D. (1991). Extrathoracic and endocrine manifestations of lung cancer. In R.A. Bordow & K.M. Moser (Eds.) ^*Manual of clinical problems in pulmonary medicine* (pp 463–465). Boston: Little, Brown and Company.

Volker, D.L. (1992). Pathophysiology of cancer. In J.C. Clark & R.F. McGee (Eds.), *Core curriculum for oncology nursing* (pp. 265–285). Philadelphia: W.B. Saunders.

Wachtel, T., Allen-Masterson, S. Reuben, D. Goldberg, R, & Mor, V. (1988). The end stage cancer patient: Terminal common pathway. *The Hospice Journal, 4*(4), 43–80.

Walsh, T.D. (1990). Symptom control in patients with advanced cancer. *American Journal of Hospice and Palliative Care, 7*(6), 20–29.

Wegmmann, J.A., & Hakius, P. (1990). Central nervous system cancers. In S.L. Groenwald, M.H. Frogge, M. Goodman, & C.H. Yarbro (Eds.), *Cancer nursing: Principles and practice* (3rd ed.) (pp. 751–773). Boston: Jones and Bartlett Publishers.

Weiss, L. (1992). Comments on hematogenous metastatic patterns in humans as revealed by autopsy. *Clinical and Experimental Metastasis, 10*(3), 191–199.

Female Reproductive Cancer (Breast, Ovarian, Uterine): Metastatic Spread/ Common Symptoms

Breast Cancer

Breast cancer is the second leading cause of cancer death among women (46,000 estimated deaths in 1992), and the third leading cause of cancer death (46,300) among women and men together (American cancer society [ACS], 1992).

About 70% of invasive breast cancers are ductal adenocarcinomas (Scanlon, 1991). Metastatic spread is often detected first in regional lymph, but distal metastases may already have occurred, or may occur, without lymph involvement (Knobf, 1991). The most common significant sites of distal metastases (on autopsy) are liver, lung, and bone (> 60%), and thyroid and brain (> 20%). Other sites include (but are not limited to), in descending order, skin, kidney, skeletal muscle, and heart. Of the cancers with the highest morbidity and mortality rates, breast cancer is the most like-

ly to metastasize to skin (19.5%). It is also, after primary bone cancer, the second most likely to metastasize to skeletal muscle (Weiss, 1992).

Pain is more common among patients with breast cancer than among patients with cancer in most other primary sites, perhaps because of its high incidence (second only to prostate cancer) of bone metastasis (Arathuzik, 1991; Wachtel, Allen-Masterson, Reuben, Goldberg, & Mor, 1988; Weiss, 1992). Breast and lung cancers and melanomas tend to be more invasive than any of the other major cancers (Piemme, 1988), and thus have at least the potential of resulting in multiple symptoms. Pain, pathological fractures, skin lesions—as well as sequelae of liver, lung, and other metastasis—present difficult clinical challenges. Uremia may also occur.

While exact figures are not available, it is known that patients with breast cancer often die from infection and, after patients with melanoma, they are also more likely to die from carcinomatosis (Inagaki, Rodriguez, and Bodey, 1974). Haskell, Giuliano, Thompson, & Zarem (1990, p. 129) report that about 50% of

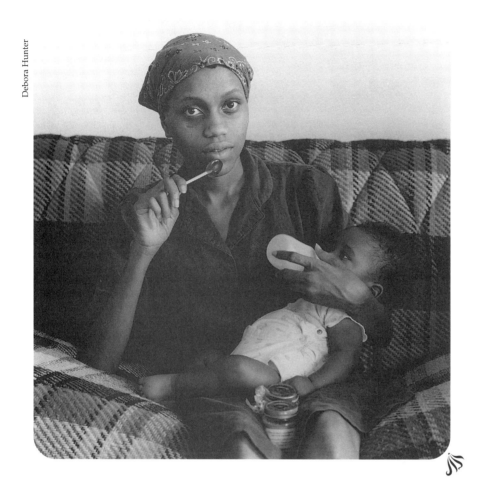

Debora Hunter

patients with breast cancer die from "the malignant process itself."

The *oncologic emergencies* most common in patients with breast cancer are **pericardial effusion, cardiac tamponade, increased intracranial pressure** (including from **carcinomatosis meningitis), spinal cord compression, airway obstruction, disseminated intravascular coagulation,** and **hypercalcemia** (Finley, 1992; Glover & Glick, 1991; Hunter, 1992). Hypercalcemia is the most common oncologic emergency in breast cancer (±9%) (Haskell et al., 1990), and patients with breast cancer are more likely than others to develop spinal cord compression (Henson & Posner, 1993).

The spread, problems, and assessments associated with breast cancer are illustrated in Table 23.1.

Ovarian Cancer

Ovarian cancer is the ninth leading cause of cancer death overall, and the fifth leading cause of cancer death in women, with total estimated 1992 deaths of 13,000. Ovarian cancer results in the greatest number of cancer deaths from gynecological cancer, but is the second most common gynecological cancer (ACS, 1992).

Eighty to ninety percent of ovarian tumors

TABLE 23.1
BREAST CANCER: SPREAD, PROBLEMS, AND ASSESSMENT

Metastatic spread	Problems	Assessment parameters
Bone	Pain	Pain is usually localized to some extent. Spinal cord compression from pathologic fracture is possible; pain may be from other processes
		Spinal cord compression: back pain may be local (somatic: Constant, dull, aching) or radicular or both; exacerbated by movement, neck flexion, straight leg raising; decreased by sitting up; tender to percussion
		Neurological deficits begin subtly and not necessarily apparent to the patient: Weakness, ataxia, stumbling; urine retention, bowel dysfunction, numbness
	Metabolic changes	**Hypercalcemia:** (Often non-specific) symptoms include fatigue, weakness, anorexia, nausea, polyuria, polydipsia, and constipation; progressing to changes in mentation, seizures, coma
Regional lymph and structures	Lymphadeno-pathy	Lymphedema: Enlarged lymph, edema, pain; cellulitis; lymphangitis
	Cardiac changes	Pericardial effusion: nonspecific cardiac symptoms, including dyspnea, cough, chest discomfort
		Cardiac tamponade: Retrosternal chest pain relieved by sitting forward; orthopnea; cough; tachypnea; tachycardia; < cardiac output (< cerebral blood, peripheral cyanosis, < systolic and pulse pressures, pulsus paradoxus; occasional nausea and vomiting and abdominal pain
Liver	Pain	Pain may be upper right abdominal or non-specific and characteristic of visceral pain; may radiate to right scapula, worsen at night
	Ascites	Abdominal distension, bulging flanks, fluid wave, weight gain, and discomfort; anorexia, early satiety, indigestion, < bowel mobility; dyspnea, orthopnea, tachypnea; weakness, fatigue; changes in color of urine, stool; pruritus
Lung(s)	Dyspnea, cough, hemoptysis	(See Table 22.1) Pleural effusion, pneumonia, **embolus, obstruction,** pre-existing conditions, ascites may cause dyspnea (Ch. 14)
Brain	CNS symptoms	**Increased intracranial pressure:** Pain usually present, more severe in the morning; progressive neurological deficits (motor, sensory, cognitive); nausea, vomiting (see chapter 13)
		Confusion, seizures: See chapter 13

(cont'd.)

	TABLE 23.1 (CONT'D.)	
Metastatic spread	**Problems**	**Assessment parameters**
Skin	Lesions	Metastatic lesions are often painful and have an unpleasant odor
Heart	Cardiac changes	Arrhythmias, congestive heart failure; see pericardial effusion and cardiac tamponade (in this table above)
Kidney	Anemia	Weakness, anorexia, headache, tachycardia
	Uremia	< urine, changes blood pressure, CHF, stomatitis, nausea and vomiting, GI bleeding, bowel changes, lethargy, changes mentation
Thyroid	Regional changes	Thyroid nodules, hoarseness, dysphagia; stridor; lymphadenopathy
Other	Various problems	Problems of therapy, e.g., opioids, corticosteroids, antidepressants, radiation, chemotherapy
		Disseminated intravascular coagulation: Fever of unknown origin (common with liver involvement)
		Infection is a frequent cause of death; carcinomatosis is more common than with any other tumor except for melanoma

are one of several epithelial cell types (Otte, 1990). Ovarian cancer is sometimes complicated by the development of breast, colon, or endometrial cancer at the same time, or shortly thereafter (Gusberg & Runowicz, 1991). Metastases is primarily through intraperitoneal seeding to the liver, diaphragm, bladder, small bowel, and large bowel. Other sites of metastases include bone, lung, kidneys, and spleen (Otte, 1990; Weiss, 1992).

Frequently encountered problems of advanced ovarian cancer include ascites and/or pleural effusion. Nutritional problems are common and patients may appear as "gaunt and alert" (Martin & Braly, 1991). Cachexia, nausea and vomiting, and constipation are common, and may be due to the extensive abdominal involvement or to more specif-

ic problems, such as intestinal obstruction (Flannery, 1992; Otte, 1990; Berek & Hacker, 1990). Some patients present with Meig's syndrome, which includes ascites, hydrothorax, and large abdominal tumor mass (Martin & Braly, 1991). Perineal pain from widespread pelvic disease may be a mix of neuropathic, visceral, and somatic pain, and thus a major challenge to manage (Stillman, 1990).

Bowel complications—e.g., obstruction and changes in peristalsis and absorption—may develop from adhesions among the bowel loops or from metastases to the mesentery, causing dysfunction of autonomic innervation (Berek, Dembo, and Ozols, 1993). In a study of patients with intestinal obstruction at St. Christopher's Hospice, patients with primary ovarian cancer exceeded all other patients com-

TABLE 23.2
OVARIAN CANCER: SPREAD, PROBLEMS, AND ASSESSMENT

Metastatic spread	Problems	Assessment parameters
Intraperitoneal seeding to large and small bowel, mesentery	Obstruction	Intestinal obstruction: Nausea and vomiting, intestinal colic, other abdominal pain, diarrhea; constipation (see section on obstruction in chapter 17)
	Other GI symptoms	Nausea and vomiting, anorexia, changes peristalsis, absorption, cachexia; changes innervation GI system
Regional lymph, other structures	Lymphadenopathy	Lymphedema: Enlarged lymph, edema (area or lower extremities); pain; cellulitis, lymphangitis
	Obstruction	**Obstructive uropathy** (ureteral): hesitancy, urgency, nocturia, frequency, < force of stream, polyuria alternating with oliguria
	Perineal pain	Severe pain; most often neuropathic, but also mixed neuropathic with visceral and/or somatic
Liver	Pain	Pain may be upper right abdominal or non-specific and characteristic of visceral pain; pain may radiate to the right scapula and worsen at night
	Ascites	Abdominal distension, bulging flanks, fluid wave, weight gain, and discomfort; anorexia, early satiety, indigestion, decreased bowel mobility (potential for obstruction); dyspnea, orthopnea, and tachypnea; weakness and fatigue; changes in color of urine and stool; pruritus
Lung(s)	Dyspnea, cough, hemoptysis	(See Table 22.1): Pleural effusion, pneumonia, **embolus, bronchial obstruction,** preexisting conditions, ascites may contribute to dyspnea (also see chapter 14)
Bone	Pain	Pain is usually localized to at least some extent. **Spinal cord compression** from pathologic fractures of the spine is possible. Pain may be associated with other processes
Other	Various problems	Problems of therapy, e.g., opioids, corticosteroids, tricyclic antidepressants, radiation, chemotherapy
		Fever of unknown origin (common with liver involvement); infection is the primary cause of death; hemorrhage more common than with other tumors
	Development of other cancers	Breast, colon, endometrial

TABLE 23.3
UTERINE OR ENDOMETRIAL CANCER: SPREAD, PROBLEMS, AND ASSESSMENT

Metastatic spread	Problems	Assessment parameters
Primary tumor growth and regional spread via extension and/or seeding	Perineal pain	Severe pain, most often neuropathic, but also mixed neuropathic with visceral and/or somatic
	Pelvic structure involvement	Fistulas: Perirectal, rectovaginal, and others
		Vaginal tumors: Fungating, ulcerative, or invasive
		Abdominal pain
	Obstruction	Intestinal obstruction: Nausea and vomiting, intestinal colic, other abdominal pain, diarrhea; constipation
		Obstruction or dysfunction of other structures possible, e.g., kidney, bladder
	Lymphadenopathy	Lymphedema: Enlarged lymph, edema, pain; cellulitis, lymphangitis
Liver	Pain	Pain may be upper right abdominal or non-specific and characteristic of visceral pain; pain may radiate to the right scapula and worsen at night
	Ascites	Abdominal distension, bulging flanks, fluid wave, weight gain, and discomfort; anorexia, early satiety, indigestion, decreased bowel mobility (potential for obstruction); dyspnea, orthopnea, and tachypnea; weakness and fatigue; changes in color of urine and stool; pruritus
Lung(s)	Dyspnea, other pulmonary symptoms	(See Table 22.1): **Pleural effusion, pneumonia, embolus, obstruction, preexisting conditions, ascites** may contribute to dyspnea (also see chapter 14)
Bone	Bone	Pain is usually localized to at least some extent. **Spinal cord compression** from pathologic fractures of the spine is possible. Pain may be associated with other processes
Brain	CNS symptoms	**Increased intracranial pressure** (rare): Pain usually present, may be more severe in the morning; progressive neurological deficits (motor, sensory, cognitive); nausea, vomiting (see more complete discussion in chapter 13)
		Confusion: See chapter 13
		Seizures: See chapter 13
Other	Various problems	Problems of therapy, e.g., opioids, corticosteroids, tricyclic antidepressants, radiation, chemotherapy

bined (> 50%) in a diagnosis of obstruction (Baines, 1990).

Death is often from infection (septicemia or pneumonia), electrolyte imbalance, and cardiovascular collapse (Inagaki et al., 1974; Otte, 1990).

The *oncologic emergencies* most often associated with ovarian cancer are **obstructive uropathy (ureteral obstruction)** and **bronchial obstruction** (Glover & Glick, 1991).

The spread, problems, and assessments associated with ovarian cancer are illustrated in Table 23.2.

Uterine or Endometrial Cancer

Uterine or endometrial cancer is the 13th leading cause of cancer death overall, and the sixth leading cause of cancer death in women, with total estimated 1992 deaths of 10,000 (ACS, 1992). While uterine cancer is the most common gynecological cancer, it results in fewer fatalities than ovarian, the second most common gynecological cancer (Gusberg & Runowicz, 1991).

The most common tumor type is adenocarcinoma, and several variants exist. The tumor may spread by invasion of the myometrium (the smooth muscle coat of the uterus) to the cervix, vagina, and elsewhere; and by metastases to the peritoneum, lymph, and adnexa (ovaries and uterine tubes) (Creasman, 1993; Flannery, 1992). Kidneys, brain, bone, thyroid, and adrenals may also be involved (Weiss, 1992), as may the lungs (Piemme, 1988). Tumors other than adenocarcinoma, i.e., sarcoma, may metastasize to liver, lung, bone, and brain. (Otte, 1990).

The presence of widespread pelvic disease often presents challenges in management. Perineal pain from invasion of structures and nerve plexi may be a mix of neuropathic, visceral, and somatic pain (Stillman, 1990). Fistulas, vaginal tumors, and skin breakdown can be very difficult to manage. Bowel obstruction, ascites, and respiratory distress may develop (Berman & Berek, 1990).

There are no *oncologic emergencies* typically associated with uterine cancer (Glover & Glick, 1991; Hunter, 1992).

The spread, problems, and assessments associated with uterine or endometrial cancer are illustrated in Table 23.3.

References

American Cancer Society. (1992). Cancer facts and figures—1992. Atlanta: Author.

Arathuzik, D. (1991). Pain experience for metastatic breast cancer patients. *Cancer Nursing, 14*(1), 41–48.

Baines, M.J. (1990). Management of malignant intestinal obstruction in patients with advanced cancer. In K.M. Foley, J.J. Bonica, & V. Ventafridda (Eds.), *Advances in pain research and therapy, Volume 16: Proceedings of the Second International Congress on Cancer Pain.* (pp. 327–335). New York: Raven Press.

Berek, J.S., & Hacker, N.F. (1990). Gynecologic neoplasms: Ovary and fallopian tubes. In C.M. Haskell (Ed.), *Cancer treatment* (pp. 295–325). Philadelphia: W.B. Saunders.

Berek, J.S., Dembo, A., & Ozols, R.F. (1993). Ovarian cancer. In J.F. Holland, E. Frei, R.C. Bast, D.W. Kufe, D.L. Morton, & R.W. Weischselbaum (Eds.), *Cancer medicine* (3rd ed.) (pp. 1659–1690). Philadelphia: Lea & Febiger.

Berman, M.L., & Berek, J.S. (1990). Gynecologic neoplasms: Uterine carcinomas. In C.M. Haskell (Ed.), *Cancer treatment* (pp. 338–351). Philadelphia: W.B. Saunders.

Creasman, W.T. (1993). Adenocarcinoma of the uterine corpus. In J.F. Holland, E. Frei, R.C. Bast, D.W. Kufe, D.L. Morton, & R.W. Weischselbaum (Eds.), *Cancer medicine* (3rd ed.) (pp. 1647–1655). Philadelphia: Lea & Febiger.

Finley, J.P. (1992). Nursing care of patients with metabolic and physiological oncological emergencies. In J.C. Clark & R.F. McGee (Eds.), *Core curriculum for oncology nursing* (pp. 169–192), Philadelphia: W.B. Saunders.

Flannery, M. (1992). Reproductive cancers. In J.C. Clark & R.F. McGee (Eds.), *Core curriculum for oncology nursing* (pp. 451–469), Philadelphia: W.B. Saunders.

Glover, D., & Glick, J.H. (1991). Oncologic emergencies. In A.I. Holleb, D.J. Fink, & G.P. Murphy (Eds.), *Clinical oncology* (pp. 513–533). Atlanta: American Cancer Society.

Gusberg, S.B., & Runowicz, C.D. (1991). Gynecologic cancers. In A.I. Holleb, D.J. Fink, & G.P. Murphy (Eds.), *Clinical oncology* (pp. 481–497). Atlanta: American Cancer Society.

Haskell, C.M., Giuliano, A.E., Thompson, R.W., & Zarem, H.A. (1990). Breast cancer. In C.M. Haskell (Ed.), *Cancer treatment* (3rd ed.) (pp. 123–164). Philadelphia: W.B. Saunders Company.

Henson, J.W., & Posner, J.B. (1993). Neurological complications. In J.F. Holland, E. Frei, R.C. Bast, D.W. Kufe, D.L. Morton, & R.W. Weischselbaum (Eds.), *Cancer medicine* (3rd ed.) (pp. 2268–2286). Philadelphia: Lea & Febiger.

Hunter, J.C. (1992). Nursing care of patients with structural oncological emergencies. In J.C. Clark & R.F. McGee (Eds.), *Core curriculum for oncology nursing* (pp. 156–168), Philadelphia: W.B. Saunders.

Inagaki, J., Rodriguez, V., & Bodey, G.P. (1974). Causes of death in cancer patients. *Cancer, 33*(2), 568–573.

Knobf, M.T. (1991). Breast cancer. In S.B. Baird, R. McCorkle, & M. Grant (Eds.), *Cancer nursing* (pp. 425–451). Philadelphia: W.B. Saunders.

Martin, L.K., & Braly, P.S. (1991). Gynecologic cancers. In S.B. Baird, R. McCorkle, & M. Grant (Eds.), *Cancer nursing* (pp. 502–535). Philadelphia: W.B. Saunders.

Otte, D.M. (1990). Gynecologic cancers. In S.L. Groenwald, M.H. Frogge, M. Goodman, & C.H. Yarbro (Eds.), *Cancer nursing: Principles and Practice* (3rd ed.) (pp. 845–888). Boston: Jones and Bartlett Publishers.

Piemme, J.A. (1988). Secondary primary or metastatic cancer. In S.B. Baird (Ed.) *Decision making in oncology nursing* (pp. 20–23). Philadelphia: B.C. Decker.

Scanlon, E.F. (1991). Breast cancer. In A.I. Holleb, D.J. Fink, & G.P. Murphy (Eds.), *Clinical oncology* (pp. 177–193). Atlanta: American Cancer Society.

Stillman, M.J. (1990). Perineal pain. In K.M. Foley, J.J. Bonica, & V. Ventafridda (Eds.), *Advances in pain research and therapy, Volume 16: Proceedings of the Second International Congress on Cancer Pain.* (pp. 359–377). New York: Raven Press.

Wachtel, T., Allen-Masterson, S. Reuben, D. Goldberg, R, & Mor, V. (1988). The end stage cancer patient: Terminal common pathway. *The Hospice Journal, 4*(4), 43–80.

Weiss, L. (1992). Comments on hematogenous metastatic patterns in humans as revealed by autopsy. *Clinical and Experimental Metastasis, 10*(3), 191–199.

Gastrointestinal Cancer (Colorectal, Stomach, Esophageal, and Oral): Metastatic Spread/ Common Symptoms

Colorectal Cancer

Colorectal cancer is the second leading cause of cancer death in women and men. It occurs about equally in women and men, with total estimated 1992 deaths from colon cancer at 51,000, and from rectum cancer at 7,300 (American Cancer Society [ACS], 1992).

More than 60% of primary colon tumors are in the left or descending colon (Steele, Tepper, Motwani, & Bruckner, 1993). The most common tumor type found in the colon is adenocarcinoma; carcinoid tumors are commonly found in the appendix and rectum (carcinoid tumors are also common in the small bowel [Haskell & Guiliano, 1990]), and epidermoid or cloagenic tumors are commonly found in the anus (Beart, 1991). Metastatic spread is primarily to regional lymph (perineal, inguinal, retroperitoneal). Distal sites are primarily liver, lung, and bone

(Beart, 1991), with liver metastases nearly always preceding, and in fact "cascading" to lung (Weiss, 1992, p. 196). Adjacent structures may also be invaded, causing such problems as recto-vaginal fistulas (Boarini, 1990).

Many patients with colorectal cancer have a colostomy, and the combination of colostomy with attendant management problems, cachexia, and other processes of advanced cancer result in significant challenges in care. With or without a colostomy, bowel problems are common (Wachtel, Allen-Masterson, Reuben, Goldberg, & Mor, 1988). Bowel obstruction is most common with tumors of the descending and sigmoid colon (Strohl, 1992). Patients with colorectal cancer tend to experience less pain than do those with other primary tumors, except for brain. Yet more than 50% of patients with colorectal cancer experience pain, dyspnea, and nausea; and 80%-90% experience anorexia and weight loss (Wachtel et al., 1988). A significant number of patients with colorectal cancer develop widespread pelvic metastases to pelvic organs and nerve plexi. From this, a very difficult to manage mix of neuropathic, visceral, and somatic perineal pain may develop (Stillman, 1990).

The systemic effects of carcinoid tumors usually occur only when there is liver metastases. Symptoms, which vary according to tumor site, include flushing, diarrhea, bronchoconstrictions, and cardiac lesions (Haskell & Giuliano, 1990).

Most patients with colorectal cancer die from infections, such as, in descending order, septicemia, pneumonia, and peritonitis; and patients with colorectal cancer are more likely to die from hemorrhage than are any others (Inagaki, Rodriguez, & Bodey, 1974).

The *oncologic emergency* most often associated with colorectal tumors is **obstructive uropathy** (Glover & Glick, 1991). Some authors, e.g., Miaskowski (1991), classify bowel obstruction as an oncologic emergency. Many others do not. Bowel obstruction and other problems associated with colorectal tumors are discussed in chapter.

The spread, problems, and assessments associated with colorectal cancer are illustrated in Table 24.1.

Stomach Cancer

Stomach, or gastric, cancer is the eighth leading cause of cancer death in women and men. It occurs more often in men than in women (8:5) with 13,300 total estimated 1992 deaths (ACS, 1992).

Most stomach cancers are adenocarcinomas. Metastasis is primarily through the lymphatic system, but also directly through the stomach wall to adjacent organs (liver, pancreas, intestine, and others) or mesentery, via blood, and direct seeding of the peritoneum (Frogge, 1990). Bone and brain metastases may also occur (Weiss, 1992). The stomach is also sometimes (< 10%) the "primary and only site" for lymphoma (Lawrence, 1991, p. 246).

The major problems of stomach cancer are usually directly related to the primary tumor, and include sometimes severe abdominal pain, pain after eating, nausea and vomiting, belching, early satiety, regurgitation, dysphagia, and dyspepsia (Ehlke, 1990). Anemia, weakness, and fatigue are common (Frogge, 1990). Cachexia is common in advanced disease. Other problems of advanced disease include peritoneal and pleural effusions, high obstruction (stomach to small bowel), bleeding, and jaundice (Bruckner & Kondo, 1993). The types of paraneoplastic syndromes associated with stomach cancer include skin, central nervous system, thrombophlebitis, and hormone syndromes, e.g., Cushing's syndrome (Haskell, Selch, & Ramming, 1990b).

Causes of death are often pneumonia or lung abscess, due at least in part to immobility and malnutrition. Other causes are often related to similar effects of the cancer (Frogge, 1990).

The *oncologic emergencies* most often associated with stomach cancer are **increased intracranial pressure** and **cardiac tamponade** (Finley, 1992).

The spread, problems, and assessments associated with stomach cancer are illustrated in Table 24.2.

Esophageal Cancer

Carcinoma of the esophagus is the 14th leading cause of cancer death overall, with a male to female ratio of 3:1. The total estimated 1992 deaths from carcinoma of the esophagus is 10,000 (ACS, 1992).

The most common tumor types are squamous cell in the body of the esophagus and, increasingly, adenocarcinoma at the esophagogastric junction (Haskell, Selch, & Ramming, 1990a). These may take different forms, including malignant ulcer, circumferential stricture, or mass within the esophageal lumen (Skinner & Skinner, 1993). These are also described as ulcer-

TABLE 24.1

COLORECTAL CANCER: SPREAD, PROBLEMS, AND ASSESSMENT

Metastatic spread	Problems	Assessment parameters
Colon, regional structures	Obstruction	Intestinal obstruction: Pain (colic), nausea and vomiting, diarrhea (see section on obstruction in chapter 17)
	Constipation	May or may not be related to obstruction
Anorexia	Nausea and vomiting, anorexia	May or may not be related to obstruction
Regional lymph and structures	Lymphadeno-pathy	Lymphedema: Enlarged lymph, edema (area or lower extremities); pain; cellulitis, lymphangitis
	Obstructive uropathy	Especially from rectal tumors causing ureteral **obstruction:** hesitancy, urgency, nocturia, frequency, < force of stream, polyuria alternating with oliguria
		Fistulas
	Perineal pain	Severe pain, most often neuropathic, but also mixed neuropathic with visceral and/or somatic
Liver	Pain	Pain may be upper right abdominal or non-specific and characteristic of visceral pain; may radiate to scapula, be worse at night
	Ascites	Abdominal distension, bulging flanks, fluid wave, weight gain, and discomfort; anorexia, early satiety, indigestion, decreased bowel mobility; dyspnea, orthopnea, and tachypnea; weakness and fatigue; changes in color of urine, stool; pruritus
Lung(s)	Dyspnea, cough, hemoptysis	(See Table 22.1) Pleural effusion, pneumonia, **embolus, obstruction,** preexisting conditions, ascites may also contribute to dyspnea
Bone	Pain	Pain is usually localized to some extent; pain may be from other processes
		Spinal cord compression: Back pain may be local (somatic: Constant, dull, aching) or radicular or both; exacerbated by movement, neck flexion, straight leg raising; decreased by sitting up; tender to percussion. Neurological deficits begin subtly and not necessarily apparent to the patient: Weakness, ataxia, stumbling; urine retention, bowel dysfunction, impotence, numbness
Other	Various problems	Problems of therapy, e.g., opioids, corticosteroids, antidepressants, radiation, chemotherapy
		Skin integrity may be a major challenge if colostomy present
		Fever of unknown origin is common with liver involvement
		Infection is the most frequent cause of death; hemorrhage is more common than with other tumors

TABLE 24.2

STOMACH CANCER: SPREAD, PROBLEMS, AND ASSESSMENT

Metastatic spread	Problems	Assessment parameters
Primary tumor growth and regional spread	GI disturbances, anemai	Abdominal pain; pain after eating, dyspepsia; nausea and vomiting; belching, regurgitation; early satiety; dysphagia; diarrhea; stomach/ small bowel obstruction; cachexia; peritoneal effusions; weakness, fatigue; headache, tachypnea
Liver	Pain	Pain typically upper right abdominal or non-specific, characteristic of visceral pain; pain may radiate to right scapula and worsen at night
	Ascites	Abdominal distension, bulging flanks, fluid wave, weight gain, and discomfort; anorexia, early satiety, indigestion, < bowel mobility; dyspnea, orthopnea, tachypnea; weakness, fatigue; changes in color of urine, stool; pruritus
Regional lymph and structures	Lymphadeno-pathy	Lymphedema: Enlarged lymph, edema, obstruction adjacent organs (see obstructive uropathy in chapter 18) or structures, pain; cellulitis, lymphangitis
Lung(s)	Dyspnea, cough, hemoptysis	(See Table 22.1): Pleural effusion, pneumonia, **embolus, obstruction,** preexisting conditions, ascites; see chapters 14 and 22 for other pulmonary problems
Bone	Pain	Pain is usually localized to at least some extent. **Spinal cord compression** from pathologic fractures of the spine is possible. Pain may be associated with other processes
Brain	CNS symptoms	**Increased intracranial pressure:** Pain usually present, may be more severe in the morning; progressive neurological deficits (motor, sensory, cognitive); nausea, vomiting (see more complete discussion in chapter 13)
		Confusion: See chapter 13
		Seizures: See chapter 13
Other	Various problems	Problems of therapy, e.g., opioids, corticosteroids, tricyclic antidepressants, radiation, chemotherapy
		Pericardial effusion → Tamponade: retrosternal chest pain relieved by sitting forward; orthopnea; cough; tachypnea; tachycardia; decreased cardiac output (< cerebral blood, peripheral cyanosis, < systolic and pulse pressures, and pulsus paradoxus (weaker during inspiration)); occasional nausea and vomiting and abdominal pain
		Skin: Acanthosis nigricans, dermatomyositis, circinate erythemas, pemphigoid
		CNS: Dementia, cerebellar ataxia
		Thrombophlebitis
		Ectopic hormone syndromes, e.g., Cushing's syndrome

ative, infiltrating, and fungating (Frogge, 1990). Carcinoma of the upper (cervical) esophagus may spread by invasion of adjacent structures, including carotid arteries, pleura, recurrent laryngeal nerves, trachea, and larynx. Tumors of the middle (thoracic) esophagus may spread to the left main stem bronchus, pleura, and related structures. Tumors of the lower esophagus can invade the pericardium, aorta, diaphragm, and phrenic nerve. Lymphatic spread follows patterns similar to direct spread, with tumors of the thoracic esophagus often spreading to mediastinal and other nodes (Frogge, 1990; Haskell et al., 1990a). Hematogenous spread is commonly to liver, lungs, bone, and kidney. Brain metastases occurs in almost 20% of patients (Haskell et al., 1990a; Weiss, 1992).

The primary problem of carcinoma of the esophagus is dysphagia, which requires 90% tumor involvement (Skinner & Skinner, 1993). Dysphagia generally begins with solids, progresses to liquids, and even to saliva. Odynophagia (Painful swallowing) is present in about 50% of patients. Dysphagia leads to at least two major problems: (1) malnutrition, weight loss, and eventually cachexia; and (2) aspiration pneumonia from food spilling over. A chronic cough may point to aspiration, or a "cough-swallow sequence" (Frogge, 1990, p. 810) may point to tracheo-esophageal fistula. Hoarseness indicates laryngeal nerve involvement. Chronic hiccups and paralysis of the arm or diaphragm often indicate phrenic nerve involvement. Hemoptysis may be from an ulcerative tumor or may indicate aortic involvement. Patients with fever should be evaluated for pneumonia. Pain can arise from the primary tumor, especially if ulcerative, or from invasive or metastatic extension. (Ehlke, 1991 Frogge, 1990; Haskell et al., 1990a). Metastases to liver, lungs, bone, and brain can result in a variety of pain syndromes. Pain in the ear indicates pharyngeal metastases (Calcaterra & Juillard, 1990).

Palliative care may include surgical by-pass, esophagectomy, or intubation of an endoprosthesis (Skinner & Skinner, 1993). Prevention of complications from endoprosthesis insertion is extremely important (Frogge, 1990), and is discussed in the section on dysphagia in chapter 17.

Death commonly occurs from pneumonia; about 50% of patients have bronchial pneumonia, related to aspiration or cachexia (Ehlke, 1991).

The *oncologic emergencies* typically associated with carcinoma of the esophagus include **hypercalcemia** (25%), **superior vena cava syndrome, tracheal obstruction** and **increased intracranial pressure.** Invasion of the aorta or carotid arteries may result in massive hemorrhage (Frogge, 1990; Haskell et al., 1990a).

The spread, problems, and assessments associated with esophageal cancer are illustrated in Table 24.3.

Oral Cancer

Oral cancer is the 17th leading cause of cancer death in women and men. About twice as many men as women die from oral cancer, but the percentage of women is increasing. The total estimated 1992 deaths from oral cancer was 7,950 (ACS, 1992; Norris & Cady, 1991).

Most fatal oral cavity tumors are in the pharynx, followed by the mouth, tongue, and a very few on the lips (ACS, 1992, p. 5). The most common tumor type is squamous cell carcinoma (SCC) (Norris & Cady, 1991). Tumor spread is primarily by regional submucosal extension and, (especially when the primary tumor is deeper into the oropharynx) also by regional (especially cervical) nodes (Reese, 1991; Wolf, Lippman, Laramore, & Hong, 1993). Local invasion can include bone, nerves, and muscle, as well as submucosa and area structures, such as the tongue or soft tissue of the neck (Norris & Cady, 1991), where malignant ulceration may occur. Distant metastases via lymph also

TABLE 24.3

Metastatic spread	Problems	Assessment parameters
Primary tumor growth, regional extension	< lumen esophagus	Dysphagia: Inability to swallow solids, liquids, saliva; odynophagia
		Cachexia, weight loss
		Aspiration pneumonia from food spill-over
		Chronic cough; cough-swallow sequence from tracheo-esophageal fistula
		Hoarseness from laryngeal nerve involvement
		Chronic hiccups, paralysis arm and/or diaphragm from phrenic nerve involvement
	Pain	Pain: related to the above
	Bleeding	Hemorrhage from carotid artery or aorta involvement
		Hemoptysis from ulcerative primary tumor
		Superior vena cava syndrome: dilated neck or thoracic veins; facial edema; tachypnea; facial plethora; cyanosis; edema upper extremities; cough, hoarseness
Lung(s), pleura (regional extension or metastases)	Dyspnea, other pulmonary problems	(See Table 22.1): pleural effusion, pneumonia, embolus
		Obstruction: rapidly progressive dyspnea; hemoptysis; chronic cough; wheezing, stridor; aspiration; pneumonia
Liver	Pain	Pain may be upper right abdominal or non-specific, characteristic of visceral pain; may radiate to right scapula and worsen at night
		Abdominal distension, bulging flanks, fluid wave, weight gain, and discomfort; anorexia, early satiety, indigestion, < bowel mobility; dyspnea, orthopnea, tachypnea; weakness, fatigue; changes in color of urine, stool; pruritus
Bone	Pain	Pain is usually localized to at least some extent; **spinal cord compression** is possible; pain may be associated with other processes
	Metabolic changes	**Hypercalcemia:** (Often non-specific) symptoms include fatigue, polyuria, polydipsia, and constipation; progressing to changes in mentation, seizures, and coma
Brain	CNS symptoms	**Increased intracranial pressure** rare: Pain usually present, may be more severe in the morning; progressive neurological deficits (motor, sensory, cognitive); nausea, vomiting (see more complete discussion in chapter 13)
		Confusion: See chapter 13
		Seizures: See chapter 13
Other	Various problems	Problems of therapy e.g., opioids, corticosteroids, tricyclic antidepressants, radiation, chemotherapy

TABLE 24.4
ORAL CANCER: SPREAD, PROBLEMS, AND ASSESSMENT

Metastatic spread	Problems	Assessment parameters
Regional extension and associated damage	Pain	Pain may be neuropathic or mixed, and may result from the cancer or treatment
		Aching pain in the shoulder and neck following radical neck surgery may be significantly relieved by sling support and nerve blocks
		Deep ear pain and/or odynophagia may occur
	Dysphagia	Dysphagia may be complicated by paralysis of the tongue or other neurological complications involving swallowing, the lips, and area sensory function; as well as chronic aspiration or nasal regurgitation. Altered nutrition is common
	Chronic aspiration	Chronic aspiration results in frequent choking; and may result in pneumonia; reluctance to take fluids results in dehydration
	Tumor necrosis	Tumor necrosis, especially deep tumors, results in foul odor and taste; malignant ulceration occurs
		External (fungating) tumors present problems of pain, odor, and appearance
	Communication deficits	Communication difficulties may include hearing, vision, and speaking changes
		Hemorrhage is not uncommon. The complex of blood vessels (and nerves) found in the oropharynx and neck are subject to tumor extension and subsequent destruction of structures
Other	Various problems	Problems of therapy, e.g., opioids, corticosteroids, tricyclic antidepressants, radiation, chemotherapy
	Metabolic changes	**Hypercalcemia:** (Often non-specific) symptoms include fatigue, weakness, anorexia, nausea, polyuria, polydipsia and constipation; progressing to changes in mentation, seizures, and coma

occurs, but only in < 15% of patients with terminal disease (Wolf et al., 1993).

The problems of advanced oral cancer are classified according to the areas or structures involved, and may include pain, dysphagia, hearing loss, vision changes, difficulty speaking, trismus (trigeminal nerve dysfunction causing spasms of the masticatory muscles, resulting in lockjaw), chronic nasal regurgitation, chronic aspiration, shoulder weakness, odor (from tumor necrosis), and problems secondary to treatment (Goodman, 1990; Reese, 1991; Wolf et al., 1993). Treatment often involves surgery and radiation. Surgery, especially radical dissection, frequently results in both physical and psychosocial problems

(Goodman, 1990; Reese, 1991). Among the physical problems of surgery are neuropathic pain and dysfunction of affected sensory and motor innervation (Foley, 1991). The end results of many of the problems of oral cancer are malnutrition, and at least the potential for ineffective breathing.

Hypercalcemia is the only oncology emergency typically associated with oral cancer. Hemorrhage occurs in some cases.

The spread, problems, and assessments associated with oral cancer are illustrated in Table 24.4.

References

American Cancer Society. (1992). Cancer facts and figures—1992. Atlanta: Author.

Beart, R.W. (1991), Colorectal cancer. In A.I. Holleb, D.J. Fink, & G.P. Murphy (Eds.), *Clinical oncology* (pp. 213-218). Atlanta: American Cancer Society.

Boarini, J. 1990). Gastrointestinal cancer: Colon, rectum, and anus. In S.L. Groenwald, M.H. Frogge, M. Goodman, & C.H. Yarbro (Eds.), *Cancer nursing: Principles and practice* (3rd ed.) (pp. 792-805). Boston: Jones and Bartlett Publishers.

Bruckner, H.W., & Kondo, T. (1993). Neoplasms of the stomach. In J.F. Holland, E. Frei, R.C. Bast, D.W. Kufe, D.L. Morton, & R.W. Weischselbaum (Eds.), *Cancer medicine* (3rd ed.) (pp. 1395-1430). Philadelphia: Lea & Febiger.

Calcaterra, T.C., & Juillard, G.J.F. (1990). Head and neck neoplasms: Larynx and hypopharynx. In C.M. Haskell (Ed.), *Cancer treatment* (3rd ed.) (pp. 389-395). Philadelphia: W.B. Saunders Company.

Ehlke, G. (1991). Gastrointestinal cancers. In S.B. Baird, R. McCorkle, & M. Grant (Eds.), *Cancer nursing* (pp. 485-501). Philadelphia: W.B. Saunders.

Finley, J.P. (1992). Nursing care of patients with metabolic and physiological oncological emergencies. In J.C. Clark & R.F. McGee (Eds.), *Core curriculum for oncology nursing* (pp. 169-192), Philadelphia: W.B. Saunders.

Foley, K.M. (1991). Diagnosis and treatment of cancer pain. In A.I. Holleb, D.J. Fink, & G.P. Murphy (Eds.), *Clinical oncology* (pp. 555-575). Atlanta: American Cancer Society.

Frogge, M.H. (1990). Gastrointestinal cancer: Esophagus, stomach, liver, and pancreas. In S.L. Groenwald, M.H. Frogge, M. Goodman, & C.H. Yarbro (Eds.), *Cancer nursing: Principles and ractice* (3rd ed.) (pp. 806-844). Boston: Jones and Bartlett Publishers.

Glover, D., & Glick, J.H. (1991). Oncologic emergencies.

In A.I. Holleb, D.J. Fink, & G.P. Murphy (Eds.), *Clinical oncology* (pp. 513-533). Atlanta: American Cancer Society.

Goodman, M. (1990). Head and neck cancer. In S.L. Groenwald, M.H. Frogge, M. Goodman, & C.H. Yarbro (Eds.), *Cancer nursing: Principles and practice* (3rd ed.) (pp. 889-929). Boston: Jones and Bartlett Publishers.

Haskell, C.M., & Giuliano, A.E. (1990). Carcinoid tumors. In C.M. Haskell (Ed.), *Cancer treatment* (3rd ed.) (pp. 418-426). Philadelphia: W.B. Saunders.

Haskell, C.M., Selch, M.T., & Ramming, K.P. (1990). Gastrointestinal neoplasms: Esophagus. In C.M. Haskell (Ed.), *Cancer treatment* (3rd ed.) (pp. 207-217). Philadelphia: W.B. Saunders Company.

Haskell, C.M., Selch, M.T., & Ramming, K.P. (1990). Gastrointestinal neoplasms: Stomach. In C.M. Haskell (Ed.), *Cancer treatment* (3rd ed.) (pp. 217-229). Philadelphia: W.B. Saunders Company.

Inagaki, J., Rodriguez, V., & Bodey, G.P. (1974). Causes of death in cancer patients. *Cancer, 33*(2), 568-573.

Lawrence, W. (1991). Gastric neoplasms. In A.I. Holleb, D.J. Fink, & G.P. Murphy (Eds.), *Clinical oncology* (pp. 245-253). Atlanta: American Cancer Society.

Miaskowski, C. (1991). Oncologic emergencies. In S.B. Baird, R. McCorkle, & M. Grant (Eds.), *Cancer nursing* (pp. 885-893). Philadelphia: W.B Saunders.

Norris, C.M., & Cady, B. (1991). Head, neck, and thyroid cancer. In A.I. Holleb, D.J. Fink, & G.P. Murphy (Eds.), *Clinical oncology* (pp. 306-328). Atlanta: American Cancer Society.

Reese, J.L. (1991). Head and neck cancers. In S.B. Baird, R. McCorkle, & M. Grant (Eds.), *Cancer nursing* (pp. 567-583) Philadelphia: W.B. Saunders.

Skinner, D.B., & Skinner, K.A. (1993). Neoplasms of the esophagus. In J.F. Holland, E. Frei, R.C. Bast, D.W. Kufe, D.L. Morton, & R.W. Weischselbaum (Eds.), *Cancer medicine* (3rd ed.) (pp. 1382-1394). Philadelphia: Lea & Febiger.

Steele, G., Tepper, J., Motwani, B.T., & Bruckner, H.W. (1993). Adenocarcinoma of the colon and rectum. In J.F. Holland, E. Frei, R.C. Bast, D.W. Kufe, D.L. Morton, & R.W. Weischselbaum (Eds.), *Cancer medicine* (3rd ed.) (pp. 1493-1522). Philadelphia: Lea & Febiger.

Stillman, M.J. (1990). Perineal pain. In K.M. Foley, J.J. Bonica, & V. Ventafridda (Eds.), *Advances in pain research and therapy, Volume 16: Proceedings of the Second International Congress on Cancer Pain.* (pp. 359-377). New York: Raven Press.

Strohl, R.A. (1992). Colorectal cancers. In J.C. Clark & R.F. McGee (Eds.), *Core curriculum for oncology nursing* (pp. 470-479), Philadelphia: W.B. Saunders.

Wachtel, T., Allen-Masterson, S., Reuben, D. Goldberg, R, & Mor, V. (1988). The end stage cancer patient: Terminal common pathway. *The Hospice Journal, 4*(4), 43-80.

Weiss, L. (1992). Comments on hematogenous metastatic patterns in humans as revealed by autopsy. *Clin-*

ical and experimental metastasis, 10(3), 191-199.

Wolf, G.T., Lippman, S.M., Laramore, G.E., & Hong, W.K. (1993). Head and neck cancer. In J.F. Holland, E. Frei, R.C. Bast, D.W. Kufe, D.L. Morton, & R.W. Weischselbaum (Eds.), *Cancer medicine* (3rd ed.) (pp. 1211-1275). Philadelphia: Lea & Febiger.

Urinary Tract Cancer (Renal and Other Urinary Cancers and Bladder and Prostate Cancers): Metastatic Spread/Common Symptoms

Renal and Other Urinary Cancers

Renal and other urinary cancers, excepting bladder, are the twelfth leading cause of cancer death overall, with total estimated 1992 deaths of 10,700. They affect about twice as many men as women (ACS, 1992).

Renal cell carcinoma, usually adenocarcinomas, is the most common tumor type (Richie, 1993). Spread is via blood to liver, lungs, and bones, and also via lymph (Lind & Nakao, 1990). The contralateral kidney and ipsilateral adrenal gland may also be affected (Richie, 1993) and uremia often occurs. Metastases to the heart is found in almost 15% of patients with renal cancer (Weiss, 1992).

Problems include those common to metastatic disease in liver, lungs, and bones. Flank pain, abdominal mass, and hematuria are the "classic triad" of renal carcinoma symptoms. Anemia and weight loss are very common in advanced disease. Liver dysfunction in the absence of hepatic involvement also occurs (Lind & Irwin, 1991; Neuwirth, Figlin, & deKernion, 1990). Paraneoplastic syndromes are sometimes associated with renal cancer. These include hypercalcemia and parathyroid-like hormone production (related to Cushing's syndrome) (Lind & Nakao, 1990). Increased erythrocyte sedimentation rate, anemia, hypertension, and cachexia are common (> 30%) and fever of unknown origin also occurs (Richie, 1993).

Oncologic emergencies associated with renal cancers include **increased intracranial pressure, spinal cord compression, bronchial obstruction, ureteral obstruction,** and **hypercalcemia** (Glover & Glick, 1991; Hunter, 1992; Richie & Kantoff, 1993).

The spread, problems, and assessments associated with renal cancer are illustrated in Table 25.1.

Charles Kemp: TERMINAL ILLNESS: A GUIDE TO NURSING CARE. © 1995 J. B. Lippincott.

TABLE 25.1
RENAL CANCER: SPREAD, PROBLEMS, AND ASSESSMENT

Metastatic spread	Problems	Assessment parameters
Kidney		Weakness, anemia; anorexia; "classic triad": Flank pain, abdominal mass, hematuria
	Uremia	< urine, changes blood pressure, CHF, stomatitis, nausea and vomiting, GI bleeding, bowel changes, lethargy, changes mentation
Liver	Pain	Pain may be upper right abdominal or non-specific and characteristic of visceral pain; pain may radiate to the right scapula and worsen at night
	Ascites	Abdominal distension, bulging flanks, fluid wave, weight gain, and discomfort; anorexia, early satiety, indigestion, decreased bowel mobility (potential for obstruction); dyspnea, orthopnea, and tachypnea; weakness and fatigue; change in color of urine, stool; pruritus
Lung(s)	Dyspnea, other pulmonary symptoms	(See Table 22.1): **obstruction,** pleural effusion, pneumonia, embolus, preexisting conditions, ascites; (also see pericardial effusion (also see chapters 14 and 22)
Bone	Pain	Pain is usually localized to at least some extent, especially with metastases to bony thorax. Back pain may indicate spinal cord compression (see below and discussion in chapter 13). Pathologic fractures other than spine are possible. Pain may be associated with other processes
		Spinal cord compression: Back pain may be local (somatic: Constant, dull, aching) or radicular or both; exacerbated by movement, neck flexion, straight leg raising; decreased by sitting up; tender to percussion. Neurological deficits begin subtly and may not be apparent to the patient: Weakness, ataxia, stumbling; urine retention (frequent, small voiding); bowel dysfunction, impotence; numbness

(cont'd.)

Bladder Cancer

Bladder cancer is the 15th leading cause of cancer death overall, with total estimated 1992 deaths of 9,500, and affecting about twice as many men as women (ACS, 1992).

More than 90% of bladder cancers are transitional cell carcinoma (from the epithelium), and most of the remainder are squamous cell (Lind, 1992). Invasion of the bladder muscle and beyond is common, and metastases are most frequently found in regional lymph nodes, other lymph, followed by liver, lung, and bone (Lind, 1992; Macfarlane, Figlin, & deKernion, 1993). Weiss (1992) reports that the adrenal gland is a common site (> 34%), as is the kidney(s) (> 18%).

Extension to pelvic nerve plexi and other

TABLE 25.1 *(CONT'D.)*		
Metastatic spread	**Problems**	**Assessment parameters**
	Metabolic changes	**Hypercalcemia:** (Often non-specific) symptoms include fatigue, weakness, anorexia, nausea, polyuria, polydipsia, and constipation; progressing to changes in mentation, seizures, and coma
		See paraneoplastic syndromes below
Brain	CNS symptoms	**Increased intracranial pressure:** Pain usually present, may be more severe in the morning; progressive neurological deficits (motor, sensory, cognitive); nausea, vomiting (see more complete discussion in chapter 13)
Paraneoplastic syndromes		Hypercalcemia; parathyroid-like hormone production (similar to Cushing's syndrome); and coma
Regional lymph and structures	Lymphadenopathy	Lymphedema: Enlarged lymph, edema, pain; cellulitis, lymphangitis
Other	Various problems	Problems of therapy, e.g., opioids, corticosteroids, tricyclic antidepressants, radiation, chemotherapy
		Fever of unknown origin

structures can result in mixed somatic, visceral, and neuropathic perineal pain—a "formidable challenge" of management (Stillman, 1990, p. 364). Spread to adjacent structures, such as sigmoid colon, rectum, prostate, or vagina (Lind, 1992) can create major problems in hygiene and care. Elimination problems are prominent, and include "irritable bladder" (dysuria, frequency, urgency) and hematuria (Lind & Irwin, 1991). Uremia may also occur. Obstruction may occur at the bladder neck (low) or ureter (high) (Lind & Nakao, 1990). Gross hematuria may occur, and can be controlled with the instillation of formalin (Neuwirth, Figlin, & deKernion, 1990).

The *oncologic emergency* most commonly associated with bladder cancers is **obstructive uropathy** (Glover & Glick, 1991; Lind, 1992).

The spread, problems, and assessments associated with bladder cancer are illustrated in Table 25.2.

Prostate Cancer

Prostate cancer is the second leading cause of cancer death among men (34,000 estimated deaths in1992) and the fourth leading cause of cancer death overall (ACS, 1992). The incidence of prostate cancer surpasses that of lung cancer in men, and is expected to continue to increase as the population ages (Martin, 1990).

By far the most common site (almost 70% on autopsy) of metastases is bone (Weiss, 1992). Lymph (pelvic, abdominal, and thoracic), adjacent structures, adrenals, kidneys, lungs, liver, and other sites may also be involved (Neuwirth & deKernion, 1990; Piemme, 1988; Trump & Robertson, 1993).

In the National Hospice Study, patients with prostate and breast cancer reported a higher incidence of pain than did any others. The increased pain can be attributed to the high incidence of bone metastases (Wachtel, Allen-

TABLE 25.2
BLADDER CANCER: SPREAD, PROBLEMS, AND ASSESSMENT

Metastatic spread	Problems	Assessment parameters
Primary tumor growth and regional spread via extension and/or seeding	Perineal pain	Severe pain: Most often neuropathic, but also mixed neuropathic with visceral and/or somatic
	Pelvic structure involvement	Fistulas: Perirectal, rectovaginal, and others
		Vaginal tumors: Fungating, ulcerative, or invasive
		Abdominal pain
	Obstruction	Intestinal obstruction: Nausea and vomiting, intestinal colic, other abdominal pain, diarrhea; constipation
		Obstructive uropathy (ureteral): hesitancy, urgency, nocturia, frequency, < force of stream, polyuria alternating with oliguria
	Other elimination problems	Irritable bladder: Dysuria, frequency, urgency; incontinence; retention; hematuria
	Lymphadenopathy	Lymphedema: Enlarged lymph, edema (area or lower extremities), pain, cellulitis, lymphangitis. Extensive pelvic disease can result in neurologic impairment and/or urinary dysfunction
Liver	Pain	Pain may be upper right abdominal or non-specific, characteristic of visceral pain; may radiate to right scapula and worsen at night
	Ascites	Abdominal distension, bulging flanks, fluid wave, weight gain, and discomfort; anorexia, early satiety, indigestion, < bowel mobility; dyspnea, orthopnea, tachypnea; weakness, fatigue; changes in color of urine and stool; pruritus
Lung(s)	Dyspnea, other pulmonary symptoms	(See Table 22.1) **Pleural effusion, pneumonia, embolus, obstruction, preexisting conditions; ascites** may contribute to dyspnea (also see chapters 14 and 22)
Bone	Pain	Pain is usually localized to at least some extent. **Spinal cord compression** from pathologic fractures of the spine is possible. Pain may be associated with other processes
Kidneys	Anemia	Weakness, anorexia; also see "Obstruction," listed under "Problems," above.
	Uremia	< urine, changes blood pressure, CHF, stomatitis, nausea and vomiting, GI bleeding, bowel changes, lethargy, changes mentation
	Various problems	Problems of therapy, e.g., opioids, corticosteroids, tricyclic antidepressants, radiation, chemotherapy

TABLE 25.3
PROSTATE CANCER: SPREAD, PROBLEMS, AND ASSESSMENT

Metastatic spread	Problems	Assessment parameters
Bone	Pain	Pain is usually localized to some extent; pathologic fractures possible; pain may be from other processes
		Spinal Cord Compression: Back pain may be local (somatic: constant, dull, aching) or radicular or both; exacerbated by movement, neck flexion, straight leg raising; decreased by sitting up; tender to percussion. Neurological deficits begin subtly and not necessarily apparent to the patient: Weakness, ataxia, stumbling; urine retention, bowel dysfunction, impotence, numbness
Regional lymph, and other structures	Lymphaden-opathy	Lymphedema: Enlarged lymph, edema (area or lower extremities), pain, cellulitis, lymphangitis. Extensive pelvic disease can result in neurologic impairment and/or urinary dysfunction
	Obstruction	**Obstructive uropathy** (Ureteral): Hesitancy, urgency, nocturia, frequency, <decreased force of stream alternating with oliguria
	Perineal pain	Severe perineal pain, most often neuropathic with visceral and/or somatic aspects
Liver	Pain	Pain may be upper right abdominal or non-specific, characteristic of visceral pain; may radiate to right scapula and worsen at night
	Ascites	Abdominal distension, bulging flanks, fluid wave, weight gain, and discomfort; anorexia, early satiety, indigestion, < bowel mobility; dyspnea, orthopnea, tachypnea; weakness, fatigue; changes in color of urine, stool; pruritus
Lung(s)	Dyspnea, other pulmonary symptoms	(See Table 22.1) **obstruction; embolus;** pleural effusion; pneumonia; preexisting conditions; ascites may result in dyspnea; lymph metastases may be involved (also see chapters 14 and 22)
Kidneys	Anemia	Weakness, anorexia, headache, tachycardia, dyspnea
Other	Various problems	Problems of therapy, e.g., opioids, corticosteroids, tricyclic antidepressants, radiation, chemotherapy
		Disseminated intravascular coagulation
		Fever of unknown origin (common with liver involvement)

Masterson, Reuben, Goldberg, & Mor, 1988) and to lumbosacral invasion. Pelvic and related complications are common, and may include lower extremity edema from lymphadenopathy, urinary dysfunction (retention, dribbling, urgency, frequency, hematuria), and neurological impairment (Lind, 1992; Trump & Robertson, 1993) (Table 25.3). Anemia may also occur (Neuwirth & deKernion, 1990). While "virtually any complication of advanced malignancy can be seen in carcinoma of the prostate" (Trump & Robertson, 1993) patients "who die of metastatic prostate cancer often demonstrate excellent local control of the disease" (Frank, Graham, & Nabors, 1991, p. 283).

The *oncologic emergencies* most common in patients with prostate cancer are **spinal cord compression, obstructive uropathy, SIADH,** and **disseminated intravascular coagulation** (Finley, 1992; Trump & Robertson, 1993). Note that despite a very high incidence of bone metastases, hypercalcemia is not common.

The spread, problems, and assessments associated with prostate cancer are illustrated in Table 25.3.

References

American Cancer Society. (1992). Cancer facts and figures—1992. Atlanta: Author.

Finley, J.P. (1992). Nursing care of patients with metabolic and physiological oncological emergencies. In J.C. Clark and R.F. McGee (Eds.), *Core curriculum for oncology nursing* (pp. 169–192). Philadelphia: W.B. Saunders.

Frank, I.N., Graham, S.D., & Nabors, W.L. (1991). Urologic and male genital cancers. In A.I. Holleb, D.J. Fink, & G.P. Murphy (Eds.), *Clinical oncology* (pp. 271–289). Atlanta: American Cancer Society.

Glover, D., & Glick, J.H. (1991). Oncologic emergencies. In A.I. Holleb, D.J. Fink, & G.P. Murphy (Eds.), *Clinical oncology* (pp. 513–533). Atlanta: American Cancer Society.

Hunter, J.C. (1992). Nursing care of patients with structural oncological emergencies. In J.C. Clark & R.F. McGee (Eds.), *Core curriculum for oncology nursing* (pp. 156–168), Philadelphia: W.B. Saunders.

Lind, J.M. (1992). Genitourinary cancers. In J.C. Clark & R.F. McGee (Eds.), *Core curriculum for oncology nursing* (pp. 428–450), Philadelphia: W.B. Saunders.

Lind, J.M., & Irwin, R.J. (1991). Genitourinary cancers. In S.B. Baird, R. McCorkle, & M. Grant (Eds.), *Cancer nursing* (pp. 466–484) Philadelphia: W.B. Saunders.

Lind, J.M., & Nakao, S.L. (1990). Urologic and male genital cancers. In S.L. Groenwald, M.H. Frogge, M. Goodman, & C.H. Yarbro (Eds.), *Cancer nursing: Principles and practice* (3rd ed.) (pp. 1026–1073). Boston: Jones and Bartlett Publishers.

Macfarlane, T., Figlin, R.A., & deKernion, J.B. (1993). Neoplasms of the bladder. In J.F. Holland, E. Frei, R.C. Bast, D.W. Kufe, D.L. Morton, & R.W. Weischselbaum (Eds.), *Cancer medicine* (3rd ed.) (pp. 1546–1559). Philadelphia: Lea & Febiger.

Martin, J.P. (1990). Male cancer awareness: Impact of an employee education program. *Oncology Nursing Forum, 17*(1), 59–64.

Neuwirth, H., & deKernion, J.B. (1990). Genitourinary neoplasms: Prostate. In C.M. Haskell (Ed.), *Cancer treatment* (3rd ed.) (pp. 737–749). Philadelphia: W.B. Saunders Company.

Neuwirth, H., Figlin, R.A., & deKernion, J.B. (1990). Genitourinary neoplasms: Kidney. In C.M. Haskell (Ed.), *Cancer treatment* (3rd ed.) (pp. 769–778). Philadelphia: W.B. Saunders Company.

Piemme, J.A. (1988). Secondary primary or metastatic cancer. In S.B. Baird (Ed.) *Decision making in oncology nursing* (pp. 20–23). Philadelphia: B.C. Decker.

Richie, J.P. (1993). Renal cell carcinoma. In J.F. Holland, E. Frei, R.C. Bast, D.W. Kufe, D.L. Morton, & R.W. Weischselbaum (Eds.), *Cancer medicine* (3rd ed.) (pp. 1529–1538). Philadelphia: Lea & Febiger.

Richie, J.P., & Kantoff, P.W. (1993). Neoplasms of the renal pelvis and ureter. In J.F. Holland, E. Frei, R.C. Bast, D.W. Kufe, D.L. Morton, & R.W. Weischselbaum (Eds.), *Cancer medicine* (3rd ed.) (pp. 1539–1546). Philadelphia: Lea & Febiger.

Stillman, M.J. (1990). Perineal pain. In K.M. Foley, J.J. Bonica, & V. Ventafridda (Eds.), *Advances in pain research and therapy, Volume 16: Proceedings of the Second International Congress on Cancer Pain.* (pp. 359–377). New York: Raven Press.

Trump, D.L., & Robertson, C.N. (1993). Neoplasms of the prostate. In J.F. Holland, E. Frei, R.C. Bast, D.W. Kufe, D.L. Morton, & R.W. Weischselbaum (Eds.), *Cancer medicine* (3rd ed.) (pp. 1493–1522). Philadelphia: Lea & Febiger.

Wachtel, T., Allen-Masterson, S., Reuben, D., Goldberg, R., & Mor, V. (1988). The end stage cancer patient: Terminal common pathway. *The Hospice Journal, 4*(4), 43–80.

Weiss, L. (1992). Comments on hematogenous metastatic patterns in humans as revealed by autopsy. *Clinical and Experimental Metastasis, 10*(3), 191–199.

Blood/Lymph and Skin Cancer (Non-Hodgkin's Lymphoma, Leukemia, Multiple Myeloma, Melanoma): Metastatic Spread/Common Symptoms

Non-Hodgkin's Lymphoma

Non-Hodgkin's Lymphoma (NHL) is the fifth leading cause of cancer death for men and the seventh for women; and the sixth leading cause of cancer death overall (19,400 estimated deaths in 1992) (ACS, 1992). There is an increase in the number of patients with lymphoma secondary to acquired immune deficiency syndrome (Eyre & Farver, 1991).

Lymph involvement may be widespread, and in fact, the disease is often disseminated at diagnosis, including to extranodal sites (Sarna & Kagan, 1990). By the time curative treatment is exhausted, extranodal disease may appear virtually anywhere, including most commonly in bone marrow and liver (Freedman & Nadler, 1993), but also in gastrointestinal tract, head and neck, skin, and elsewhere (Carson & Callaghan, 1991; Sarna and Kagan, 1990). Many patients with NHL, especially those with AIDS, are immunosuppressed, hence susceptible to common and uncommon infections, including herpes zoster and *Pneumocystis carinii* pneumonia (Yarbro, 1990).

Death is usually from infection or hemorrhage, resulting from decreased bone marrow function (Yarbro, 1990).

The *oncologic emergencies* most common in patients with lymphoma are **superior vena cava syndrome** (NHL is the 2nd most likely cancer to cause SVCS), **spinal cord compression, ureteral obstruction,** and **increased intracranial pressure** (from carcinomatous meningitis), and **hyperuricemia** (Glover & Glick, 1991; Yarbro, 1990).

The spread, problems, and assessments associated with non-Hodgkin's lymphoma are illustrated in Table 26.1.

Charles Kemp: TERMINAL ILLNESS: A GUIDE TO NURSING CARE. © 1995 J. B. Lippincott.

TABLE 26.1
NON-HODGKIN'S LYMPHOMA: SPREAD, PROBLEMS, AND ASSESSMENT

Metastatic spread	Problems	Assessment parameters
Bone marrow	< bone marrow function	Immunosupression: increased infection Bleeding disorders
Liver	Pain	Pain may be upper right abdominal or non-specific and characteristic of visceral pain; pain may radiate to the right scapula and worsen at night
	Ascites	Abdominal distension, bulging flanks, fluid wave, weight gain, and discomfort; anorexia, indigestion, decreased bowel mobility; dyspnea, orthopnea, and tachypnea; weakness, fatigue; changes in color of urine and stool; pruritus
Lymph, often widespread	Lymphaden-opathy	Lymphedema: enlarged lymph, edema (area or lower extremities); pain; cellulitis, lymphangitis Dyspnea from lymphangitis carcinomatosis, pulmonary edema
	Obstruction	**Obstructive uropathy** (ureteral): ureteral obstruction: hesitancy, urgency, nocturia, frequency, < force of stream, polyuria alternating with oliguria
GI tract	GI disturbances	Diarrhea, constipation, abdominal pain; intestinal obstruction
Lung(s)	Dyspnea, cough, hemoptysis	(See Table 22.1) Pleural effusion, **embolus,** pneumonia, preexisting conditions, ascites; see lung (also see chapters 14 and 22) for other pulmonary problems; lymph metastases may be involved; dyspnea may occur without pulmonary involvement
Skin	Skin lesions	Pain, odor
Other	Various problems	**Superior vena cava syndrome:** Dilated neck or thoracic veins; facial edema, plethora; tachypnea; cyanosis; edema upper extremities; cough, hoarseness
		Spinal cord compression: Back pain may be local (somatic: constant, dull, aching) or radicular or both; exacerbated by movement, neck flexion, straight leg raising; decreased by sitting up; tender to percussion. Neurological deficits begin subtly and may not be apparent to the patient: Weakness, ataxia, stumbling; urine retention (frequent, small voiding); bowel dysfunction, impotence; numbness
		Increased intracranial pressure: Pain usually present, may be more severe in the morning; progressive neurological deficits (motor, sensory, cognitive); nausea, vomiting (see more complete discussion in chapter 13)
		Problems of therapy, e.g., opioids, corticosteroids, tricyclic antidepressants, radiation, chemotherapy
		Fever of unknown origin (common with liver involvement)

Leukemia

Leukemia is the seventh leading cause of cancer death in women and men, and is about evenly divided between the sexes in occurrence (ACS, 1992). Leukemia is the leading cause of death from cancer in children (Ransohoff, Koslow, & Cooper, 1991).

The most common types of leukemias in Western counties are acute lymphoblastic leukemia (ALL), acute myelogenous leukemia (AML), acute nonlymphocytic leukemia (ANLL), chronic lymphocytic leukemia (CLL), and chronic myelogenous leukemia (CML) (Carson & Callaghan, 1991; Mitus & Rosenthal, 1991). The ALL leukemia is the most common form of childhood leukemia (ACS, 1992). While all leukemias are similar in many respects, some differences also exist.

Infection, bleeding, fatigue, and pain are among the most serious and common problems of advanced leukemia. Infections may include perirectal abscess, pneumonia, septicemia, urinary tract infection, and cellulitis; infections may be viral or bacterial, and some may be opportunistic (Berenson & Gale, 1990; Foon, Champlin, & Gale, 1990). Because infection is generally associated with neutropenia, typical signs and symptoms may be absent; the first sign is usually fever (Wujcik, 1991). Anemia is almost universal (Berenson & Gale, 1991), and bleeding may be found in the skin, mucous membranes, and GI or GU tracts (Carson & Callaghan, 1991). Fatigue and weakness may be related to anemia or to other processes. The course of leukemia is most often slow with much treatment, and patients may thus be physically and emotionally exhausted by the end-stages. Bone or joint pain is common, and may resemble arthritic pain (Berenson & Gale, 1990). Headache or other neurologic changes may herald increased intracranial pressure (Wujcik, 1991; Mitus & Rosenthal, 1991).

Other problems found frequently in patients with leukemia are increased intracra-nial pressure, lymphadenopathy, abdominal pain, weight loss, and testicular swelling (Maguire-Eisen and Edmonds, 1992). Patients with advanced disease may also be liable to late effects of therapy, including cardiomyopathy (with congestive failure and pericarditis) and neuropsychiatric symptoms (Maguire-Eisen & Edmonds, 1992). Change in mentation, especially when accompanied by shortness of breath, may signal leukostasis—white blood cell clotting in microvasculature (Mitus & Rosenthal, 1991). CNS involvement is more common in patients with ALL (Schiffer, 1993).

The later stages of chronic myelogenous leukemia may be marked by the occurrence of "blast crisis," characterized by fever of unknown origin, increased anemia and thrombocytopenia, and decreased response to any therapy. A good response to therapy in a blast crisis may result in meningeal leukemia (Silver, 1993).

The *oncologic emergencies* most common in patients with leukemia are **increased intracranial pressure** (including from **cerebral hemorrhage** and **carcinomatosis meningitis**), **obstructive uropathy, cardiac tamponade, hyperuricemia, and hypercalcemia** (Finley, 1992; Glover & Glick, 1991; Mitus & Rosenthal, 1991; Wujcik, 1990).

The spread, problems, and assessments associated with leukemia are illustrated in Table 26.2.

Multiple Myeloma

Multiple myeloma (MM) is the 16th leading cause of cancer death for women and men, and occurrence is about equally divided between the two groups. Estimated 1992 deaths were 9,200 (ACS, 1992). MM occurs about twice as often in blacks as in whites (Lichtenstein & Berenson, 1990).

MM, along with Waldenström's macroglobulinemia and heavy chain disease, is a plasma cell dyscrasia. Proliferation of plasma cells occurs most commonly in bones, and also in

		TABLE 26.2
		LEUKEMIA: SPREAD, PROBLEMS, AND ASSESSMENT
Metastatic spread	**Problems**	**Assessment parameters**
Bone marrow dysfunction	Bleeding	Thrombocytopenia: Bleeding occurs in skin, mucus membranes, and GI or GU tracts
	Infection	Leukocytopenia, neutropenia: Signs and symptoms of infection may be absent; infections may be bacterial or viral; may include perirectal abscess, GI or GU tract, cellulitis, pneumonia, septicemia
		Fever of unknown origin
	Fatigue	Erythrocytopenia results in anemia: Weakness, fatigue, tachycardia, headache
Lymph	Lymphadenopathy	Lymphedema: Enlarged lymph, edema, obstruction adjacent organs (see "Obstructive uropathy," below, under "Assessment Parameters") or structures, pain; cellulitis, lymphangitis
Liver	Pain	Pain may be upper right abdominal or non-specific and characteristic of visceral pain; pain may radiate to the right scapula and worsen at night
	Ascites	Abdominal distension, bulging flanks, fluid wave, weight gain, and discomfort; anorexia, indigestion, decreased bowel mobility; dyspnea, orthopnea, and tachypnea; weakness, fatigue; changes in color of urine and stool; pruritus
GI tract	GI disturbances	Hemorrhage, ulceration, bleeding; abdominal pain

(cont'd.)

bone marrow and extraosseous sites, such as kidneys and heart (Bubley & Schnipper, 1991; Cook, 1990).

Bone pain, often extreme, is the most common problem of MM. Pathologic fractures are common, and may occur in the spine, ribs, skull, pelvis, and proximal long bones. Central nervous system involvement is primarily spinal cord compression. Hypercalcemia develops in 20%–40% of patients with MM. Hypercalcemia and bone pain may become synergistic with pain and/or pathological fractures, leading to immobility, with immobility leading to hypercalcemia and increased likelihood of pathologic fractures. These processes also contribute to the development of pneumonia. Bone marrow involvement leads to anemia, manifested by fatigue and weakness; to thrombocytopenia and attendant bleeding; and to neutropenia, which (along with treatment) predisposes patients to recurrent and refractory infections (Anderson, 1993; Bubley & Schnipper, 1991; Cook, 1990; Lichtenstein & Berenson, 1990).

Renal involvement occurs in 50%–75% of patients, and acute renal failure may be pre-

TABLE 26.2 (CONT'D.)		
Metastatic spread	**Problems**	**Assessment parameters**
Bones, joints	Pain	Pain and swelling are common
Lung(s)	Dyspnea, cough, hemoptysis	(See Table 22.1): pleural effusion, pneumonia, embolus, preexisting conditions, ascites may contribute to dyspnea (see chapters 22 for other pulmonary problems); lymph involvement common
Kidney	Obstruction	**Obstructive uropathy** (ureteral): Hesitancy, urgency, nocturia, frequency, < force of stream, polyuria alternating with oliguria
Skin	Skin lesions	Infection, pain, odor
Brain	CNS symptoms	**Increased intracranial pressure:** (May be from cerebral hemorrhage or meningeal leukemia); pain usually present, may be more severe in the morning; progressive neurological deficits (motor, sensory, cognitive); nausea, vomiting (see more complete discussion in chapter 13)
		Changes in mentation + shortness of breath may indicate leukostasis
Other	Various problems	Problems of therapy, e.g., opioids, corticosteroids, tricyclic antidepressants, radiation, chemotherapy; late effects of therapy include cardiomyopathy with congestive failure and pericarditis; neuropsychiatric complications of therapy
		Pericardial effusion → tamponade: Retrosternal chest pain relieved by sitting forward; orthopnea; cough, tachypnea; tachycardia; decreased cardiac output (< cerebral blood, peripheral cyanosis, < systolic and pulse pressures, and pulsus paradoxus (weaker during inspiration)); occasional nausea and vomiting and abdominal pain
	Metabolic changes	**Hypercalcemia:** (Often non-specific), symptoms include fatigue, weakness, anorexia, nausea, polyuria, polydipsia, and constipation; progressing to changes in mentation, seizures, and coma

cipitated most commonly by dehydration, and also by infection, hyperuricemia, pyelonephritis, hypercalcemia, "myeloma kidney," and deposits of calcium and amyloid in the heart, blood vessels, and gastrointestinal tract. Hydration must therefore be aggressive (Anderson, 1993; Bubley & Schnipper, 1991).

Hyperviscosity syndrome may lead to decreased circulation with intermittent claudication and, if progressive, to visual disturbances, gangrene, and neurological impairment (Cook, 1990).

Cardiac failure is relatively common and is due primarily to infiltration of myocardium with amyloids, hyperviscosity syndrome, and/or anemia (Anderson, 1993).

Death is usually from infection or renal failure.

The *oncologic emergencies* most common in patients with MM are **hypercalcemia, spinal cord compression,** and **hyperuricemia** (Cook, 1990; Glover & Glick, 1991).

The spread, problems, and assessments associated with multiple myeloma are illustrated in Table 26.3.

TABLE 26.3
MULTIPLE MYELOMA: SPREAD, PROBLEMS, AND ASSESSMENT

Metastatic spread	Problems	Assessment parameters
(Proliferation of plasma cells) in bones	Pain	From pressure; pathologic fractures are common; primary sites are spine, ribs, skull, pelvis, proximal long bones
		Spinal cord compression: Back pain may be local (somatic: constant, dull, aching) or radicular or both; exacerbated by movement, neck flexion, straight leg raising; decreased by sitting up; tender to percussion. Neurological deficits begin subtly and may not be apparent to the patient: Weakness, ataxia, stumbling; urine retention (frequent, small voiding); bowel dysfunction, impotence; numbness
	Metabolic changes	**Hypercalcemia:** (Often non-specific), symptoms include fatigue, weakness, anorexia, nausea, polyuria, polydipsia, and constipation; progressing to changes in mentation, seizures, and coma
	Immobility	Related to or influenced by pain, pathologic fractures, hypercalcemia. Evaluate for pneumonia
Marrow involvement	Bleeding	Thrombocytopenia
		Neutropenia (frequent infections, especially pneumonia)
	Anemia	Fatigue, weakness, headache, tachypnea
Kidney	Weakness	Anemia; anorexia
		Acute renal failure related to dehydration, infection, pyelonephritis, hypercalcemia, "myeloma kidney," and systemic amyloid deposits. Symptoms include oliguria, fluid retention, engorged neck veins, bounding pulse, first a decrease, then an increase in blood pressure, electrolyte abnormalities, GI symptoms. Renal failure may be irreversible
Heart	Cardiac failure	Due to amyloid infiltration of myocardium, hyperviscosity syndrome, or anemia
		Hyperviscosity syndrome: Decreased circulation, intermittent claudication, visual disturbances, gangrene
Other	Various problems	Problems of therapy, e.g., opioids, corticosteroids, tricyclic antidepressants, radiation, chemotherapy

TABLE 26.4
MELANOMA: SPREAD, PROBLEMS, AND ASSESSMENT

Metastatic spread	Problems	Assessment parameters
Regional lymph	Lymphaden-opathy	Lymphedema: Enlarged lymph, edema (area or lower extremities), pain, cellulitis, lymphangitis. Extensive pelvic disease can result in neurologic impairment and/or urinary dysfunction
Skin, subcutaneous tissue	Lesion	Pain, odor, other cosmetic issues
Primary tumor	Ulceration	Pain, odor, other cosmetic issues
Lung(s)	Dyspnea	See Carcinomatosis, below (also see chapters 14 and 22)
GI system	GI disturbances	See colorectal cancer in chapter 24; bowel obstruction in chapter 17
Heart	Cardiac symptoms	Arrhythmia; congestive heart failure
Carcino-matosis	Multiple problems	**Spinal cord compression:** Back pain may be local (somatic: constant, dull, aching) or radicular or both; exacerbated by movement, neck flexion, straight leg raising; decreased by sitting up; tender to percussion. Neurological deficits begin subtly and may not be apparent to the patient: Weakness, ataxia, stumbling; urine retention (frequent, small voiding); bowel dysfunction, impotence; numbness Pleural effusion: Cough; trachea displaced; absent, decreased fremitus; may increase near top of effusion; percussion dull to flat; absent, decreased breath sounds; adventitious sounds, possible pleural rub

(cont'd.)

Melanoma

Cutaneous Melanoma (CM) is the 18th leading cause of cancer death, with total estimated 1992 deaths of 6,700. It affects about twice as many men as women (American Cancer Society [ACS], 1992). Incidence is increasing worldwide, and in the United States, has doubled in the past ten years (Loeschner & Booth, 1990).

Primary sites of metastases of melanoma are regional lymph, then skin, subcutaneous tissue, and lung (Singletary & Balch, 1991). Other sites of metastases include liver, bone, and brain (Piemme, 1988). Gastrointestinal metastases occur, and may lead to small bowel obstruction or to chronic bleeding (Morton, Wong, Kirkwood, & Parker, 1993). Less common is metastasis to the heart (Chernecky & Krech, 1991). Melanoma is significantly more likely than any other tumor to spread to almost all vital organs, resulting in carcinomatosis (Inagaki, Rodriguez, & Bodey, 1974), and thus

TABLE 26.4 *(CONT'D.)*

Metastatic spread	Problems	Assessment parameters
Carcino-matosis	Multiple problems	Pneumonia: Elevated temperature; purulent sputum (not always present); percussion affected area dull; decreased breath sounds; pleural effusion; immobility, ineffective breathing
		Lymphangitis carcinomatosis: Dyspnea from pulmonary edema
		Pulmonary embolus: Chest pain; hemoptysis; tachypnea; cough; tachycardia
		Pericardial effusion → tamponade: Retrosternal chest pain relieved by sitting forward; orthopnea; cough, tachypnea; tachycardia; decreased cardiac output (< cerebral blood, peripheral cyanosis, < systolic and pulse pressures, and pulsus paradoxus (weaker during inspiration)); occasional nausea and vomiting and abdominal pain; upper extremities; cough, hoarseness
		Obstuction: Rapidly progressive dyspnea; hemoptysis; chronic cough; wheezing, stridor; aspiration; pneumonia
		Respiratory muscle weakness: General weakness; anorexia, cachexia; paraneoplastic syndromes
		Increased intracranial pressure; Pain usually present, may be more severe in the morning; progressive neurological deficits (motor, sensory, cognitive); nausea, vomiting (see more complete discussion in chapter 13)
		Confusion: See chapter 13
		Seizures: See chapter 13
		Problems of therapy, e.g., opioids, corticosteroids, tricyclic antidepressants, radiation, chemotherapy
		Fever of unknown origin (common with liver involvement)

presents a vast array of symptoms. Ulceration of the primary tumor may occur (Morton et al., 1993), resulting in odor and in other challenges in care. Symptoms from a single distal site of metastasis can sometimes be palliated surgically (Morton et al., 1993).

The course of CM is "highly variable" and the occurrence of spontaneous regression of melanoma is well-documented, even at times in the presence of metastases (Morton, Cochran, & Lazar, 1990, p. 506).

The *oncologic emergencies* commonly associated with melanoma include: **pericardial effusion, spinal cord compression, increased intracranial pressure** from brain metastases or from **carcinomatosis meningitis** (along with lung and breast cancer, melanoma is one of the malignancies most likely to metastasize to the brain), *airway obstruction, hemorrhage* from small bowel obstruction, and *disseminated intravascular coagulation [DIC]* (Glover & Glick, 1991; Miaskowski, 1991; Morton et al., 1993; Tabbarah and Casciato, 1990).

The spread, problems, and assessments associated with melanoma are illustrated in Table 26.4.

References

American Cancer Society. (1992). Cancer facts and figures—1992. Atlanta: Author.

Anderson, K. (1993). Plasma cell tumors. In J.F. Holland, E. Frei, R.C. Bast, D.W. Kufe, D.L. Morton, & R.W. Weischselbaum (Eds.), *Cancer medicine* (3rd ed.) (pp.

2075–2092). Philadelphia: Lea & Febiger.

Berenson, J.R., & Gale, R.P. (1990). Acute lymphoblastic leukemia. In C.M. Haskell (Ed.), *Cancer treatment* (3rd ed.) (pp. 606–620). Philadelphia: W.B. Saunders Company.

Bubley, G.J., & Schnipper, L.E. (1991). Multiple myeloma. In A.I. Holleb, D.J. Fink, & G.P. Murphy (Eds.), *Clinical oncology* (pp. 397–409). Atlanta: American Cancer Society.

Carson, C., & Callaghan, M.E. (1991). Hematopoietic and immunologic cancers. In S.B. Baird, R. McCorkle, & M. Grant (Eds.), *Cancer nursing* (pp. 536–566). Philadelphia: W.B. Saunders.

Chernecky, C., & Krech, R. L. (1991). Complications of advanced disease. In S.B. Baird, R. McCorkle, & M. Grant (Eds.), *Cancer nursing: A comprehensive textbook* (pp 885–893). Philadelphia: W.B Saunders.

Cook, M.B. (1990). Multiple myeloma. In S.L. Groenwald, M.H. Frogge, M. Goodman, & C.H. Yarbro (Eds.), *Cancer nursing: Principles and practice* (3rd ed.) (pp. 990–998). Boston: Jones and Bartlett Publishers.

Eyre, H.J., & Farver, M.L. (1991). Hodgkin's disease and non-Hodgkin's lymphomas. In A.I. Holleb, D.J. Fink, & G.P. Murphy (Eds.), *Clinical oncology* (pp. 377–396). Atlanta: American Cancer Society.

Finley, J.P. (1992). Nursing care of patients with metabolic and physiological oncological emergencies. In J.C. Clark & R.F. McGee (Eds.), *Core curriculum for oncology nursing* (pp. 169–192), Philadelphia: W.B. Saunders.

Foon, K.A., Champlin, R.E., & Gale, R.P. (1990). Acute myelogenous leukemia and the myelodysplastic syndromes. In C.M. Haskell (Ed.), *Cancer treatment* (3rd ed.) (pp. 589–606). Philadelphia: W.B. Saunders Company.

Freedman, A.S., & Nadler, L.M. (1993). Non-Hodgkin's lymphoma. In J.F. Holland, E. Frei, R.C. Bast, D.W. Kufe, D.L. Morton, & R.W. Weischselbaum (Eds.), *Cancer medicine* (3rd ed.) (pp. 2028–2068). Philadelphia: Lea & Febiger.

Glover, D., & Glick, J.H. (1991). Oncologic emergencies. In A.I. Holleb, D.J. Fink, & G.P. Murphy (Eds.), *Clinical oncology* (pp. 513–533). Atlanta: American Cancer Society.

Inagaki, J., Rodriguez, V., & Bodey, G.P. (1974). Causes of death in cancer patients. *Cancer, 33*(2), 568–573.

Lichtenstein, A., & Berenson, J.R. (1990). Myeloma, macroglobulinemia, and heavy chain disease. In C.M. Haskell (Ed.), *Cancer treatment* (3rd ed.) (pp. 636–655). Philadelphia: W.B. Saunders Company.

Loeschner, L.J., & Booth, A. (1990). Skin cancer. In S.L. Groenwald, M.H. Frogge, M. Goodman, & C.H. Yarbro (Eds.), *Cancer nursing: Principles and practice* (3rd ed.) (pp. 999–1014). Boston: Jones and Bartlett Publishers.

Maguire-Eisen, M., & Edmonds, K.S. (1992). Leukemias. In J.C. Clark & R.F. McGee (Eds.), *Core curriculum for oncology nursing* (pp. 480–487), Philadelphia: W.B. Saunders.

Miaskowski, C. (1991). Oncologic emergencies. In S.B. Baird, R. McCorkle, & M. Grant (Eds.), *Cancer nursing* (pp. 885–893). Philadelphia: W.B Saunders.

Mitus, A.J., & Rosenthal, D.S. (1991). Adult leukemias. In A.I. Holleb, D.J. Fink, & G.P. Murphy (Eds.), *Clinical oncology* (pp. 410–432). Atlanta: American Cancer Society.

Morton, D.L., Cochran, A.J., & Lazar, G. (1990). Melanoma. In C.M. Haskell (Ed.), *Cancer treatment* (pp. 500–512). Philadelphia: W.B. Saunders.

Morton, D.L., Wong, J.H., Kirkwood, J.M., & Parker, R.G. (1993). Malignant melanoma. In J.F. Holland, E. Frei, R.C. Bast, D.W. Kufe, D.L. Morton, & R.W. Weischselbaum (Eds.), *Cancer medicine* (3rd ed.) (pp. 1793–1824). Philadelphia: Lea & Febiger.

Piemme, J.A. (1988). Secondary primary or metastatic cancer. In S.B. Baird (Ed.) *Decision making in oncology nursing* (pp. 20–23). Philadelphia: B.C. Decker.

Ransohoff, J., Koslow, M., & Cooper, P.R. (1991). Cancer of the central nervous system and pituitary. In A.I. Holleb, D.J. Fink, & G.P. Murphy (Eds.), *Clinical oncology* (pp. 329–337). Atlanta: American Cancer Society.

Sarna, G.P., & Kagan, A.R. (1990). Non-Hodgkin's lymphoma. In C.M. Haskell (Ed.), *Cancer treatment* (3rd ed.) (pp. 682–718). Philadelphia: W.B. Saunders Company.

Schiffer, C.A. (1993). Acute myeloid leukemia in adults. In J.F. Holland, E. Frei, R.C. Bast, D.W. Kufe, D.L. Morton, & R.W. Weischselbaum (Eds.), *Cancer medicine* (3rd ed.) (pp. 1907–1933). Philadelphia: Lea & Febiger.

Silver, R.T. (1993). Chronic myeloid leukemia. In J.F. Holland, E. Frei, R.C. Bast, D.W. Kufe, D.L. Morton, & R.W. Weischselbaum (Eds.), *Cancer medicine* (3rd ed.) (pp. 1934–1946). Philadelphia: Lea & Febiger.

Singletary, S.E., & Balch, C.M. (1991). Malignant melanoma. In A.I. Holleb, D.J. Fink, & G.P. Murphy (Eds.), *Clinical oncology* (pp. 263–270). Atlanta: American Cancer Society.

Tabbarah, H.J., & Casciato, D.A. (1990). Malignant effusions. In C.M. Haskell (Ed.), *Cancer treatment* (pp. 815–825). Philadelphia: W.B. Saunders.

Wujcik, D. (1991). Leukemia. In S.L. Groenwald, M.H. Frogge, M. Goodman, & C.H. Yarbro (Eds.), *Cancer Nursing: Principles and practice* (3rd ed.) (pp. 930–950). Boston: Jones and Bartlett Publishers.

Yarbro, C.H. (1990). Lymphomas. In S.L. Groenwald, M.H. Frogge, M. Goodman, & C.H. Yarbro (Eds.), *Cancer nursing: Principles and practice* (3rd ed.) (pp. 974–989). Boston: Jones and Bartlett Publishers.

V | Management of Other Terminal Illnesses

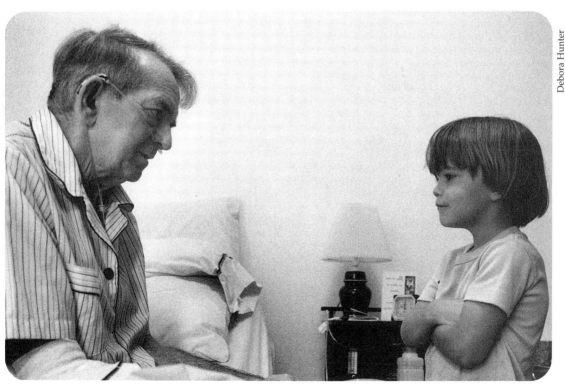

✍

Introduction

ancer is the most commonly seen disease in hospice and palliative care settings, primarily because it is relatively easy to determine when curative treatment is futile and because advanced cancer presents a relatively predictable and short course of illness. Other diseases are less predictable, but still, many patients with diseases other than cancer benefit from palliative care. Diseases discussed in this section of the book include:

- Acquired immunodeficiency syndrome (AIDS);
- degenerative neurological disorders (multiple sclerosis [MS], Parkinson's disease, amyotrophic lateral sclerosis, myasthenia gravis);
- Alzheimer's disease; and
- cardiovascular and chronic obstructive pulmonary disease;

Care for patients who are dying from these diseases is often complicated by one of two factors:

1. In several of these—e.g., AIDS and heart disease—there exists an uncertain trajectory. In many cases, it is difficult to determine with certainty that curative treatment should be withdrawn and palliative treatment instituted.
2. In other diseases—e.g., Alzheimer's and MS—the disease process is extremely slow, and satisfactory systems of care do not exist to any significant extent.

In this section of the book, approaches to the problems of these diseases are explored.

The concept of palliative care for patients with cancer is generally applicable to patients with other diseases as well. For example, although pain syndromes of AIDS or MS differ in some respects from those of cancer, the general approach to assessment and treatment is quite similar. Approaches to gastrointestinal, urinary tract, and other problems are also similar. Moreover, *it is not always necessary to draw a line between curative and palliative care. Competent curative treatment of an illness should never preclude competent management of symptoms.*

Psychosocial issues for the diseases in this section, although similar in many respects to the psychosocial issues common in cancer, are different in other respects. AIDS, for example, carries at least the potential for several unique psychosocial problems, including the potential for transmission, and the presence in the minds of family, caretakers, etc., of negative implications about how the patient may have contracted the disease—e.g., through IV drug use or homosexual activity.

In the case of slow, neurodegenerative disorders, these diseases often bring unimaginable physical, psychological, and spiritual stress to caregivers. Still, many of the basic principles of care remain similar.

Acquired Immunodeficiency Syndrome

The worldwide spread of acquired immunodeficiency syndrome (AIDS) and its causative agent, human immunodeficiency virus type 1 (HIV-1), is the most dramatic health problem of the modern world. In the United States alone, more than 113,000 persons died from AIDS in the first ten years of the pandemic (1981–1991) (Centers for Disease Control [CDC], 1991).

Epidemiology and Characteristics of the Disease

Worldwide, between 38 million and 110 million adults, and more than 10 million children, are expected to be infected with HIV-1 by the year 2000 (Ehrhardt, 1992). Barring an unforeseen breakthrough in treatment, all of these infected individuals will develop AIDS. In the United States, the epidemiology of AIDS is shifting from a population composed mainly of homosexual and bisexual men, and of IV drug users, to a more diverse grouping. HIV-infected individuals now include steadily increasing numbers of children and of heterosexual women and men. African Americans and Hispanic Americans account for a disproportionate

share of cases of both AIDS and HIV infection (CDC, 1992a). It is estimated that, as of this year (1994), about 57% of patients with AIDS will be homosexual or bisexual men who contract the infection through sex, about 4% will be homosexual or bisexual men who are infected from injecting drugs with contaminated needles, about 27% will be women and heterosexual men who are infected from injecting drugs with contaminated needles, and about 13% will be women and men contracting the disease from heterosexual contact. (CDC, 1992b).

Patients with AIDS present several major challenges to practitioners involved with terminal, palliative, or hospice care (National Commission on Acquired Immune Deficiency Syndrome [NCAIDS], 1991; Stephany, 1992; Swan, Benjamin, & Brown, 1992). Some of these challenges are described in the following list.

- The severity and unpredictability of AIDS means that caring for patients with advanced disease becomes an emotional and clinical challenge of the highest order.

Charles Kemp: TERMINAL ILLNESS: A GUIDE TO NURSING CARE. © 1995 J. B. Lippincott.

- A host of psychosocial problems surrounds AIDS—not the least of which is the fact that this is a transmissible disease, which may strike fear into those attending the patient.
- The trajectory of the disease is different from all others discussed in this book. While AIDS is clearly fatal, there is difficulty in ascertaining when the patient is actively dying.
- Disagreement exists among health care workers about which treatments are palliative and which are curative. Treatment of opportunistic infections presents troubling questions to some staff in programs dedicated to palliative care.

While many factors are involved in attaining quality care for AIDS patients—the extent of disease, the problems inherent in it, practitioner orientation or expertise, organizational philosophy, traditional attitudes and values in the area where care is given—it is clear that one of the basic requirements is the coordination of a continuum of services (Morrison, 1993; NCAIDS, 1991). Care also demands enormous flexibility on the part of providers. Regardless of how carefully guidelines for palliative care are developed (e.g., von Gunten, Martinez, Weitzman, & Von Roenn, 1991), the fact remains that patients with AIDS are extremely difficult to categorize in terms of life expectancy.

More than 85% of patients with AIDS present with an opportunistic infection and, in general, the more frequent or varied the infections, the poorer the prognosis (Hanson, Horsburgh, Fann, Havlik, & Thompson, 1993; Hughes & Schofferman, 1991). Almost 90% of all deaths from AIDS are due to opportunistic infections, and as treatment methods improve for different complications of HIV infection, other fatal complications emerge (Masur, 1990). The degree of immunosuppression in AIDS patients is related to disease progression and to the incidence of infection—although immunosuppression does not *always* result in infection

or disease progression. Immunosuppression is best measured by the quantity of circulating CD4+ lymphocytes, or helper T cells (U.S. Public Health Service [USPHS], 1993). The greatest risk of death occurs with decreased CD4 cell count, diagnosis of wasting syndrome, *Mycobacterium avium-intracellulare* complex infection (MAC), or lymphoma. Other conditions indicating reduced survival time include *Pneumocystis carinii* pneumonia, Kaposi's sarcoma, toxoplasmosis, cryptococcosis, cryptosporidiosis, and esophageal candidiasis (Hanson et al., 1993).

Transmission Precautions

Regardless of the specifics of infection transmission, in all cases it is essential to practice universal precautions (Mocsny, 1993) and to instruct and aid others, especially all those who are themselves immunosuppressed, in avoiding infection. See Figure 27.1 for a description of universal precautions against infection transmission.

Treatment of AIDS

The present concepts for treating patients with AIDS include several basic tenets:

- Assessments are comprehensive: CD4+ counts and other lab values are regularly taken. However, The character of assessments changes according to disease progression. As CD4+ counts decrease and complications increase in number and severity, the need for lab values and other intrusive or painful diagnostic procedures diminishes.
- Treatment is organized according to five axes of care:
  1. The psychosocial and spiritual health of the patient, and of his or her significant others, is addressed throughout the course of illness.

FIGURE 27.1
Universal Precautions

The fear of contracting HIV infection probably exceeds the likelihood of infection. From 1981–1992, a total of 12 cases of occupationally acquired HIV infection of nurses have been documented (Centers for Disease Control, 1992c). Nevertheless, practitioners must always protect themselves *and* others from disease transmission. The following is a summary of blood and other body fluids precautions that does not substitute for the current policies and procedures that every health care organization should have. Policies and procedures should be based on Centers for Disease Control guidelines. Note that the best means of protecting oneself from the most common, lethal means of transmission of HIV—needlestick—is to pay careful attention to what one is doing. Note also that patients with advanced AIDS have other infections, many of which are transmitted in the same manner as HIV. Tuberculosis is not transmitted in the same way as are most of the other opportunistic infections: TB is most often contracted by inhalation of airborne droplets.

- Gloves are worn when contact with a patient's body fluids, mucus membranes, or non-intact skin may occur; and whenever needles are handled. Gloves reduce the transfer or exposure volume of blood in hollow-bore needles (Mast, Woolwine, & Gerberding, 1993). Gloves are unnecessary for bathing or for casual contact with a patient.
- Handwashing is essential before and after each patient contact. Use disposable paper towels to dry and turn water on and off.
- Gowns or aprons are not routinely necessary. They are best used when there is the possibility of contact with body fluids that might get on the practitioner's clothing, i.e., when changing dressings with heavy drainage or during procedures involving splashes.
- Masks and protective eyewear or face shields should be used when splashing body fluids are anticipated, e.g., suctioning, bronchoscopy, surgery, and debridement.
- Needle and sharps use and disposal require careful, compulsive attention by practitioners. Disposal is immediate and into a rigid, puncture-proof container.

2. Nutrition and exercise are especially important early on in the process of HIV/AIDS. In the terminal stage, the ability to exercise or take in nutrition diminishes.
3. Prevention of deterioration is emphasized primarily in the early stages. Avoidance of complications is increasingly difficult as CD4+ counts decrease.
4. The patient and family are educated about the illness in general, and especially about which changes in symptoms require urgent attention.

5. Medical therapy and nursing measures related to it are generally directed to: (a) anti-HIV measures; (b) prophylaxis of opportunistic infections; (c) treatment of specific conditions; and (d) management of symptoms.
- Complications—including the progression of current problems and the development of new problems—are prevented or identified early and/or their effects are minimized. Thus, practitioners must anticipate possibilities throughout the course of care. Antiretroviral therapy (e.g., zidovudine

[AZT]) is part of the effort to prevent or minimize complications, although it is often discontinued during therapy for major opportunistic infections. Other treatment may be a combination of curative and palliative care, or may be designed only to slow wasting. Many medications used to treat AIDS and its associated infections are likely to produce toxic effects. The balance between desired and untoward effects is often difficult to establish. (See Table 27.1

for a listing of commonly used drugs for patients with AIDS, the indications for their use, and common side effects and toxcities.)

- Practitioners must protect themselves (and others) from HIV and associated infections.

AIDS treatment is in a state of rapid development. Numerous studies are underway, and readers who regularly work with patients with AIDS are strongly encouraged to consult cur-

TABLE 27.1
COMMONLY USED DRUGS FOR PATIENTS WITH AIDS

Drug Name	Indications	Common Side Effects, Toxicities
Acyclovir (Zovirax)	Herpes zoster/simplex	Oral: Headache, nausea, vomiting, diarrhea, vertigo, hematuria. Parenteral: Lethargy, potential for renal dysfunction, confusion, coma
Didanosine (ddl) (Videx)	Advanced HIV infection and intolerance to, or deterioration during zidovudine (AZT) therapy	Seizures, headache, peripheral neuropathy cardiomyopathy, chills, fever, diarrhea, abdominal pain, pancreatitis. Signs of pancreatitis should be reported promptly. Patients at risk for pancreatitis (independently of ddl use) should be closely monitored.
Epoetin alfa (Procrit)	Anemia in AZT-treated patients	Hematocrit may rapidly increase and thus cause clotting. Side effects include hypertension, chest pain, shortness of breath, diarrhea, nausea, fatigue, fever. Seizures may occur, especially if dosage is rapidly increased
Fluconazole (Diflucan)	Cryptococcal meningitis, candidiasis	Abnormal liver function, nausea, abdominal pain, dizziness, headache, skin rash
Foscarnet sodium Sodium (Foscavir)	CMV retinitis	Renal failure, seizures, polydipsia, nausea, anorexia, electrolyte imbalances (Ca, phosphatemia), fatigue, irritability
Ganciclovir (Cytovene)	CMV retinitis; disseminated CMV	Cytopenic changes, abnormal liver function, phlebitis, nausea, abdominal pain, anorexia, headache, changes in mentation, skin rash
Interferon alfa- 2a recombinant (Intron-A, Roferon-A)	Kaposi's sarcoma	Leukopenia, congestive cardiomyopathy, liver enzyme changes, weight loss, flu-like symptoms, alopecia, fatigue

(cont'd.)

rent AIDS journals for the latest guidelines and developments in regard to patient care.

Practitioners should also be aware that alternative healing practices are used by some patients with AIDS. Buyer's clubs are found in most large cities, and some medications and herbal preparations specifically developed for alternative AIDS treatment are available through the mail. Some are benign and possibly helpful. Others involve powerful chemical-biological agents—such as compound Q—that may have difficult-to-predict, adverse effects. In addition, some medications available by prescription—e.g., itraconazole, ddc, etc.—are also obtainable through buyer's clubs. Some herbs, such as comfrey, contain toxic alkaloids. It is essential for the practitioner to determine what medications/agents or herbs patients are taking. However, in order to make this determination, it is important that care givers approach patients free of judgements and prejudices of their own. Alternative healing practices are

TABLE 27.1 (CONT'D.)		
Drug Name	**Indications**	**Common Side Effects, Toxicities**
Itraconazole (Sporanox)	Histoplasmosis, blastomycosis	Nausea, fatigue, rash, K depletion, edema
Ketoconazole (Nizoral)	Candidiasis	Hepatitis, nausea, diarrhea, headache, dizziness, drowsiness, skin rash, photophobia
Pentamidine isethionate-aerosol (NebuPent)	PCP Prophylaxis	Chest pain, coughing, congestion, dyspnea, pharyngitis, skin rash, pneumothorax
Pentamidine isethionate —IV and IM (Pentam)	PCP treatment	Blood dyscrasias, hyper or hypoglycemia, hypotension, changes in heart rate and rhythm, skin rash
Pyrimethamine (Daraprim)	Toxoplasmosis treatment	Folic acid deficiency (including bleeding, diarrhea, stomatitis, dysphagia), seizures, nausea, fever, anorexia, fatigue, skin rash, motor dysfunction. Leucovorin is sometimes given in conjunction with pyrimethamine to prevent bone marrow suppression.
Trimethoprim & sulfa-methoxazole (Bactrim, Septra)	PCP treatment, salmonella	Leukopenia, thrombocytopenia, hepatitis, fever, skin rash, changes in urine, muscle and joint pain, dysphagia, diarrhea, nausea, dizziness, headache
Zalcitabine (HIVID, ddC)	Used in combination with AZT to treat adults with decreased CD4+ count and significant deterioration	Peripheral neuropathy, pancreatitis
Zidovudine (AZT) (Retrovir)	HIV infection	Leukopenia, anemia, neutropenia, changes in platelet count, diarrhea, nausea, fever, dizziness, skin rash, headache, insomnia, myopathy

Note: Reproduced with permission from Pharmaceutical Manufacturers Association, 1992.

evaluated on the basis of whether they are *harmful.* Safe practices can be encouraged, while steering patients away from harmful ones.

Physical Problems of AIDS

Disease-related problems of AIDS may be classified (Chaisson & Volberding, 1990) according to the following categories:

- acute retroviral syndrome;
- persistent generalized lymphadenopathy (PGL);
- hematologic manifestations;
- constitutional disease;
- oral and other candidiasis;
- other oral complications;
- neuromuscular and related complications;
- skin manifestations;
- gastrointestinal syndromes (esophageal, stomach, small bowel, and enterocolitis);
- renal disease;
- pulmonary disease (Pneumocystis carinii pneumonia, mycobacterial infections, histoplasmosis, and coccidioidomycosis);
- neurologic complications (cryptococcal meningitis, cytomegalovirus, toxoplasmic encephalitis, AIDS dementia); and
- AIDS-related cancers.

Each of these problems is discussed below. However, only the most common problems and infections are covered in this chapter. Many others occur in AIDS, e.g., bacterial pneumonia, heart disease, other sexually transmitted diseases, etc. (See Table 27.2 for an outline of frequent clinical findings—and potential clinical significance—of symptoms in HIV-seropositive patients.) Symptom management of problems specific to AIDS (as listed above) is addressed in this chapter, but readers should also make use of the chapters with information on specific diseases, their symptoms, and management, found throughout this book.

ACUTE RETROVIRAL SYNDROME

Acute retroviral syndrome, or primary HIV infection, is non-specific and similar to mononucleosis, with common manifestations of fever, night sweats, malaise, myalgia, sore throat, anorexia, nausea, diarrhea, large liver and spleen, lymphadenopathy, and rash. Treatment is symptomatic and supportive, and the syndrome resolves in weeks to months (Chaisson & Volberding, 1990; Tindall, Imrie, Donovan, Penny, & Cooper, 1990).

PERSISTENT GENERALIZED LYMPHADENOPATHY (PGL)

PGL may begin with the primary HIV infection and persist throughout the course of the disease as lymphadenopathy syndrome (LAS). In the context of AIDS, lymphadenopathy is not a major problem, except that it may be a sign of other complications, such as syphilis, Hodgkin's disease, lymphoma, Kaposi sarcoma, or mycobacterial infection.

HEMATOLOGIC MANIFESTATIONS

Hematologic manifestations, or problems, of AIDS commonly include anemia, leukopenia, and/or thrombocytopenia. Etiologies include infections, possibly nutritional deficiencies, cancer, and medications (Hambleton & Abrams, 1990; Northfelt & Mitsuyasu, 1992). Anemia is very common in patients with AIDS, and worsens as the disease progresses (Caron, Jacobson, & Walsh, 1992). Transfusing packed red blood cells may be necessary for anemia (Hambleton & Abrams, 1990). Administration of hematopoietic growth factors may result in improvement of bone marrow suppression (Caron et al., 1992). HIV-related immune thrombocytopenia (ITP), as well as thrombocytopenia from other etiologies, is common in patients with AIDS. Treatment with zidovu-

TABLE 27.2
FREQUENT CLINICAL FINDINGS IN THE *HIV-SEROPOSITIVE* PATIENT

Examination	Clinical finding	Potential clinical significance
Vital signs and appearance	Weight loss Muscle wasting Fever	HIV-related wasting syndrome If no localizing symptoms, consider infections with MAI, TB, CMV, and occult sinusitis or prostatitis
Eye	White, indistinct retinal spots White retinal exudates and hemorrhages	Cotton wool spots; no known significance CMV retinitis
	Visual field defects	Unilateral: Optic neuritis, CMV, or Toxoplasma retinitis Bilateral: CNS mass lesion (lymphoma, toxoplasmosis, PML)
Oral cavity	White plaques Oral ulcers Gingivitis/periodontitis Purple lesion	Oral candidiasis, oral hairy leukoplakia HSV, CMV, aphthous ulcers, disseminated histoplasmosis HIV-associated gingivitis/periodontitis Kaposi's sarcoma
Lymph nodes	Persistent (>3 mo), generalized (two or more extrainguinal sites) lymphadenopathy (PGL) Lymphadenopathy in which individual nodes are either tender, large, or inflamed	Persistent, generalized lymphadenopathy Lymphoma, toxoplasmosis, tuberculosis, syphilis
Abdomen	Hepatosplenomegaly Perirectal ulcer	MAI, tuberculosis, lymphoma, histoplasmosis HSV, CMV, histoplasmosis
Genitalia	Genital sores	Syphilis, HSV, chancroid warts
Nervous system	Cognitive difficulties Sensory-motor deficits	HIV encephalopathy, stroke, depression, vitamin B_{12} deficiency CNS lymphoma, CNS toxoplasmosis, cryptococcal meningoencephalitis, syphilis, progressive multifocal leukoencephalopathy, HIV-associated neuropathy, nucleoside toxicity
Skin	Purple macule or papule Scaling rash Purpura Vesicular rash	Kaposi's sarcoma, cat-scratch disease Seborrheic dermatitis, fungal infection, psoriasis HIV-associated thrombocytopenia Herpes zoster, HSV, drug reaction

Note: From *Therapeutic Approach to the HIV Seropositive Patient* by S.L. Boswell, and M.S. Hirsch. In V.T. DeVita, S. Hellman, & S.A. Rosenberg (Eds.). *AIDS: Etiology, Diagnosis, Treatment, and Prevention* (3rd ed.), 1992, Philadelphia: J.B. Lippincott Company. Reprinted by permission.

dine is usually successful (Rarick et al., 1991). Patients with bleeding disorders should avoid medications that are associated with increasing bleeding, such as acetylsalicylic acid and other aspirin products, anticoagulants (e.g., heparin), dipyridamole (Persantine), and alcohol. Patients should avoid trauma, tight or constrictive clothing, and constipation. Nutrition and hydration should be maintained.

CONSTITUTIONAL DISEASE

Constitutional disease is usually a long-standing condition in earlier stages of HIV infection, and is characterized by low-grade fevers, fatigue, intermittent diarrhea, and other problems or complaints (Chaisson & Volberding, 1990).

ORAL AND OTHER CANDIDIASIS

Oral candidiasis is the most common oral fungal infection in patients with AIDS, occurring in about 70% of persons who are HIV positive (Dodd et al., 1991; Smith, Midgley, Allan, Connolly, & Gazzard, 1991). Prevalence increases as CD4 counts decrease (Feigal et al., 1991). Vaginal and/or perineal candidiasis is common in women with AIDS. Esophageal candidiasis indicates advanced disease and CD4 counts below 100 (Polis & Kovacs, 1992). The incidence of systemic candidiasis is increasing, and often results in death from sepsis (Finley, Joshi, & Neill, 1992). Symptoms of oropharyngeal candidiasis include removable white ("cottage cheese") plaques, or flat red lesions with no removable plaques, pain, and dysphagia. The pain and unpleasant taste contribute to difficulty in eating and subsequent malnutrition. Perineal or vaginal candidiasis is characterized by pain, pruritus, discharge, and red lesions. Esophageal candidiasis symptoms include dysphagia, odynophagia, feeling of obstruction and/or retrosternal, burning pain (Dodd et al., 1991; Hughes & Schofferman, 1991; Polis & Kovacs, 1992). Treatment includes topi-

cal agents (nystatin or clotrimazole) and systemic anti-fungals (itraconazole, fluconazole, or ketaconazole), with the latter two indicated in resistant or esophageal infections (Greenspan & Greenspan, 1992; La Brooy, 1993; Polis & Kovacs, 1992). Most patients have a recurrence of candidiasis within three months (Smith et al., 1991).

OTHER ORAL COMPLICATIONS

Oral disorders other than from candidiasis include oral hairy leukoplakia, herpes simplex, oral warts, recurrent aphthous ulcers, periodontal disease, and lesions due to opportunistic infections and cancer (Boswell & Hirsch, 1992; Greenspan & Greenspan, 1992). Lesions from opportunistic infections (cytomegalovirus and disseminated histoplasmosis), and cancer associated with AIDS, also occur.

Candidiasis and oral hairy leukoplakia are sometimes mistaken for one another. The latter is associated with less morbidity and clinical significance. Oral hairy leukoplakia is characterized by white, non-removable plaques on the tongue, and is sometimes mixed with Candida albicans. The condition may respond to some extent to topical anti-fungals because of the presence of Candida. Otherwise, anti-fungals are ineffective and treatment is not indicated (Azizi & Epstein, 1992).

Herpes simplex lesions tend to be larger and last longer in patients with AIDS than in other patients. Topical acyclovir is used for lesions on the lip and systemic acyclovir for intraoral lesions. Foscarnet is used for resistant infections (Berger, 1990).

Oral warts are sometimes large and may spread through the oral cavity. They may be removed surgically, but tend to recur (Greenspan, Greenspan, & Winkler, 1990).

Recurrent aphthous ulcers (or stomatitis) are the most common type of oral ulceration (Schooley, 1992) and tend to be larger in patients with AIDS than in others (Greenspan & Greenspan, 1992).

Periodontal disease includes rapidly progressive gingivitis with ulcers, bleeding, and pain, as well as very rapidly progressive periodontal disease, including bone lesions and necrosis. Treatment includes surgical débridement and topical antiseptics, and sometimes metronidazole (Flagyl) (Greenspan et al., 1990).

Neuromuscular and Related Complications

Neuromuscular complications include peripheral neuropathies, autonomic neuropathies, and myopathies. Peripheral neuropathies are common at all stages of HIV infection and AIDS. They may be due to HIV infection or to unknown causes, opportunistic infections (especially cytomegalovirus [CMV] or herpes), or medications (Galantino, 1991).

Peripheral neuropathies are the most common cause of pain in patients with AIDS (Schofferman & Brody, 1990). (Please see the section on Neuropathic Pain in chapter 12.) The most common neuropathy is distal symmetrical (painful sensory) polyneuropathy (DSP), which begins early in HIV infection (Brew, 1993). DSP is characterized by progressive bilateral distal paresthesias, beginning in the feet. Pain, sensory loss, weakness, and muscle atrophy may occur (Simpson & Wolfe, 1991).

An important neuropathy is the ascending radiculopathy caused by CMV. This progressive sensorimotor neuropathy is characterized by early bowel and bladder dysfunction (Price, Brew, & Roke, 1992). Without early treatment (with ganciclovir), death may occur within several weeks (Simpson & Wolfe, 1991) Other peripheral neuropathies exist, but are less common than those described here.

Autonomic neuropathies may be manifested by impotence, bowel and bladder impairment, abnormal sweating, and presyncope (Simpson & Wolfe, 1991). Loss of bowel and bladder control is common in AIDS dementia complex (Koppel, 1992).

Myopathies include progressive muscle weakness and myalgia, especially of the thighs (Simpson & Wolfe, 1991). Long-term zidovudine use may result in wasting of buttock muscles and lower extremity weakness (Brew, 1993).

Skin Manifestations

Common skin disorders in patients with AIDS include: noninfectious problems, such as seborrheic dermatitis, and drug reactions; and infectious disorders, or manifestations of infectious disorders, such as acute exanthem of HIV infection, herpes zoster, herpes simplex, molluscum contagiosum infection, human papillomavirus infections, syphilis, and bacterial infections (e.g., folliculitis, impetigo, furuncles, and conjunctivitis). Skin disorders such as candidiasis, oral herpes simplex, and hairy leukoplakia are discussed above under Other Oral Complications. Skin disorders related to CMV, to *Pneumocystis carinii* infection, and to mycobacterial infections, are discussed in the sections below; and skin disorders of Kaposi's sarcoma are discussed in the section below on AIDS-Related Cancers.

Seborrheic dermatitis is the most common noninfectious skin disorder found in patients with AIDS. It is characterized by erythema, or fine white scaling without erythema, usually on the scalp, face, eyebrows, back, axillae, and groin. Treatment is difficult; there is poor response to topical agents (e.g., glucocorticoids) and limited response to ketoconazole (Safai & Schwartz, 1992). Drugs whose use commonly results in skin reactions are trimethoprim-sulfamethoxazole, zidovudine, and fluconazole (Safai & Schwartz, 1992).

Acute exanthem is an early manifestation of HIV infection, and consists of small pink macules and papules on the trunk and extremities, fever, and pharyngitis (Cockerell, 1992).

Herpes zoster usually occurs early in the disease, and is characterized by painful vesicles that appear in areas of the neurodermatome. High oral doses, or intravenous doses, of acyclovir are used to prevent or treat lesions in or associated with the eyes (Greenspan & Greenspan, 1992) or to treat severe infections elsewhere (Cockerell, 1992). Pain is treated as described in the section on Neuropathic Pain in chapter 12. Herpes simplex infections are sometimes disseminated, in which case vesicles may be found everywhere on the skin surface. Anogenital infections may also be found, and sometimes result in necrotic lesions. Perineal care and prevention of further infection is a challenge in such cases (Cockerell, 1992). Molluscum contagiosum infections are characterized by spreading, rounded papules. The infection is not life-threatening, and is difficult to treat.

Human papillomavirus infections may result in resistant warts and/or condyloma, often anogenital, whose growth can result in anal obstruction (Cockerell, 1992).

Syphilis, like other infections in patients with AIDS, may have more severe symptoms, including a number of atypical skin changes (Cockerell, 1992).

Folliculitis, usually staphylococcal, is characterized by pruritic erythema, pustules, and/or papules on the face, trunk, or groin. Lesions may progress to abscesses, furuncles, or carbuncles. Treatment is with penicillinase-resistant antibiotics (Berger, 1990).

Impetigo is due to staphylococcus or streptococcus infection, and in patients with AIDS is usually found in the inguinal or axillary regions. Typically, painful red macules progress to bullae, which eventually rupture. Treatment is with topical or systemic antibiotics (Cockerell, 1992).

GASTROINTESTINAL SYNDROMES

Common gastrointestinal (GI) problems of patients with AIDS include problems of the esophagus, nausea, vomiting, hematemesis, early satiety, anorexia, abdominal pain, diar-

rhea, and weight loss (Chaisson & Volberding, 1990; Dworkin, 1992). This section is divided broadly into discussions of esophageal disease, infections, diarrhea, and nutrition. Gastrointestinal problems resulting from cancer are discussed in the section on AIDS-Related Cancers. Symptom control specific to patients with AIDS is discussed at appropriate points in this section; additional material on symptom control can be found in previous chapters on specific problems.

Esophageal pathology is characterized by dysphagia, odynophagia, retrosternal pain, nausea, anorexia, and/or weight loss. Esophagitis is most commonly secondary to candidiasis, herpes simplex, or CMV infection. Other causes include reflux esophagitis, Kaposi's sarcoma lesions, lymphoma, or peptic ulcer disease (Chaisson & Volberding, 1990; La Brooy, 1993).

GI infections in patients may be bacterial, viral, fungal, or protozoal. The more common infections are due to CMV, disseminated *Mycobacterium avium-intracellulare* complex (MAC), salmonella, and Cryptosporidium (Cello, 1990). Microsporidia is emerging as a potentially important cause of GI symptoms, but the extent of its presence is not yet known. Other, less common, GI infections include giardiasis, amebiasis, Shigella, and various systemic fungal infections (Cello, 1990, Dworkin, 1992; Kotler, 1992). Only salmonella, Cryptosporidium, and Microsporidia are discussed at any length here under GI infections; the other common infections are discussed more fully in the sections below on opportunistic infections.

GI problems associated with CMV extend from one end of the gut to the other. Among the syndromes found in CMV GI infection are esophagitis, gastritis, intestinal ulcers, ileitis, intestinal perforation, colitis, hepatitis, pancreatitis, cholangitis, and wasting (Kotler, 1992). Involvement of the colon is characterized by abdominal pain, diarrhea, and rectal bleeding (Dworkin, 1992). See the section on CMV below for indications in treatment of the infection.

MAC in the GI tract usually involves the small bowel, but infection may occur anywhere in the GI tract (Dworkin, 1992). Disseminated MAC infection is characterized by fever, wasting, debilitation, and, in many cases, diarrhea (Kotler, 1992). See the section on *Mycobacterium avium-intracellulare* below for indications in treatment of the infection.

Salmonella and other bacterial infections in patients with AIDS are characterized by recurrence and by a high incidence of bacteremia (Kotler, 1992). The small and/or large bowel may be affected and diarrhea is usually profuse and accompanied by cramping, bloating, nausea, and weight loss (Chaisson & Volberding, 1990). Once begun, the infection may require life-long antibiotic therapy (Dworkin, 1992).

Cryptosporidium (a protozoan) is a common enteric pathogen of patients with AIDS. Cryptosporidiosis is a chronic infection characterized by diarrhea and a wasting syndrome known in Africa as "slim disease" (Kotler, 1992). Fever, nausea and vomiting, and abdominal cramping, especially after meals, may also occur (Hughes & Schofferman, 1991). Some patients develop severe secretary diarrhea, with massive and rapid fluid loss. More than 20% of patients with cryptosporidiosis may have a spontaneous remission lasting for as long as two months, and probably related to increased lymphocyte counts (McGowan, Hawkins, & Weller, 1993). Treatment of diarrhea from cryptosporidiosis is difficult. Antibiotics and combined agents (e.g., tinidazole, thiabendazole, and co-trimoxazole) are ineffective (Kelly & Buve, 1993; La Brooy, 1993). Varied results are reported with the use of parenteral octreotide (La Brooy, 1993; Manfredi et al., 1993; Romeu et al., 1991). Antidiarrheal agents to reduce stool volume and narcotics to decrease motility may provide limited relief. Fluid supplements for patients with cryptosporidiosis should be low-fat, lactose free, high calorie, and high protein. Supplements with large amounts of fats and sugar may increase diarrhea and cause bloating (Kotler, 1992).

Microsporidia infection appears to be a significant cause of diarrhea in patients whose GI problems are not attributable to another cause (La Brooy, 1993; Kotler, 1992).

Diarrhea is an overwhelming problem for many patients with AIDS. AIDS complicated by chronic diarrhea is almost twice as expensive to treat as AIDS not complicated by chronic diarrhea, and the patient's quality of life is significantly reduced (Lubeck, Bennett, Mazonson, Fifer, & Fries, 1993). Despite tremendous effort in research and among practitioners, symptom management is challenging and sometimes unsuccessful (Stephany, 1992). The somatostatin analogue octreotide has shown some promise in managing refractory diarrhea (Manfredi et al., 1993). However, octreotide is not effective in most cases (La Brooy, 1993). Management is thus directed primarily to treating the infection causing the diarrhea and trying other measures discussed here and in chapter 17.

Progressive, involuntary weight loss occurs in almost all patients with AIDS and is due to factors such as reduced intake, alterations in metabolism, and malabsorption (Keithley, Zeller, Szeluga, & Urbanski, 1992). Malnutrition and decreased immune response are mutually exacerbating (Andrassy, 1990). In the United States, wasting syndrome, characterized by profound weight loss and chronic diarrhea or chronic weakness, occurs in more than 20% of patients with AIDS. As with other forms of cachexia, wasting syndrome in patients with AIDS does not respond to nutritional therapy (Nahlen et al., 1993). Less severe wasting, may, however, respond to nutritional therapy. In general, when there is weight loss and diarrhea, supplements or diet should be isotonic, lactose-free, high calorie, high protein, low fat (e.g., Vivonex), and taken in small and more frequent amounts (Kotler, 1992; Weaver, 1992). Lactose and polymeric supplements are usually better-tolerated in the absence of diarrhea. However, there is significant variation in response to diet and experimentation, and an individual patient's response is often necessary to correctly gauge treatment modality (Graf, Beal, & Steele, 1992; Smerko, 1990). Because of frequency of complications, especially infection, total parenteral nutrition (TPN) is seldom indicated (Dworkin, 1992; Graf et al., 1992). Enteral feeding (e.g., NG tube) is preferred over TPN (Andrassy, 1990). Because there is enormous variation in content of nutritional supplements, it is wise to utilize the expertise of a registered dietician in examining dietary alternatives.

RENAL DISEASE

Renal disease occurs in 10%–30% of patients with AIDS and is most often found in patients who are African American, and who have a history of injecting drugs (Chaisson & Volberding, 1990). Some of the more common medications used in patients with AIDS (e.g., sulfa drugs, pentamidine, acyclovir, foscarnet, and others) are associated with renal complications (Balow, 1992), as are infections such as MAC and fungal infections (Chaisson & Volberding, 1990). Nephropathy is characterized by rapid progression, few treatment options, and early demise (Balow, 1992).

PULMONARY DISEASE

Pneumocystis carinii pneumonia (PCP)
PCP is either a protozoan or fungal infection, and is the most common life-threatening opportunistic infection in patients with AIDS (Henry & Holzemer, 1992). As a result of advances in treatment, deaths from PCP have declined since 1985 (Mansur, 1990). While PCP may progress rapidly, the onset is often insidious, with fever, weight loss, and fatigue gradually developing for as long as several months. The three most common physical symptoms are unexplained fever, non-productive cough, and shortness of breath progressive from on-exertion to at-rest. Physical examination is

often complicated by wasting and other effects of the disease and respiratory findings may be unremarkable. Dry rales may be present, but consolidation is uncommon, except in far-advanced stages (Henry & Holzemer, 1992). Cutaneus PCP occasionally occurs and is manifested by dome-shaped nodules around the ears and nasopharynx (Cockerell, 1992). Sputum examination using saline mist inhalation ("induced sputum") is currently the best, non-invasive means of diagnosis (Lewis, 1991).

Primary therapy for PCP is currently either Trimethoprim/ sulfamethoxazole (TMP/SMX) or pentamidine, both given intravenously to patients with severe PCP (Klein et al., 1992). Symptoms may worsen for several days after initiation of therapy. Patients with mild to moderately severe disease can take oral TMP and SMX (Hopewell, 1990). TMP may also be given in an aerosol combination with diaminodiphenylsulfone (Dapsone). Other medications for PCP include: (1) trimetrexate; and (2) clindamycin and primaquine (Hopewell, 1990). Treatment of PCP is characterized by adverse effects of medications, which may subsequently have to be discontinued (Klein et al., 1992). TMP/SMX may also be taken prophylactically, preferably orally, but also in an aerosol for primary or secondary prophylaxis. Pentamidine may be taken in an aerosol (USPHS, 1993) but the resultant metallic taste is disliked by most patients. Although corticosteroids are recommended by some (e.g., Levine, 1991), the incidence of secondary infections increases with their use (Hopewell, 1990; Nelson, Erskine, Hawkins, & Gazzard, 1993). Problems of PCP include dyspnea, fever, fatigue, alterations in nutrition, treatment side effects, and problems related to chronic AIDS (Henry & Holzemer, 1992; Rolston & Bodey, 1993). Other respiratory infections, such as CMV, cryptococcal, or other pneumonia, may coexist with PCP. Supportive care is similar to that described under specific problems in earlier chapters, except that practitioners should understand that significant relief occurs through treatment of the

PCP rather than symptom control. Supplemental oxygen, and sometimes ventilation, may be necessary as temporary measures (Hopewell, 1990).

Tuberculosis

Tuberculosis (TB) is caused by *Mycobacterium tuberculosis*. The prevalence of TB in the United States is increasing, in part due to tuberculosis in patients with AIDS (White, 1990). TB infection is a distinct threat to health care workers and to others who come into contact with infected patients; guidelines for protection and regular testing are available from Centers for Disease Control (Wallace & Lasker, 1993). In patients with AIDS, skin tests may give false negative results because of compromised immune response (Makulowich, 1991), and normal chest radiographs may also be negative (Pedro-Botet, Gutierrez, Miralles, & Rubies-Prat, 1992). The situation is further complicated by an increasing incidence of multidrug resistant TB (MDR-TB) (Wallace & Lasker, 1993). In patients with AIDS, TB often presents as a pulmonary infection with a rapid clinical course; or as a disseminated, systemic illness. In either case, the prognosis is poor (Chaisson & Volberding, 1990). Primary symptoms of pulmonary TB include weight loss, night sweats, fatigue, anorexia, fever, and persistent cough (Makulowich, 1991). Other common symptoms are hemoptysis, pleuritic chest pain, and dyspnea (O'Grady & Frasier, 1992; Pitchenik & Fertel, 1992). Extrapulmonary TB is common among patients with AIDS, manifested according to the affected organ system, and commonly includeing lymphadenopathy (Pitchenik & Fertel, 1992).

As with treatments for other AIDS infections, treatment for TB is constantly developing. Treatment is based on susceptibility or resistance (of the mycobacterium). Isoniazid (INH) or rifampin (RIF) are the most effective medications. For resistant and MDR-TB, a number of trials are underway in which INH and/or RIF are combined with pyridoxine, pyrazinamide (PZA), ethambutol (ETH), fluoroquinolones, and/or aminoglycoside antibiotics (e.g., streptomycin) (Wallace & Lasker, 1993). Staff who work with patients who have, or are suspected to have, TB should be tested at regular intervals.

Mycobacterium Avium-Mycobacterium Intracellulare Complex Infection (MAI or MAC)

MAI or MAC, in its disseminated form, is the most commonly reported bacterial infection in patients with AIDS (Friedland & Klein, 1992). MAC is associated with a poor prognosis, and with survival of three-to-seven months after infection (Carr, Penny, & Cooper, 1993, p. s58). Symptoms of MAC, in its pulmonary form, are similar in onset to TB (O'Grady & Frasier, 1992). Disseminated MAC symptoms often include high fever, night sweats, fatigue, anorexia, malaise, anemia and weight loss, along with symptoms specific to the affected system(s), except that pulmonary symptoms are uncommon (Pitchenik & Fertel, 1992). A common site of infection is the gastrointestinal system, with symptoms of abdominal pain, diarrhea, debility, and progressive wasting (Friedland & Klein, 1992; Kotler, 1992, p. 267). The only body tissues that are not frequently infected are the brain, bone, and muscle (Young & Inderlied, 1990). Unlike TB, MAC is not communicable to the general population (Pitchenik & Fertel, 1992).

Treatment involves multidrug regimes, often with high toxicity and modest results, except for some reduction of symptoms (Friedland & Klein, 1992; Pitchenik & Fertel, 1992). Fever and constitutional symptoms may respond to prostaglandin inhibitors (Kotler, 1992).

Histoplasmosis and Coccidioidomycosis

Histoplasmosis and coccidioidomyosis are fungal infections with relatively similar manifestations, including fever, weight loss, and respiratory complications. Both diseases may present in disseminated forms, including central nervous system involvement, hematologic abnormalities, and skin lesions. Treatment for both is amphotericin or ketaconazole; with itraconazole and fluconazole showing promise (Polis & Kovacs, 1992; Sharkey-Mathis, Velez, Fetchick, & Graybill, 1993).

NEUROLOGIC COMPLICATIONS

Cryptococcosis
Cryptococcus infection commonly presents as a CNS disorder, and also as pulmonary, and/or disseminated disease; and is the primary cause of meningitis in patients with AIDS (Finley et al., 1992; Polis and Kovacs, 1992). The infection begins in the lungs via inhalation of spores and spreads through the bloodstream to the meninges. Headache and fever are the most frequently reported initial symptoms. Other, less frequent manifestations include nausea and vomiting, changes in mental status, and meningeal signs (e.g., stiff neck) (Hughes & Schofferman, 1991; Panther & Sande, 1990; Mocsny, 1992a; Polis & Kovacs, 1992). If unchecked, disease progression may include disseminated disease, with problems occurring according to the affected system, as well as CNS manifestations, such as altered mental status and hydrocephalus (Diamond, 1990). Therapy includes amphotericin B and flucytosine, followed by frequently successful suppressive therapy (Polis & Kovacs, 1992).

Cytomegalovirus
Cytomegalovirus (CMV) is the second most common infection in patients with AIDS (Finley, Joshi, & Neill, 1992), but seldom causes symptoms until AIDS is relatively advanced and the immune system seriously compromised (Schooley, 1992). CMV occurs frequently in the lower GI tract, characteristically with symptoms of diarrhea, fever, abdominal pain, rebound tenderness, and no other stool pathogens present (Hutman, 1991a). CMV colitis is associated with extreme wasting (Hutman, 1991b). CMV also commonly appears in the esophagus, respiratory system, and may be disseminated (Finley et al., 1992). CMV is the most common cause of retinitis and is a common cause of death from respiratory infection (Mansur, 1990). Disseminated CMV is common on autopsy, but may not be clinically diagnosed (Hutman, 1991b; Mohar et al., 1992). In part, the incidence of CMV is increasing because of advances in therapy for PCP (Carr et al., 1993), and increasing awareness of the importance of CMV in AIDS (Yarrish, 1992). Development of CMV is sometimes associated with use of systemic corticosteroids for other disorders, such as idiopathic thrombocytopenia purpura, PCP, or cerebral edema (Nelson et al., 1993).

In patients diagnosed with CMV, secondary prophylaxis with ganciclovir or foscarnet against retinitis is "mandatory," with the latter giving longer survival (Carr et al., 1993). Ganciclovir or foscarnet are the main treatment options (Harb, Bacchetti, & Jacobson, 1991; Schooley, 1992). Unfortunately, CMV is increasingly resistant to ganciclovir, and, to a lesser extent, to foscarnet (Mansur, 1990). The problem of extensive or complete adventitious vision loss is best approached with specialty care from a rehabilitation therapist or similar professional, and from a volunteer working with the blind. Major problems to address are safety at home or in the treatment facility, promoting independence (including bathing, grooming, dressing, medicating, eating, and toileting), and minimizing sensitivity to light (Ungvarski, 1992).

Toxoplasmosis
Toxoplasmosis is a latent protozoan infection, usually of the central nervous system (CNS). Toxoplasmic encephalitis is the most commonly treated CNS AIDS disorder. It develops over several days from initial symptoms to neurological deficits (Price et al., 1992). Toxoplasmosis is manifested initially by dull, constant headache and subtle alteration in mental status (Mocsny, 1992b). Symptoms of progression include fever,

headache, altered mental status (including confusion, lethargy, delusions, fatigue, cognitive impairment, anomia, coma), seizures, or focal neurologic signs (most commonly hemiparesis, but including ataxia, movement disorder, aphasia, and visual changes) (Israelski, Dannemann, & Remington, 1990; Mocsny, 1992b). Cognitive deficits from this infection may not be correctable (Mocsny, 1993). Toxoplasmosis also occurs in the respiratory system, heart, peritoneum, pancreas, liver, colon, and testes. Definitive diagnosis is possible only by brain biopsy, so diagnosis is through characteristic findings on various neurologic and other studies, plus response to therapy (Israelski et al., 1990).

Primary therapy is usually a combination of pyrimethamine and sulfadiazine or trisulfapyrimidines orally. Toxicity is common, especially bone marrow suppression, which induces thrombocytopenia, granulocytopenia, or megaloblastic anemia. Folinic acid (leucovorin calcium) is given orally or parenterally to prevent or treat marrow toxicity (Hughes & Schofferman, 1991; Price et al., 1992). Other treatments are being investigated. Toxoplasmic encephalitis may be complicated by syndrome of inappropriate antidiuretic hormone secretion (see the section on Paraneoplastic Syndromes in chapter 20) (Hughes & Schofferman, 1991). Primary therapy is followed by lifelong maintenance therapy on anti-toxoplasmosis agents (Mocsny, 1993). Supportive care includes providing and teaching seizure precautions, providing and teaching how to create a stress-reduced environment to aid in the treatment of headache, and responding appropriately to any cognitive or other neurological deficits (Moscny, 1992b). Please refer to the section, Confusion: Delirium and Dementia, in chapter 13.

AIDS Dementia Complex

AIDS dementia complex (ADC) is a complex of cognitive, motor, and behavioral dysfunction that tend to develop slowly late in the course of HIV infection, often after several major opportunistic infections (Brew, 1993; Price et al., 1992). To a lesser extent, ADC sometimes exists in the absence of other manifestations of AIDS (Scharnhorst, 1992). ADC, sometimes known as HIV encephalopathy, may be a result of HIV, or CMV, or HIV and CMV infection of the CNS (Sotrel & Multani, 1992). While there are subgroups of disorders of ADC, and variations among individuals, there are generally common clinical features of the disorder. Cognitively, patients gradually deteriorate from slightly slowed thinking, difficulty concentrating, and forgetfulness, to confusion, amnesia, mutism, and global dementia. Motor dysfunction often begins with poor handwriting, tremors, unsteady gait, poor balance (especially with fast head turns), and lower extremity weakness. Eventually a cane is needed to walk, then a walker, and finally the patient is bedfast and incontinent. Behavior varies, but it is common for patients to become withdrawn and apathetic. Some patients, however, have manic behavior. Insight decreases late in the process, and thus patients are often aware of their mental deterioration. The condition is complicated by all the psychosocial features common to AIDS: depression, anxiety, fear, isolation, etc. (Brew, 1993; Price & Sidtis, 1992; Worth, Savage, Baer, Esty, & Navia, 1993).

Treatment and/or prophylaxis of ADC is with zidovudine and results are generally encouraging (Brew, 1993). Susceptibility to side effects of antipsychotics—e.g., extrapyramidal symptoms—is increased in patients with ADC, and probably in other patients with HIV infection. Please see chapters 13, 28, and 29 for further information on assessing and caring for patients with related problems.

AIDS-RELATED CANCER

Kaposi's Sarcoma

Kaposi's sarcoma (KS) is the most common neoplasm among patients with HIV infection, and is significantly more common among homosexual and bisexual men with AIDS than in any other

AIDS population (Boyle, Sewell, Milliken, Cooper, & Penny, 1993). For unknown causes, the incidence of KS as an index AIDS diagnosis is decreasing. At the same time, success in treating other manifestations of AIDS has meant that KS is a greater problem in immunosuppressed patients (Gompels et al., 1992). KS usually presents as painless, slightly raised or nodular, reddish skin lesions (darker in dark-skinned patients) of varied size (0.5–2 cm) that may be associated with area edema. Lesions grow in size and become more tumorous or nodular, and/or coalesce to form larger lesions that may ulcerate. In advanced disease, the oral cavity, gastrointestinal tract, and respiratory system may be involved, and to a lesser extent, other areas (Kaplan & Volberding, 1993; Levine, Gill, & Salahuddin, 1992). Except for those with pulmonary involvement, patients with KS are more likely to die from infection than KS. Skin lesions may become painful and serve as sites for secondary infection. Facial or lower extremity edema secondary to lymphatic obstruction is common (Kaplan & Volberding, 1993). GI involvement may result in considerable visceral pain.

Treatment includes radiation to reduce skin or other troublesome lesions (e.g., oral, pharyngeal) and systemic therapy for advanced disease (Boyle et al., 1993; Gompels et al., 1992; Kaplan & Volberding, 1993). Systemic therapy presents a variety of treatment problems.

Non-Hodgkin's Lymphoma

Although not as common as KS in patients with AIDS, Non-Hodgkin's lymphoma (NHL) is increasing in incidence overall, and is found in all populations of patients with AIDS (Boyle et al., 1993). AIDS-associated NHL is characterized by lymphadenopathy and extranodal disease, most commonly involving the central nervous system, bone marrow, gastrointestinal tract, and liver; and a poor prognosis (Kaplan & Volberding, 1993). Most patients with AIDS-related NHL present with systemic symptoms, such as unexplained fever, drenching night

sweats, and/or weight loss (Levine et al., 1992). Symptoms of advanced disease are related to involved sites, which may be extensive. Primary CNS lymphoma may result in a wide variety of neurologic symptoms and is associated with the poorest prognosis of any site (Levine, 1992). Treatment involves multiple and varied protocols, all of which are complicated by the toxicity of the more effective agents (Boyle et al., 1993). Although the prognosis for patients with AIDS-related non-Hodgkin's lymphoma is markedly poorer than for those without AIDS, the discussion of NHL in section IV of this book is also relevant to patients with AIDS.

Children With AIDS

As increasing numbers of women are infected with HIV (CDC, 1992b), so, too, will increasing numbers of infants be infected by mother-infant transmission. Some children and adolescents also will be increasingly infected as a secondary effect of IV drug use and homosexual and heterosexual contacts, as well as through sexual abuse. Transmission via transfusion, which devastated young hemophiliacs, is not currently a problem of large dimension, as it was before universal testing was initiated in blood banks. From 1981–1990, 1,449 children age 14 or younger died from AIDS (CDC, 1991b). (An approximately equal number of children are projected to die from cancer in 1992 [American Cancer Society, 1992]). The suffering of children with AIDS is compounded by the frequency with which entire families are infected (Butler & Pizzo, 1992).

While many aspects of AIDS are similar in children and adults, there are some important age-specific characteristics. Infants who are symptomatic before age 12 months tend to develop more opportunistic infections, contract HIV-related encephalopathy, and have a poorer prognosis. Infection may be manifested by failure to thrive, lymphadenopathy, organomegaly, and increased incidence of common childhood illness. Infections, e.g., PCP, may be more severe in children than in adults. CNS involvement is also more common in children than in adults (Grubman, Conviser, & Oleske, 1992). As in other highly specialized situations, practitioners should seek current and specialized resources to help in understanding children with AIDS. Please see the recommended readings listed below.

Recommended Reading

DeVita, V.T., Hellman, S. & Rosenberg, S.A. (Eds.). (1992). *AIDS: Etiology, diagnosis, treatment, and prevention* (3rd ed.). Philadelphia: J.B. Lippincott Company.

Flaskerud, J.H. & Ungvarski, P.J. (Eds.). (1992). *HIV/AIDS: A guide to nursing care*. Philadelphia: W.B. Saunders Company.

Sande, M.A. & Volberding, P.A. (Eds.). (1990). *The Medical management of AIDS* (2nd ed.). Philadelphia: W.B. Saunders Company.

Wormser, G.P. (Ed.). (1992). *AIDS and other manifestations of HIV infection* (2nd ed.). New York: Raven Press.

References

American Cancer Society. (1992). *Cancer facts and figures—1992*. Atlanta: Author.

Andrassy, R.J. (1990). Nutrition and immunocompromise. *AIDS Patient Care*. 4(Supplement 1), s9–s12.

Azizi, B., & Epstein, J.B. (1992). Oral hairy leukoplakia in immunocompromised patients. *AIDS Patient Care*, 6(3), 118–122.

Balow, J.E. (1992). Renal complications. In V.T. DeVita, S. Hellman, & S.A. Rosenberg (Eds.), *AIDS: Etiology, diagnosis, treatment, and prevention* (3rd ed.) (pp. 334–336). Philadelphia: J.B. Lippincott Company.

Berger, T.G. (1990). Dermatologic care in the AIDS patient: A 1990 update. In M.A. Sande & P.A. Volberding (Eds.) *The Medical Management of AIDS* (2nd ed.) (pp. 114–130). Philadelphia: W.B. Saunders Company.

Boswell, S.L., & Hirsch, M.S. (1992). Therapeutic approaches to the HIV-seropositive patient. In V.T. DeVita, S. Hellman, & S.A. Rosenberg (Eds.), *AIDS: Etiology, diagnosis, treatment, and prevention* (3rd ed.) (pp. 417–433). Philadelphia: J.B. Lippincott Company.

Boyle, M.J., Sewell, W.A., Milliken, S.T., Cooper, D.A., & Penny, R. (1993). HIV and Malignancy. *Journal of Acquired Immune Deficiency*, 6 (Supplement 1), s5–s9.

Brew, B.J. (1993). HIV-1-related neurological disease. *Journal of Acquired Immune Deficiency Syndromes*, 6 (Supplement 1), s10–s15.

Butler, K.M., & Pizzo, P.A. (1992). HIV infection in children. In V.T. DeVita, S. Hellman, & S.A. Rosenberg (Eds.), *AIDS: Etiology, diagnosis, treatment, and prevention* (3rd ed.) (pp. 285–312). Philadelphia: J.B. Lippincott Company.

Caron, D., Jacobson, D., & Walsh, C. (1992). Hematologic findings in HIV infection. In G.P. Wormser (Ed.), *AIDS and other manifestations of HIV infection* (2nd ed.) (pp. 455–461). New York: Raven Press.

Carr, A., Penny, R., & Cooper, D.A. (1993). Prophylaxis of opportunistic infections in patients with HIV infection. *Journal of Acquired Immune Deficiency Syndrome*, 6 (Supplement 1), s56–s60.

Cello, J.P. (1990). AIDS-associated Gastrointestinal disease. In M.A. Sande & P.A. Volberding (Eds.) *The Medical Management of AIDS* (2nd ed.) (pp. 145–160). Philadelphia: W.B. Saunders Company.

Centers for Disease Control. (1991). Mortality attributable to HIV infection/AIDS—United States, 1981–1990, *Morbidity and Mortality Weekly Report*, 40(3), 41–44.

Centers for Disease Control. (1992a). The second 100,000 cases of acquired immunodeficiency syndrome—United States, June 1981–December 1991. *Morbidity and Mortality Weekly Report*, 41(2), 28–29.

Centers for Disease Control. (1992b). Projections of the number of persons diagnosed with AIDS and the number of immunosuppressed HIV-infected persons—United States, 1992–1994. *Morbidity and Mortality Weekly Report*, 41(18), 1–26.

Centers for Disease Control. (1992c). Surveillance for occupationally acquired HIV infection—United States, 1981–1992. *Morbidity and Mortality Weekly Report*, 41(43), 823–825.

Chaisson, R.E., & Volberding, P.A. (1990). Clinical manifestations of HIV infection. In G.L. Mandell, R.G. Douglas, & J.E. Bennett (Eds.), *Principles and practices of infectious diseases* (3rd ed.) (pp. 1059–1092). New York: Churchill Livingston.

Cockerell, C.J. (1992). Cutaneous and histologic signs of HIV infection other than Kaposi's sarcoma. In G.P. Wormser (Ed.), *AIDS and other manifestations of HIV infection* (2nd ed.) (pp. 463–476). New York: Raven Press.

Diamond, R.D. (1990). Cryptococcus neoformans. In G.L. Mandell, R.G. Douglas, & J.E. Bennett (Eds.), *Principles and practices of infectious diseases* (3rd ed.) (pp. 1980–1989). New York: Churchill Livingston.

Dodd, C.L., Greenspan, D., Katz, M., Westonhouse, J.L., Feigal, D.W., & Greenspan, J.S. (1991). Oral candidiasis in HIV infection: Pseudomembranous and erythematous candidiasis show similar rates of progression to AIDS. *AIDS*, 5(11), 1339–1343.

Dworkin, B.M. (1992). Gastrointestinal manifestations of AIDS. In G.P. Wormser (Ed.), *AIDS and other manifestations of HIV infection* (2nd ed.) (pp. 419–432). New York: Raven Press.

Ehrhardt, A.A. (1992). Trends in sexual behavior and the HIV pandemic. *American Journal of Public Health, 82*(11), 1459–1461.

Feigal, D.W., Katz, M.H., Greenspan, D., Westonhouse, J., Winklestein, W., Lang, W., Samue, M., Buchbinder, S.P., Hessol, N.A., Lifson, A.R., Rutherford, G.W., Moss, A., Osmond, D., Shiboski, S., & Greenspan, J.S. (1991). The prevalence of oral lesions in HIV-infected homosexual and bisexual men: Three San Francisco epidemiological cohorts. *AIDS, 5*(5), 519–525.

Finley, J.L., Joshi, V.V., & Neill, J.S.A. (1992). General pathology of HIV infection. In G.P. Wormser (Ed.), *AIDS and other manifestations of HIV infection* (2nd ed.) (pp. 499–541) New York: Raven Press.

Friedland, G., & Klein, R. (1992). Tuberculosis and other bacterial infections. In V.T. DeVita, S. Hellman, & S.A. Rosenberg (Eds.), *AIDS: Etiology, diagnosis, treatment, and prevention* (3rd ed.) (pp. 180–193). Philadelphia: J.B. Lippincott Company.

Galantino, M.L. (1991). Pain management and neuromuscular reeducation for the HIV patient. *AIDS Patient Care, 5*(2), 81–85.

Gompels, M.M., Hill, A., Jenkins, P., Peters, B., Tomlinson, D., Harris, J.R.W., Stewart, S., & Pinching, A.J. (1992). Kaposi's sarcoma in HIV infection treated with vincristine and bleomycin. *AIDS, 6*(10), 1175–1180.

Graf, L.J., Beal, J., & Steele, S. (1992). Management of chronic weight loss with an elemental formula. *AIDS Patient Care, 6*(2), 50–51.

Greenspan, J.S., & Greenspan, D. (1992). Oral lesions associated with HIV infection. In G.P. Wormser (Ed.), *AIDS and other manifestations of HIV infection* (2nd ed.) (pp. 489–498). New York: Raven Press.

Greenspan, J.S., Greenspan, D., & Winkler, J.R. (1990). Diagnosis and management of the oral manifestations of HIV infection and AIDS. In M.A. Sande & P.A. Volberding (Eds.) *The Medical Management of AIDS* (2nd ed.) (pp. 131–144). Philadelphia: W.B. Saunders Company.

Grubman, S., Conviser, R., & Oleske, J. (1992). HIV infection in infants, children, and adolescents. In G.P. Wormser (Ed.), *AIDS and other manifestations of HIV infection* (2nd ed.) (pp. 201–216). New York: Raven Press.

Hambleton, J., & Abrams, D.I. (1990). Hematologic manifestations of HIV infection. In M.A. Sande & P.A. Volberding (Eds.), *The Medical Management of AIDS* (2nd ed.) (pp. 182–194). Philadelphia: W.B. Saunders Company.

Hanson, D.L., Horsburgh, C.R., Fann, S.A., Havlik, J.A., & Thompson, S.E. (1993). Survival prognosis of HIV-infected patients. *Journal of Acquired Immune Deficiency Syndrome, 6*(6), 624–629.

Harb, G.E., Bacchetti, P., & Jacobson, M.A. (1991). Survival of patients with AIDS and cytomegalovirus disease treated with ganciclovir or foscarnet. *AIDS, 5*(8), 959–965.

Henry, S.B., & Holzemer, W.L. (1992). Critical care management of the patient with HIV infection who has *Pneumocystis carinii* pneumonia. *Heart & Lung, 21*(3), 243–249.

Hopewell, P.C. (1990). *Pneumocystis carinii* pneumonia. In M.A. Sande & P.A. Volberding (Eds.), *The Medical Management of AIDS* (2nd ed.) (pp. 209–240). Philadelphia: W.B. Saunders Company.

Hughes, A.M., & Schofferman, J. (1991). AIDS and the spectrum of HIV disease. In S.B. Baird, R. McCorkle, & M. Grant (Eds.), *Cancer nursing: A comprehensive textbook* (pp. 647–663). Philadelphia: W.B Saunders.

Hutman, S. (1991a). CMV gastrointestinal disease. *AIDS Patient Care, 5*(6), 282–285.

Hutman, S. (1991b). CMV Colitis. *AIDS Patient Care, 5*(6), 282–285.

Israelski, D.M., Dannemann, B.R., & Remington, J.S. (1990). Toxoplasmosis in patients with AIDS. In M.A. Sande & P.A. Volberding (Eds.) *The Medical Management of AIDS* (2nd ed.) (pp. 241–264). Philadelphia: W.B. Saunders Company.

Kaplan, L.D., & Volberding, P.A. (1993). Neoplasms in acquired immunodeficiency syndrome. In J.F. Holland, E. Frei, R.C. Bast, D.W. Kufe, D.L. Morton, & R.W. Weischselbaum (Eds.), *Cancer medicine* (3rd ed.) (pp. 2105–2120). Philadelphia: Lea & Febiger.

Keithley, J.K., Zeller, J.M., Szeluga, D.J., & Urbanski, P.A. (1992). Nutritional alterations in persons with HIV infection. *Image, 24*(3), 183–189.

Kelly, P., & Buve, A. (1993). Chemotherapy of African AIDS diarrhoea. *AIDS, 7*(1), 91–93.

Klein, N.C., Duncanson, F.P., Lenox, T.H., Forszniak, C., Sherer, C.B., Quentzel, H., Nunez, M., Suarez, M., Kawwaff, O., Pitta-Alvarez, A., Freeman, K., & Wormser, G.P. (1992). Trimethoprim-sulfamethoxazole versus pentamidine for *Pneumocystis carinii* pneumonia in AIDS patients: Results of a large prospective randomized treatment trial. *AIDS, 6*(3), 301–305.

Koppel, B.S. (1992). Neurological complications of AIDS and HIV infection: An overview. In G.P. Wormser (Ed.), *AIDS and other manifestations of HIV infection* (2nd ed.) (pp. 315–348). New York: Raven Press.

Kotler, D.P. (1992). Gastrointestinal manifestations of HIV infection and AIDS. In V.T. DeVita, S. Hellman, & S.A. Rosenberg (Eds.), *AIDS: Etiology, diagnosis, treatment, and prevention* (3rd ed.) (pp. 259–283). Philadelphia: J.B. Lippincott Company.

La Brooy, J.T. (1993). Enteropathy in HIV infection. *Journal of Acquired Immune Deficiency Syndromes, 6* (Supplement 1), s16–s19.

Levine, A.M. (1992). Lymphoma and other miscellaneous cancers. In V.T. DeVita, S. Hellman, & S.A. Rosenberg (Eds.), *AIDS: Etiology, diagnosis, treatment, and prevention* (3rd ed.) (pp. 225–235). Philadelphia: J.B. Lippincott Company.

Levine, S.J., & Shelhamer, J.H. (1992). Pulmonary complications. In V.T. DeVita, S. Hellman, & S.A.

Rosenberg (Eds.), *AIDS: Etiology, diagnosis, treatment, and prevention* (3rd ed.) (pp. 320–334). Philadelphia: J.B. Lippincott Company.

Levine, D. (1991). Treating PCP with corticosteroids. *AIDS Patient Care, 5*(1), 28–30.

Lewis, J.L. (1991). The diagnosis of *Pneumocystis carinii* pneumonia by induced sputum. *Aids Patient Care, 5*(5), 237–241.

Lubeck, D.P., Bennett, C.L., Mazonson, P.D., Fifer, S.K., & Fries, J.F. (1993). Quality of life and health service use among HIV-infected patients with chronic diarrhea. *Journal of Acquired Immune Deficiency Syndromes, 6*(5), 478–484.

Makulowich, G.S. (1991). The new challenges of controlling tuberculosis transmission. *AIDS Patient Care, 5*(5), 244–248.

Manfredi, R., Vezzadini, P., Costigliola, P., Ricchi, E., Pia Fanti, M., & Chiodo, F. (1993). Elevated plasma levels of vasoactive intestinal peptide in AIDS patients with refractory idiopathic diarrhoea. Effects of treatment with octreotide. *AIDS, 7*(20, 223–226.

Mansur, H. (1990). The changing face of opportunistic infections for the nineties. *AIDS Patient Care, 4*(5), 25–29.

Mast, S.T., Woolwine, J.D., & Gerberding, J.L. (1993). Efficacy of gloves in reducing blood volumes transferred during simulated needlestick injury. *Journal of Infectious Diseases, 168*(12), 1589–1592.

Mc Gowan, I., Hawkins, A.S., & Weller, I.V.D. (1993). The natural history of Cryptosporidium diarrhoea in HIV-infected patients. *AIDS, 7*(3), 349–354.

Mocsny, N. (1992a). Cryptococcal meningitis in patients with AIDS. *Journal of Neuroscience Nursing, 24*(5), 265–268.

Mocsny, N. (1992b). Toxoplasmic encephalitis in patients with AIDS. *Journal of Neuroscience Nursing, 24*(1), 30–33.

Mocsny, N. (1993). Toxoplasmic encephalitis in the AIDS patient. *Rehabilitation Nursing, 18*(1), 20–22,25.

Mohar, A., Romo, J., Salido, F., Jessurun, J., Ponce de Leon, S., Reyes, E., Volkow, P., Larraza, O., Peredo, M.A., Cano, C., Gomez, G., Sepulveda, J., & Mueller, N. (1992). The spectrum of AIDS in a consecutive series of autopsied patients in Mexico. *AIDS, 6*(5), 467–473.

Morrison, C. (1993). Delivery systems for the care of persons with HIV infection and AIDS. *Nursing Clinics of North America, 28*(2), 317–332.

Nahlen, B.L., Chu, S.Y., Nwanyanwu,, O.C., Berkelman, R.L., Martinez, S.A., & Rullan, J.V. (1993). HIV wasting syndrome in the United States. *AIDS, 7*(2), 183–188.

National Commission on Acquired Immune Deficiency Syndrome. (1991). *America living with AIDS.* Washington, DC: Author.

Nelson, M.R., Erskine, D., Hawkins, D.A., & Gazzard, B.G. (1993). Treatment with corticosteroids—a risk factor for the development of clinical cytomegalovirus disease in AIDS. *AIDS, 7*(3), 375–378.

Northfelt, D.W., & Mitsuyasu, R.T. (1992). Hematologic complications of HIV infection. In V.T. DeVita, S. Hellman, & S.A. Rosenberg (Eds.), *AIDS: Etiology, diagnosis, treatment, and prevention* (3rd ed.) (pp. 337–345). Philadelphia: J.B. Lippincott Company.

O'Grady, S.M., & Frasier, K.E. (1992). Recognizing and managing mycobacterial diseases in clients with AIDS. *Nurse Practitioner, 17*(7), 41–45.

Panther, L.A., & Sande, M.A. (1990). Cryptococcal meningitis in AIDS. In M.A. Sande & P.A. Volberding (Eds.) *The Medical Management of AIDS* (2nd ed.) (pp. 265–279). Philadelphia: W.B. Saunders Company.

Pedro-Botet, J., Gutierrez, J., Miralles, R., & Rubies-Prat, J. (1992). Pulmonary tuberculosis in HIV-infected patients with normal chest radiographs. *AIDS, 6*(1), 91–93.

Pharmaceutical Manufacturers Association. (1992). *AIDS medicines.* Author: Washington, DC.

Pitchenik, A.E., & Fertel, D. (1992). Mycobacterial disease in patients with HIV infection. In G.P. Wormser (Ed.), *AIDS and other manifestations of HIV infection* (2nd ed.) (pp. 277–313). New York: Raven Press.

Polis, M.A., & Kovacs, J.A. (1992). Fungal infections in patients with acquired immunodeficiency. In V.T. DeVita, S. Hellman, & S.A. Rosenberg (Eds.), *AIDS: Etiology, diagnosis, treatment, and prevention* (3rd ed.) (pp. 167–180). Philadelphia: J.B. Lippincott Company.

Price, R.W., & Sidtis, J.J. (1992). The AIDS dementia complex. In G.P. Wormser (Ed.), *AIDS and other manifestations of HIV infection* (2nd ed.) (pp. 373–382). New York: Raven Press.

Price, R.W., Brew, B.J., & Roke, M. (1992). Central and peripheral nervous system complications of HIV-1 infection and AIDS. In V.T. DeVita, S. Hellman, & S.A. Rosenberg (Eds.), *AIDS: Etiology, diagnosis, treatment, and prevention* (3rd ed.) (pp. 237–257). Philadelphia: J.B. Lippincott Company.

Rarick, M.U., Espina, B., Montgomery, T., Easley, A., Allen, J., Levine, A.M. (1991). The long-term use of zidovudine in patients with severe immune-mediated thrombocytopenia secondary to infection with HIV. *AIDS, 5*(11), 1357–1361.

Rolston, K.V.I., & Bodey, G.P. (1993). Infections in patients with cancer. In J.F. Holland, E. Frei, R.C. Bast, D.W. Kufe, D.L. Morton, & R.W. Weischselbaum (Eds.), *Cancer medicine* (3rd ed.) (pp. 1285–1337). Philadelphia: Lea & Febiger.

Romeu, J., Miro, J.M., Sirera, G., Mallolas, J., Arnal, J., Valls, M.E., Tortosa, F., Clotet, B., & Foz, M. (1991). Efficacy of octreotide in the management of chronic diarrhoea in AIDS. *AIDS, 5*(12), 1495–1499.

Safai, B., & Schwartz, J.J. (1992). Noninfectious organ-specific complications of HIV infection. In V.T. DeVita, S. Hellman, & S.A. Rosenberg (Eds.), *AIDS: Etiology, diagnosis, treatment, and prevention* (3rd ed.) (pp. 313–319). Philadelphia: J.B. Lippincott Company.

Scharnhorst, S. (1992). AIDS dementia complex in the elderly. *Nurse Practitioner, 17*(8), 37, 41–43.

Schofferman, J., & Brody, R. (1990). Pain in far advanced AIDS. In K.M. Foley, J.J. Bonica, & V. Ventafridda (Eds.), *Advances in pain research and therapy, Volume 16: Proceedings of the Second International Congress on Cancer Pain.* (pp. 379–386). New York: Raven Press.

Schooley, R.T. (1992). Herpesvirus infection in individuals with HIV infection. In V.T. DeVita, S. Hellman, & S.A. Rosenberg (Eds.), *AIDS: Etiology, diagnosis, treatment, and prevention* (3rd ed.) (pp. 193–207). Philadelphia: J.B. Lippincott Company.

Sharkey-Mathis, P.K., Velez, J., Fetchick, R., & Graybill, J.R. (1993). Histoplasmosis in the acquired immunodeficiency syndrome (AIDS): Treatment with itraconazole and fluconazole. *Journal of Acquired Immune Deficiency, 6*(7), 809–819.

Simpson, D.M., & Wolfe, D.E. (1991). Neuromuscular complications of HIV infection and its treatment. *AIDS, 5*(8), 917–926.

Smerko, A. (1990). Oral nutritional products for the HIV outpatient. *AIDS Patient Care, 4*(Supplement 1), s17–s22.

Smith, D.E., Midgley, J., Allan, M., Connolly, M., & Gazzard, B.G. (1991). Itraconazole versus ketaconazole in the treatment of oral and esophageal candidiasis in patients infected with HIV. *AIDS, 5*(11), 1367–1371.

Sotrel, A., & Multani, P. (1992). Pathology of the nervous system in HIV-infected patients. In G.P. Wormser (Ed.), *AIDS and other manifestations of HIV infection* (2nd ed.) (pp. 543–584). New York: Raven Press.

Stephany, T.M. (1992). AIDS does not fit the cancer model of hospice care. *American Journal of Hospice and Palliative Care, 9*(1), 13–14.

Swan, J.H., Benjamin, A.E., & Brown, A. (1992). Skilled nursing facility care for persons with AIDS: Comparison with other patients. *American Journal of Public Health, 82*(3), 453–455.

Tindall, B., Imrie, A., Donovan, B. Penny, R., & Cooper, D.A. (1990). Primary HIV infection: Clinical, immunologic and serologic aspects. In M.A. Sande & P.A. Volberding (Eds.) *The Medical Management of AIDS* (2nd ed.) (pp. 68–84). Philadelphia: W.B. Saunders Company.

U.S. Public Health Service. (1993). Recommendations for prophylaxis against *Pneumocystis carinii* pneumonia for persons infected with human immunodeficiency virus. *Journal of Acquired Immune Deficiency Syndromes, 6*(1), 46–55.

Ungvarski, P.J. (1992). Nursing management of the adult client. In J.H. Flaskerud & P.J. Ungvarski (Eds.), *HIV/AIDS: A guide to nursing care* (2nd ed.) (pp. 146–198). Philadelphia: W.B. Saunders Company.

von Gunten, C.F., Martinez, J., Weitzman, S.A., & Von Roenn, J. (1991). AIDS and hospice. *American Journal of Hospice and Palliative Care, 8*(4), 17–19.

Wallace, B., & Lasker, J. (1993). Tuberculosis and HIV infection: An overview. *AIDS Patient Care, 7*(2), 78–81.

Weaver, K. (1992). Reversible malnutrition in AIDS. *American Journal of Nursing, 91*(9), 25–31.

White, K. (1990). HIV and tuberculosis. *AIDS Patient Care, 4*(6), 16–19.

Worth, J.L., Savage, C.R., Baer, L., Esty, E.K., & Navia, B.A. (1993). Computer-based neuropsychological screening for AIDS dementia complex. *AIDS, 7*(5), 677–681.

Yarrish, R.L. (1992). Cytomegalovirus infections in AIDS. In G.P. Wormser (Ed.), *AIDS and other manifestations of HIV infection* (2nd ed.) (pp. 249–268). New York: Raven Press.,

Young, L.S., & Inderlied, C.B. (1990). Mycobacterium avium complex infections. *AIDS Patient Care, 4*(5), 10–19.

Degenerative Neurological Disorders

While not listed among the fifteen leading causes of death in the United States (Centers for Disease Control [CDC], 1990), degenerative neurological disorders are the primary diagnosis in some patients receiving palliative care. The physiological decline of terminally ill patients with neurological disorders is dissimilar in some respects to that of patients suffering from other major illness , but pneumonia, the sixth leading cause of death (CDC, 1990), is a common ending. Common also, is the enormous physical, psychosocial, and spiritual stress placed on family caregivers as they work to care for a suffering family member.

This chapter examines the most widespread degenerative neurological disorders: multiple sclerosis, Parkinson's disease, amyotrophic lateral sclerosis, and myasthenia gravis. (Alzheimer's disease is discussed on its own, in chapter 29.) Each disorder is discussed individually and unique aspects are identified. Problems shared by these disorders, and by Alzheimer's disease and other cognitive impairment illnesses, are discussed instead in the following chapter, along with recommendations for related care and treatment.

Multiple Sclerosis

Multiple sclerosis (MS) is a complex chronic degenerative neurological disorder with unknown cause and cure (Morgante, Madonna, & Pokoluk, 1989). Several forms, or patterns, of MS exist and not all are fatal (Hainsworth, Burke, Lindgren, & Eakes, 1993). MS usually begins between the ages of 20 and 40 (Adams & Victor, 1989, p. 758) and has a trajectory, or course of illness, lasting as long as thirty or more years (Kassirer & Osterberg, 1987). Disabilities from MS include both sensory and motor impairment. In the later stages of the fatal disease pattern, these are usually: (1) a mix of signs, including cerebella ataxia, optic nerve neuritis, and brainstem and spinal cord dysfunction; or (2) a "spinal cord form" of MS (Adams & Victor, 1989).

Cerebellar ataxia is characterized by slurred or scanning speech (i.e., speech in which there are regular pauses), nystagmus, loss of coordi-

Charles Kemp: TERMINAL ILLNESS: A GUIDE TO NURSING CARE. © 1995 J. B. Lippincott.

nation, and sometimes very severe intentional tremors. Involvement of the optic nerve is common, and results in optic neuritis, a partial or total and often temporary or improving loss of vision in one or both eye(s). Diplopia is also common. Brainstem involvement can be characterized by facial paralysis or myokymia (brief muscle contractions), loss of hearing, tinnitus, unformed auditory hallucinations, vertigo, and vomiting. Quadriplegia may also occur. Lower spinal cord involvement is manifested by paresis, spastic ataxia, lower extremity sensory changes, sexual dysfunction, constipation, and urinary dysfunction, including urinary hesitancy, urgency, frequency, and incontinence. Seizures or tetanic spasms occur in some patients (Adams & Victor, 1989; Dewis & Thornton, 1989; Hickey, 1992).

Fatigue is a common chronic symptom of MS, and increases as the disease progresses. "MS fatigue" does not always have an apparent etiology, other than the disease itself (Hubsky & Sears, 1992).

Emotional distress is common in all chronic disease, but seems to occur in MS to a greater degree than in other similarly degenerative diseases, e.g., amyotrophic lateral sclerosis (Buelow, 1991). While the euphoria sometimes found in patients with MS has received much attention, depression is far more common (Acorn & Andersen, 1990; Adams and Victor, 1989). Depression has been inconclusively studied as a response, a sign or symptom, and as a precipitating factor in MS (Acorn & Andersen, 1990). Bipolar disorder may also be disproportionately represented among patients with MS (Miller & Hens, 1993). Isolation, helplessness, hopelessness, and increased dependence are hallmarks of advanced MS, and with the lengthy trajectory of the disease, fit well with the concept of chronic sorrow (Gulick & Bugg, 1992; Hainsworth et al., 1993).

MS dementia occurs in later stages of the disease, and is characterized by euphoria, emotional lability, and depression. Cognitive dysfunction is not necessarily profound, and may

be primarily an inability to utilize new information (Mitchell, 1989). However, global dementia, or a confused psychosis, may also occur (Adams & Victor, 1989).

Treatment of MS is palliative and experimental (Hickey, 1992; Morgante et al., 1989). Steroids are commonly used during periods of exacerbation and muscle relaxants or tranquilizers are often used for spasticity or related symptoms (Hickey, 1992). Clinical trials of other treatments are routinely conducted (Morgante et al., 1989).

Pain is a more common problem in patients with MS—especially in far advanced disease—than is reflected in the literature. The most common pain is neuropathic and is characterized by sharp burning and tingling in the extremities. Headache and painful spasms of the extremities are also common, as is dull, aching lower back pain (Gulick & Bugg, 1992; Kassirer & Osterberg, 1987). Please refer to part II of this book, in particular to discussions of neuropathic pain in chapters 11 and 12.

The primary cause of death in patients with MS is, predictably, pneumonia. The second leading cause of death is more startling: In one study, 28.6% of MS deaths were attributed to suicide by (in descending order) overdose, gunshot, and starvation (Sadovnick, Eisen, Ebers, & Paty, 1991). Severe urinary tract infections are common in the later stages, and may constitute a frequent cause of death (Hickey, 1992).

Parkinson's Disease

Parkinson's disease (PD) is a chronic, degenerative, slowly progressive disease of the basal ganglia (Hickey, 1992) with disease onset most frequently around age 60 years (Adams & Victor, 1989). The primary characteristics of PD are muscle rigidity, resting tremors, bradykinesia (slow movement), and stooped and unstable posture (Vernon, 1989). Secondary characteristics include general weakness and fatigue, mask-like facies, monotone voice, blurred vision, and cognitive changes. Autonomic changes include drooling, oily skin, dysphagia, increased perspiration, constipation, orthostatic hypotension, and urinary frequency and hesitation (Hickey, 1992). As the disease progresses, all movement is slowed, including chewing, swallowing, and speaking, and the patient becomes increasingly immobile. Vision may blur and the ability to speak diminishes. About 10% to 30% of patients are likely to have moderate to severe dementia (Adams & Victor, 1989; Vernon, 1989).

Depression, with prevalence rates as high as 50%, is common in patients with PD. It is not known whether the depression is a reaction to PD or is a part of the disease (Bunting & Fitzsimmons, 1991; Habermann-Little, 1991). Beside depression, delirium and dementia are the most common psychological problems of patients with PD. Hallucinations, usually nonthreatening and visual, are a common side-effect of anti-Parkinson medications, but may also be due to the disease itself, or to depression. In the latter cases, hallucinations may be auditory, and are distressing to the patient (Bunting & Fitzsimmons, 1991). Frustration, often accompanied by irritation and anger, is almost universal among patients with PD (Marr, 1991).

L-dopa, especially Sinemet, in combination with carbidopa, remains the mainstay of drug treatment, particularly in advanced disease. Bromocriptine (Parlodel) and pergolide (Permax) are similar to L-dopa. Changes in blood levels result in the "on-off phenomenon," in which the patient suddenly becomes immobile. Adverse effects of medications are common and very troublesome to many patients (Marr, 1991, p. 326). Involuntary movements, including dyskinesias, dystonia, choreoathetosis, and restlessness sometimes result from long-term L-dopa and related medication use. (Adams & Victor, 1989; Hickey, 1992; Vernon, 1989). It is important that caregivers understand the limitations and implications of L-dopa use, and the measures necessary for safe administration.

These include eliminating vitamin B_6 supplements, decreasing alcohol intake, decreasing protein intake, taking medications with meals, taking measures to relieve dry mouth (see chapter 16), wearing elastic stockings, and monitoring for depression (Hickey, 1992).

The degenerative nature of PD, the physical and psychological demands of caregiving, decreased social interaction, and other stressors all play a role in the significant and stressful burden the disease places on caregivers (Marr, 1991). By the end-stage, the family caregiver is likely to be globally exhausted.

Amyotrophic Lateral Sclerosis

Amyotrophic lateral sclerosis (ALS), or motor neuron disease, is a rapidly progressive and degenerative disease of the motor neurons of the spinal cord and/or brain stem (Kim, 1989). Onset is usually after age 50, and the time from onset to death is three to six years. There is currently no cure (Hickey, 1992).

Typically, ALS is manifested initially by difficulty with using first one hand, and then the other. Hand and forearm atrophy and weakness spreads to the upper arms and shoulders. In later stages, ALS is characterized by lower extremity spasticity, and hyperreflexia. Fasciculations (small muscle contractions) occur in most patients. The atrophy and weakness spread to the neck and tongue, with resultant dysarthria, dysphagia, drooling, and wasting and tremors of the tongue. Muscles of the trunk and lower extremities eventually deteriorate. Muscle cramps are frequent and patients may feel aching pain or a sense of coldness in the affected areas. Involvement of chest and shoulder muscles contributes to dyspnea. Swallowing and managing secretions becomes increasingly difficult and aspiration often results. ALS does not affect vision, hearing, intellectual ability, or bladder or bowel function (Adams & Victor, 1989; Bingham, 1990; Hickey, 1992; Ho & Connors, 1983; Stone, 1987).

Psychologically, ALS is a devastating disease. The patient experiences, *with intact intellect,* an inexorable decline, including steadily increasing difficulty in breathing. Social isolation, anger, and depression are common. Many patients with ALS are emotionally labile, and outbursts of crying or laughing may occur. Stresses on the family are similar to those on families of patients with any fatal degenerative neurological disease (Hickey, 1992; Kim, 1989).

Treatment of ALS is symptomatic and supportive (Adams & Victor, 1989). Medications for symptoms include diazepam (Valium) for spasticity, quinidine for cramps, and various medications to reduce salivation (Hickey, 1992). Reducing salivation results in xerostomia. Other measures include tracheostomy and gastrostomy (Stone, 1987). Since choking and aspiration are inevitable, there should be suction equipment available (Welnetz, 1983).

Because of the patient's inability to hold his or her head or otherwise move, manage secretions, or breath adequately, the end stages of ALS require intensive patient care. Intake of food, fluids, and medications becomes a major challenge. Some patients eventually resist food and fluid for fear of choking (Welnetz, 1983). Small amounts of morphine (e.g., 2.5 mg PO every 4 hours) can be given for severe hunger pangs (Oliver, 1989).

Unless the patient gives specific directions to the contrary, mechanical ventilation is likely. Once ventilation is started, it cannot be discontinued without significant respiratory distress (Makielski, 1992; Stone, 1987); i.e., the patient usually dies. It is wise and humane to give an opioid before a patient is removed from a ventilator.

Myasthenia Gravis

Myasthenia Gravis (MG) is a chronic, progressive autoimmune neuromuscular disease characterized by muscle weakness, which partially improves with rest (Hickey, 1992; Hood,

1990). Onset in women is frequently between the ages of 20 and 30 years; and for men, around age 60. The course of MG is variable. With stable ocular myasthenia, the disease may never generalize, and with mild generalized MG, the disease is responsive to medications. With moderate generalized MG, the response to medications is less satisfactory, and with acute fulminating MG, there is poor drug response and high mortality (Adams & Victor, 1989). The progression of MG also varies widely (Hickey, 1992).

Typically, repeated activity of a muscle group results in loss of contractile power and progressive paresis. MG usually begins with chronic fatigue, but in some cases, rapid onset occurs, often following an upper respiratory infection or emotional distress (Adams & Victor, 1989). While symptoms vary among different patients, a more or less usual course of a more severe form of MG includes progressive weakness of voluntary muscles (extremities, facial, chewing, speaking, and swallowing), drooping eyelids, visual disturbances, and distortion of the face. The effects of weakened respiratory muscles and decreased tidal volume and vital capacity are complicated by difficulties swallowing and managing secretions. The end result is often aspiration pneumonia (Hood, 1990; Litchfield & Noroian, 1989).

Two sorts of crises occur with some frequency in patients with MG. Myasthenic crisis is a sudden escalation of MG symptoms, and even with increased medications, may result in respiratory paralysis. Intubation and respiratory support are necessary, and when the crisis is resolved, these are removed. Cholinergic crisis is characterized by slowly developing weakness, increased secretions, and decreased respiratory function; all often preceded by abdominal cramping and diarrhea. Cholinergic crisis is managed similarly to myasthenic crisis. (Hickey, 1992; Hood, 1990).

Psychological responses to MG are similar to responses to other degenerative illness. Isolation, helplessness, anger, and depression are familiar to most patients with MG—and to their families.

Treatment of advanced MG includes anticholinesterase drugs and corticosteroids. Plasmapheresis is used for severe disease and provides improvement for as long as six weeks. Patients with severe MG require the same intensive care as patients with other severe neuromuscular diseases.

Problems of End-Stage Degenerative Neurological Diseases

Common problems of end-stage degenerative neurological diseases are discussed in the following chapter. The below problems should, however be discussed here.

- Dysphagia is common in all degenerative neurological diseases. Intake of food, fluids, and medications becomes a major challenge. While there is variation among individuals, semi-solid or soft foods, and finally, supplements like Carnation Instant Breakfast, are best. It is essential that the patient be sitting up with head bowed slightly forward (likely requiring support) for all oral intake. Distractions during mealtimes should be minimized. Straws should not be used by patients whose lips do not function well. Smaller and smaller bites and sips are necessary over longer periods of time as the disease progresses. (Rubin-Terrado & Linkenheld, 1991; Welnetz, 1983).
- Pneumonia may result from aspiration and/or immobility. Maintaining mobility, or at least range of motion, in a long-term, bedfast patient is a major challenge, especially when, as in the case of some neuromuscular diseases, activity further exacerbates disease symptoms.
- Isolation is common in all chronic illness. The degenerative neurological diseases are perhaps more isolating because of their lengthy trajectory, the inability of patients to communicate, and the sometimes off-putting symptoms, such as drooling, facial distortion, frequent choking, and so on. Socially, end-stage disease is usually characterized by either long-term care or by caregiving provided by one family member, often a physically and emotionally exhausted elderly spouse, who provides both care and the patient's sole social contact (O'Brien, 1993). Since social support and hope are strongly related (Foote, Piazza, Holcombe, Paul, & Daffin, 1990), the reality of patient and caregiver is often grim. Psychosocial care and support take on increased importance. Each family should receive case management services, including carefully planned, intentional psychosocial support, preferably in a coordinated team effort.
- Caregiver exhaustion is common, and is compounded by caregivers frequently ignoring their own health (O'Brien, 1993). Regular monitoring of caregiver health is thus indicated. Respite services help, but as noted elsewhere, intermittent services may not receive the enthusiasm expected by some health providers. It is well to remember that these caregivers are nearly always in the midst of an unimaginably difficult and painful marathon that lasts for *years*. For those able or willing to leave the patient, disease-specific support groups are usually helpful.

For more information, please see the section, Providing Care, in chapter 29.

References

Acorn, S., & Andersen, S. (1990). Depression in multiple sclerosis: Critique of the research literature. *Journal of Neuroscience Nursing, 22*(4), 209–214.

Adams, R.D., & Victor, M. (1989). *Principles of Neurology*. New York: McGraw-Hill Information Services Company.

Bingham, E. (1990). Motor neuron disease. *Nursing Times, 86*(19), 28–31.

Buelow, J.M. (1991). A correlational study of disabilities, stressors and coping methods in victims of multiple sclerosis. *Journal of Neuroscience Nursing, 23*(4), 247–252.

Bunting, L.K., & Fitzsimmons, (1991). Depression in Parkinson's disease. *Journal of Neuroscience Nursing, 21*(5), 158–164.

Centers for Disease Control. (1990). Mortality Patterns. *Morbidity and Mortality Weekly Report, 39*(12), 193–195.

Dewis, M.E., & Thornton, N.G. (1989). Sexual dysfunction in multiple sclerosis. *Journal of Neuroscience Nursing, 21*(3), 175–179.

Foote, A.W., Piazza, D., Holcombe, J., Paul, P., & Daffin, P. (1990). Hope, self-esteem and social support in persons with multiple sclerosis. *Journal of Neuroscience Nursing, 22*(3), 155–159.

Gulick, E.E., & Bugg, A. (1992). Holistic health patterning in multiple sclerosis. *Research in Nursing and Health, 15*(3), 175–185.

Habermann-Little, B. (1991). An analysis of the prevalence and etiology of depression in Parkinson's disease. *Journal of Neuroscience Nursing, 21*(5), 165–169.

Hainsworth, M.A., Burke, M.L., Lindgren, C.L. & Eakes, G.G. (1993). Chronic sorrow in multiple sclerosis. *Home Healthcare Nurse, 11*(2), 9–13.

Hickey, J.V. (1992). *The clinical practice of neurological and neurosurgical nursing.* Philadelphia: J.B. Lippincott.

Ho, L., & Connors, J. (1983). Amyotrophic lateral sclerosis. *Canadian Nurse, 79*(3), 35.

Hood, L.J. (1990). Myasthenia gravis: Regimens and regimen-associated problems in adults. *Journal of Neuroscience Nursing, 22*(6), 358–354.

Hubsky, E.P., & Sears, J.H. (1992). Fatigue in multiple sclerosis: Guidelines for nursing care. *Rehabilitation Nursing, 17*(4), 176–180.

Kassirer, M.R., & Osterberg, D.H. (1987). Pain in chronic multiple sclerosis. *Journal of Pain and Symptom Management, 2*(2), 95–97.

Kim, T-S. (1989). Hope as a mode of coping in amy-otrophic lateral sclerosis. *Journal of Neuroscience Nursing, 21*(6), 342–347.

Litchfield, M., & Noroian, E. (1989). Changes in selected pulmonary functions in patients diagnosed with myasthenia gravis. *Journal of Neuroscience Nursing, 21*(6), 375–381.

Makielski, M. (1992). Administering pain medications for a terminal patient. *Dimensions of Critical Care Nursing, 11*(3), 157–161.

Marr, J. (1991). The experience of living with Parkinson's Disease. *Journal of Neuroscience Nursing, 23*(5), 325–330.

Miller, C.M., & Hens, M. (1993). Multiple sclerosis: A literature review. *Journal of Neuroscience Nursing, 25*(3), 174–179.

Mitchell, M. (1989). *Neuroscience nursing: A nursing diagnosis approach.* Baltimore: Williams & Wilkens.

Morgante, L.A., Madonna, M.G., & Pokoluk, R. (1989). Research and treatment in multiple sclerosis: Implications for nursing practice. *Journal of Neuroscience Nursing, 21*(5), 285–289.

O'Brien, M.T. (1993). Multiple sclerosis: Health-Promoting behaviors of spousal caregivers. *Journal of Neuroscience Nursing, 25*(2), 105–112.

Oliver, D. (1989). Motor neuron disease. In T.D. Walsh (Ed.), *Symptom control* (pp. 477–484). Oxford: Blackwell Scientific Publications.

Rubin-Terrado, M., & Linkenheld, D. (1991). Don't choke on this: A swallowing assessment. *Geriatric Nursing, 12*(6), 288–291.

Sadovnick, A.D., Eisen, K., Ebers, G.L., & Paty, D.W. (1991). Causes of death in patients attending multiple sclerosis clinics. *Neurology, 41*(8), 1193–1196.

Stone, N. (1987). Amyotrophic lateral sclerosis: A challenge for constant adaptation. *Journal of Neuroscience Nursing, 19*(3), 166–173.

Vernon, G.M. (1989). Parkinson's disease. *Journal of Neuroscience Nursing, 21*(5), 273–282.

Welnetz, K. (1983). Maintaining adequate nutrition and hydration in the dysphagic ALS patient. *Canadian Nurse, 79*(3), 30–34.

Alzheimer's Disease and Other Cognitive Impairment Illnesses

Alzheimer's disease (AD) and similar neurodegenerative diseases affect approximately 4,000,000 Americans, and with about 100,000 deaths annually, constitute the fourth leading cause of death among adults. The incidence of AD in the population over 65 years of age is about 10%, and in the population over age 85, it is more than 45% (Alzheimer's Disease and Related Disorders Association [ADRDA], 1990). While some specifics may differ slightly, the care discussed under Alzheimer's disease applies also to other dementing illnesses.

Characteristics

Alzheimer's disease is characterized by progressive and insidious deterioration of memory and other cognitive, psychosocial, and physical functions (Abraham & Neundorfer, 1990; Foreman & Grabowski, 1992). AD may or may not be complicated by delirium, delusions, and/or depression (Abraham & Neundorfer, 1990). Distinguishing between AD, delirium, and depression is sometimes difficult (Foreman & Grabowski, 1992). The AD process averages

about 7.5 years from onset to death, but may last anywhere from three to twenty years (Brechling & Kuhn, 1989).

Alzheimer's disease is manifested by such problems as memory loss, catastrophic reactions (exaggerated response to a situation), demanding behavior, night waking, hiding articles, and decreased ability to communicate (Lee, 1991). It is important to understand that while cognitive loss in general is predictable, each patient losses different abilities at different times (Danner, Beck, Heacock, & Modlin, 1993). Use of the brief Mini-Mental State Examination (Folstein, Folstein, & McHugh, 1975) is a recommended means of assessing cognitive function in patients with AD (Foreman & Grabowski, 1992; Lee, 1991). The brief Mini-Mental State Examination is included in chapter 13 (Figure 13.1). To be most meaningful, the examination should be conducted at regular intervals, preferably by the same person.

Charles Kemp: TERMINAL ILLNESS: A GUIDE TO NURSING CARE. © 1995 J. B. Lippincott.

In most patients, the ability to communicate is profoundly affected, to the extent that by the end-stage, meaningful communication is completely lost. This, and other deficits, result in increased isolation for the patient, and frustration in family and professionals—which tends to further increase isolation (Lee, 1991).

In general, AD progresses from forgetfulness, to increasing confusion, to "ambulatory dementia," and finally to a severe, increasingly vegetative state (Hall, 1988; Jacob Perlow Hospice, 1991). While these are not clearly defined stages, they are fairly typical. The stage characterized by ambulatory dementia, i.e., Alzheimer's dementia, is very troublesome for all concerned and in many cases, is the stage at which the family is no longer able to care for the patient at home (Foreman & Grabowski, 1992; Wilson, 1989). Agitation and other restless behavior, such as wandering, cursing, threatening, repetitive statements or questions, are common (Chrisman, Tabar, Whall, & Booth, 1991), especially late in the day ("sundowning").

Each stage brings its unique difficulties and also contributes to a crescendo of deterioration in the patient and pain for the family (Austrom & Hendrie, 1990). In the end-stage, patients are unable, for the most part, to recognize others, familiar objects, and even body parts. Patients may be unable to eat, chew, or swallow (Hall, 1988). Rather than speak, patients may groan or scream (ADRDA, 1989). The end-stage of AD is characterized by inability to speak more than six words, to walk, stand, sit up, smile, or hold the head up; finally, coma ensues (Jacob Perlow Hospice, 1991). This end-stage is more difficult for some caregivers to tolerate than earlier, disruptive stages (Miller, 1990).

Caregivers

A key characteristic of the disorder is the unrelenting, but painfully slow nature of the deterioration and the concomitant, steadily increasing load on the patient's family. In a very real sense, Alzheimer's disease becomes a global family disease that often affects the physical, psychosocial, and spiritual health of all concerned (Austrom & Hendrie, 1990; Brechling & Kuhn, 1989; Cleary, 1992).

Physical problems for caregivers center around exhaustion and its consequences. Most are relatives—either a spouse (usually the wife), or the daughter; and most are > 60 years of age (Austrom & Hendrie, 1990). The care is demanding and increases in difficulty as the disease progresses. Regardless of disease stage, there is always something to do. The physical work of cleaning and caring for the patient is compounded by need for constant vigilance to prevent the consequences of demented decisions and behaviors. As the patient deteriorates, total patient care becomes necessary. Caregivers are thus at risk themselves for physical deterioration.

Psychosocial problems are legion. Finances/medical bills are often an unresolved problem operating in the background. Caregiving in general is stressful (Sayles-Cross, 1993). To risks inherent in the caregiving role, caring for a relative with AD brings additional liabilities. Social isolation and ambivalence toward the object of loss, both key factors in grief and morbidity (Parkes, 1978), are frequently operational in caregivers of patients with AD. Social isolation occurs, at least in part, because of the never-ending care demands. Ambivalence is related to caregiver role changes and to negative changes in the patient's personality and behavior. Ambivalent feelings—such as love for the person that was and anger, disgust, or death wishes for the person that is—may result in terrible guilt. Grief is profound, and is complicated by the death of the personality before the body, by the lack of time (psychological space) in which to grieve, and by a lack of social sanction and support in grieving. In a caregiver with previously inadequate coping skills or other risk factors for complicated grief, there is significant risk of developing chronic sorrow (Lindgren, Burke, Hainsworth, & Eakes, 1992). Caregiver health is compromised by fatigue, and this further complicates the psychological state. Family conflict is almost inevitable. Caregivers are also confronted with "negative choices," or dilemmas, for which there is no good answer; only choices that inevitably bring pain. Current and anticipated financial burdens complete the picture.

Applying the concept of spiritual needs to caring for a relative with Alzheimer's disease shows the clear potential for encountering unmet needs. What is the *meaning* in this deterioration and loss of dignity? What *hope* is there? What *relatedness* does the patient have with God? How angry with God is the caregiver? Is anyone involved *transcending* anything? Answers to these questions do not come easily when a loved one has Alzheimer's disease. Ultimately, through giving care as long and as well as possible, they are answered to at least some extent. (See later discussion of caregiver spiritual issues.)

Providing Care

INTRODUCTION

In the early stages, most patients are cared for at home, while in later stages, most are institutionalized—a classic "negative choice" (Willoughby & Keating, 1991; Wilson, 1989). The key issue in where care is given is not, however, the level of cognitive and physical deterioration, but socioeconomic factors (Ford, Roy, Haug, Folmar, & Jones, 1991). Factors leading to staying in the community rather than being institutionalized include living with children, being male (i.e., increased likelihood of having a caregiver), and higher income (Ford, et al., 1991).

Regardless of where care is given, there is often a reluctance to ask for help or even to let others help with the care (Robinson, 1989). Many caregivers approach the task with the realization that community support is inadequate and that there is nobody better able than themselves to give the care. While such an attitude might be attributed to guilt, "martyring," or to other such processes, the reality is that in many instances, these caregivers are correct in their assessment of the situation. When one has been at the job for five years and is looking at possibly another five years, then the two-four months of two hours/day, three days/week services covered by medicare may not seem that significant.

Hospice programs have generally been reluctant to admit patients with AD. Reasons for this include the slow deterioration (uncertain prognosis) of patients with AD vs. those with cancer, and the inability of patients to communicate. Professional inexperience and knowledge deficit with respect to end-stage AD also plays a significant role (Brechling & Kuhn, 1989). The potential for obligation to provide long-term care is daunting to most hospice programs.

PHYSICAL PROBLEMS

Physical problems in the end-stage (see above) are due in large part to immobility, and may include a general deterioration in functional ability, skin breakdown, decreased range of motion, decreased strength, metabolic imbalances, and impaired cardiovascular, urinary, gastrointestinal, and respiratory functions (Hall, 1988; Maas, 1991; Mobily and Kelley, 1991). Dysphagia is also common. Each of these is discussed below, preceded by general guidelines for and discussions of dementia, communications, and agitation. Care for caregivers is also discussed.

General Guidelines
A guiding principle throughout the course of Alzheimer's disease is consistency in caregivers and routine (Harvis, 1990; Stolley, Buckwalter, & Shannon, 1991). While consistency does not

by any means insure a trouble-free situation, a lack of consistency does guarantee difficulties. The patient usually has to be repeatedly reminded of even the regular caregiver's identity.

Dementia

While the confusion of earlier stages usually gives way to an increasingly vegetative state, there may be periods of cognitive (dys)function. Measures used in earlier stages should be continued. Validation therapy, i.e., attempting to understand the meaning of the patient's attempts at communication, should be continued as a way to make emotional contact—even if it is a one-way attempt. Communication is continued as discussed below.

Communication Difficulties

When possible, sensory aides such as hearing aides and eye glasses should be kept on and in working order. Other helpful suggestions include: using simple instructions; speaking slowly, distinctly, repeating phrases, and speaking in short sentences; and demonstrating instructions or actions (e.g., cleaning dentures) (Danner et al., 1993; Harvis, 1990). Of course, the patient with end-stage AD is seldom responsive to these measures. Nevertheless, they are not harmful, and one never knows what is going on in the patient; the natural question to ask oneself, then, is "Why not try?" A significant issue in communication is that the patient is unable to report pain or other problems to others. In contradistinction to many other patients, pain in patients with AD is usually detected by behavioral clues, such as being quiet instead of the more usual moaning, changes in eating habits, flushed or pale skin, perspiration, guarding, or sudden changes in behavior (ADRDA, 1989; Marzinski, 1991).

Agitation

Although agitation, or its expression, decreases in the final stage of AD, measures should be continued or instituted to reduce anxiety and other causes of agitation or delirium. A calm environment with minimal visual, audio, and other stimuli helps prevent or reduce anxiety (Harvis, 1990). Some patients are calmed by television and some are not. The patient's response should be determined and action based on the response. It is easy enough to monitor patient responses to the presence and absence of a television or other stimulus. Audiotapes of music appropriate for the patient are a better choice for some than television. If the patient has a history of sundowning, stimuli should be further decreased in the evening. A light should be left on and the presence of the caregiver may help. Agitation may not necessarily be due to Alzheimer's disease. Other potential causes include hyponatremia, hypoglycemia, hypercalcemia, medications, pain, sleep deprivation, and fecal impaction or urinary retention (Martin, 1990). Haloperidol is the medication most commonly used for delirium because it results in less orthostatic hypotension and has a lower seizure threshold than do other similar medications. Martin (1991) recommends starting with 2–5 mg bid and titrating to effect, similarly to using morphine for patients with pain. Please also see chapter 13.

Dysphagia

Difficulty swallowing manifested by drooling or retaining or spitting out food may be due to lip, tongue or jaw impairment; while coughing or choking after or while swallowing indicate pharyngeal problems. Interventions for dysphagia include giving small meals and small bites of food, giving adequate time to chew and swallow, reminding the patient to swallow, and giving (in most instances) liquids with thicker consistencies (Rubin-Terrado & Kinkenheld, 1991). Care should be taken when giving oral medications. Large tablets, in particular, are difficult to swallow (Walsh, 1990). Dysphagia may also be due to problems other than progression of Alzheimer's disease. Bacterial, fungal, or viral infection, as well as esophageal cancer, may cause dysphagia and/or odynophagia or painful swallowing (Roubein & Levin, 1993). Family members should be taught what measures to take in case of choking. Readers are encouraged to refer to chapter 17.

Decreased Range of Motion and Strength
Passive range of motion sometimes seems futile to families who associate exercise with rehabilitation. In this case, however, the purpose is not rehabilitation, but prevention of contractures and their sequelae of further decreased range of motion, pain, and skin breakdown (Mobily & Kelley, 1991). Decreased range of motion also affects strength, as discussed below. In the end-stage, there is little that can be done about decreased strength other than whatever small gain occurs through passive range of motion. As noted above, passive range of motion in end-stage AD is not a rehabilitation effort, but preventive—in this case, limited prevention of cardiovascular deterioration. Immobility also decreases skeletal strength and increases the likelihood of stress or pathological fracture (Mobily & Kelley, 1991), and thus may further decrease mobility.

Skin Breakdown
This problem is related to immobility, incontinence, and nutritional deficits. Preventive measures include regular assessment, frequent turning, meticulous hygiene, reduction of mechanical factors (wrinkles, crumbs, etc. on the sheet), adequate hydration and nutrition, and use of egg crate mattress, special bed, sheepskin, and other protective devices (deConno, Ventafridda, & Saita, 1991; Walsh & Brescia, 1990). Treatment of decubitus ulcers includes: ensuring that all staff use the same means of measuring and assessing; relieving pressure (with Clinitron bed, for example); and treatment of ulcers, as discussed in chapter 15.

Metabolic Imbalances
Negative nitrogen balance from immobility and decreased intake, and hypercalcemia from calcium loss are both possible in advanced AD. (Mobily & Kelley, 1991). See the section on Paraneoplastic Syndromes in chapter 20 for a discussion of hypercalcemia.

Impaired Cardiovascular Function
Lying immobile and recumbent significantly increases cardiac workload, especially in the presence of extant cardiac disease (Maas, 1991). Edema, often found in the sacral area, contributes to skin breakdown. Other problems include orthostatic hypotension and risk for thrombosis (Mobily & Kelley, 1991).

Impaired Urinary Functions
Problems of impaired urinary function include urinary tract infections, perineal infections, renal calculi, and increased likelihood of skin breakdown (Maas, 1991; Mobily & Kelley, 1991). Adequate fluids (except for diuresing fluids, like coffee or tea) help prevent the first three, but contribute, perhaps, to the last problem. Use of urinary catheters virtually insures urinary tract infection (Fainsinger, MacEachern, Hanson, & Bruera, 1992) but is necessary in many cases. Unless contraindicated, patients should receive up to 3,000 cc of fluids during the day. Diuretics are best given in the morning (Harvis, 1990), especially if there is no catheter. Toileting schedules should be designed around the patient's elimination schedule (ADRDA, 1989). See also chapter 18.

Impaired Gastrointestinal Functions
Incontinence or constipation are common, and there is a potential for impaction. A bowel routine is essential. See the sections on Constipation and Diarrhea in chapter 17. As the patient deteriorates and consumes less food, bowel movements also decrease.

Impaired Respiratory Functions
Lung capacity decreases, secretions thicken and increase, and expectoration decreases, with a net result of increased risk for pneumonia. Use of sedatives also contributes to the risk. Pneumonia is characterized by elevated temperature, purulent sputum, decreased breath sounds, dullness to percussion at the affected area, and the presence of pleural effusion. Please refer to chapter 14.

Caring for the Caregiver

By the end-stage, nearly all caregivers are physically and emotionally exhausted from countless "36 hour days" (Mace & Rabins, 1981). They have worked hard and, at times, been reviled for their work by the patient, seen their sense of security vanish like smoke, kept on through days and weeks and months of despair, lost friends and friendships of family members, seen services that they thought would be helpful come—and go, grieved and grieved again for the patient and themselves, and looked to a grim future. Thus, when we as practitioners offer our help to these caregivers, it should be with the understanding that we are offering help to heroes.

In 20 years of work, I have known many people like this. In the traditional sense of heroism—with fear and uncertainty as their only companions; standing "alone in the night" against an implacable enemy; wounded in body and spirit; true to their vows—*they are heroes*. Most are also experts in caregiving.

Practitioners working with end-stage Alzheimer's patients may profit from an approach that combines a certain sense of humility with respect and honor toward these heroic caregivers, rather than one in which the health care worker arrives on the scene as the "expert," controlling all the services that can make the big difference. The fundamental objective for practitioners should be to fit their care with the needs and situation of patient and family.

It should also be borne in mind that, for many caregivers, turning over their responsibilities to another is extremely difficult (Wilson, 1989). When their role is relinquished, partially or completely, the caregiver often hovers in the room or frets in the next room. Some health care providers have difficulty with this behavior. Rather than resist it, however, it is better for practitioners to enlist caregivers' help, to ask them to teach us what they know about the needs and functioning of that particular patient. Once they are satisfied that care is adequate, caregivers are more likely to give up some part of their responsibility, and to experience a subsequent sense of relief from anxiety.

Psychosocial care also often centers around finances/medical bills, stress, and grief. In fact, all three are pressing issues for most patients and families, and they should be addressed in relation to their importance. Readers are referred to the information on this subject in chapter 2, Psychosocial Care and Issues: The Family.

Specific caregiver problems having to do with AD, and with other long-term neurological diseases, include the following issues.

- The organization needed to pay medical bills is often neglected in favor of utilizing the time for providing physical care to the patient, thus creating a sense of financial dread in the family that serves as a background to all their other problems. Helping the family to sort bills and arrange payment schedules is often immensely beneficial, and also serves to establish a working relationship between the practitioner and the caregiver(s).
- Caregivers' sense of social isolation is difficult, if not impossible, to resolve. For most people, the situation is inherently isolating and, in fact, time spent away from the patient may seem even more stressful than their duties themselves. Apart from family and friends, two helpful means of social support are: (1) Alzheimer's disease caregiver groups, set up in many locations across the country; and (2) church groups or other religiously oriented organizations. Part of the purpose of social contact is to establish a pattern of social interaction and support for the present and the future. Too often, an opposite pattern—of almost complete isolation—exists, which is extremely difficult to break, even after the patient dies.
- Ambivalence (e.g., love and hate) toward the patient is common and natural, but also dif-

ficult for the caregiver to accept or address. Guilty feelings often result from recognition of anger. At least two people are represented in the person with AD: the person who was and the demented, sometimes abusive and even violent person who is. The latter person may be viewed as responsible for destroying the life and the feelings created by the former. The reality is that the exhaustion and despair of the caregiver would not exist if not for the person with AD. It is helpful to caregivers if their (in most cases inevitable) anger is acknowledged, without judgement, by an objective source like the practitioner. The optimal situation for expressing and acknowledging these and other inevitable feelings surrounding the care of AD patients is within an organized Alzheimer's disease caregiver group.

- Grief is a major issue, and includes grief for what is already lost in the patient, for the altered relationship that exists between patient and caregiver, and for oneself. There is also anticipatory grief for what the future will bring in relation to these situations. Grief in the context of AD is complicated by the nature of the disease: The personality dies, but not the body (Austrom & Hendrie, 1990). Chronic sorrow may exist.

- Fatigue is probably inevitable, even when part—or even all—the care is given over to others; respite care and intermittent services organizations, in addition to regular nursing or personal care services, can help provide needed support. Physical help, however, is only part of the solution, and it must be supplemented by psychological support and appreciation for the immensity of the job done by the caregiver.

- Family conflict (excluding the patient) is common, and often includes guilt and blaming. "Help-rejecting complaining" is common on the part of the caregiver. Communications are influenced by old, unresolved issues, and complicated by the caregiver's physical and emotional exhaustion.

The value of a family meeting facilitated by a skilled family mental health professional helps clarify needs and improve communications. Such meetings can have a significantly positive effect on the family, especially if the facilitator is truly skilled and is not a regular health provider (who might thus be viewed as "taking sides").

- Spiritual issues are sometimes incompletely addressed. Although chapters 3 and 4 offer a more complete discussion of these needs, several questions should be addressed here in the context, not of supplying universal answers to suit every situation, but rather of providing some frame of reference.

What, for example, is the meaning in this deterioration and loss of dignity inherent in the situation of the AD patient? The meaning may not be found so much in what is happening to the patient, as in what the caregiver is doing. In other words, a better question may be, "What is the meaning of this level of love, devotion, or just plain hard-headedness?" Another question is, "What hope is there?" Again, if the focus is more on the caregiver, we can ask questions such as, "What hope is there in a person, family, or society that works this hard to do the right thing in the face of despair and of certain defeat of the flesh?" Finally, caregivers may question the patient's relationship with God, while their own relationships, instead, can be fairly predictable, generally falling into one of three phases, according to the situation of the moment: either they depend on God, they question the existence of God, or they are very angry with God. It is very helpful if practitioners are able to support and understand caregivers throughout all these phases. Involving a chaplain, minister, or religious advisor of some kind should also be considered. It should be clear to the outsider that most caregivers are transcending themselves in giving care. This is not, however, transcendence in a happy sense. It is a grim, hard transcendence—but transcendence nonetheless.

In all cases, families should be linked with community resources, such as the Alzheimer's Disease and Related Disorders Association. Experience, however, teaches health care providers that some people can have negative experiences with organizations in general, and are reluctant to try to utilize them. Health care providers may need to act as advocates, or to otherwise assist families in finding and receiving services.

The Alzheimer's Disease and Related Disorders Association is currently located at 70 East Lake Street, Chicago, IL 60601-5997. Their current phone number outside Illinois is 1-800-621-0379, and in Illinois, 1-800-572-6037.

References

Abraham, I.L., & Neundorfer, M.M. (1990). Alzheimer's: A decade of progress, a future of nursing challenges. *Geriatric Nursing, 11*(3), 116–120.

Alzheimer's Disease and Related Disorders Association. (1989). *Care for advanced Alzheimer's disease.* Chicago: Author.

Alzheimer's Disease and Related Disorders Association. (1990). *Alzheimer's Disease Statistics.* Chicago: Author.

Austrom, M.G., & Hendrie, H.C. (1990). Death of the personality: The grief response of the Alzheimer's disease family caregiver. *American Journal of Alzheimer's Care and Related Disorders and Research, March/April, 1990,* 16–27.

Brechling, B.G., & Kuhn, D. (1989). A specialized hospice for dementia patients and their families. *American Journal of Hospice Care, 6*(3), 27–30.

Chrisman, M., Tabar, D., Whall, A.L., & Booth, D.E. (1991). Agitated behavior in the cognitively impaired elderly. *Journal of Gerontological Nursing, 17*(12), 9–13.

Cleary, B.L. (1992). Alzheimer's disease: Stressors and strategies associated with caregiving. In S.G. Funk, E.M. Tornquist, M.T. Champagne, & R.A. Wiese (Eds.), *Key aspects of elder care* (pp. 320–327). New York: Springer Publishing Company.

Danner, C., Beck, C., Heacock, P., & Modlin, T. (1993). Cognitively impaired elders: Using research findings to improve nursing care. *Journal of Gerontological Nursing, 19*(4), 5–11.

deConno, F., Ventafridda, V., & Saita, L. (1991). Skin problems in advanced and terminal cancer patients. *Journal of Pain and Symptom Management, 6*(4), 247–256.

Fainsinger, R., MacEachern, T., Hanson, J., & Bruera, E. (1992). The use of urinary catheters in terminally ill cancer patients. *Journal of Pain and Symptom Management, 7*(6), 333–338.

Folstein, M.F., Folstein, S.E., & McHugh, P.R. (1975). Mini-mental state: A practical method for grading the cognitive state of patients for the clinician. *Journal of Psychiatric Research, 12,* 189–198.

Ford, A.B., Roy, A.W., Haug, M.R., Folmar, S.J., & Jones, P.K. (1991). Impaired and disabled elderly in the community. *American Journal of Public Health, 81*(9), 1207–1209.

Foreman, M.D., & Grabowski, R. (1992). Diagnostic dilemma: Cognitive impairment in the elderly. *Journal of Gerontological Nursing, 18*(9), 5–12.

Hall, G.R. (1988). Care of the patient with Alzheimer's disease living at home. *Nursing Clinics of North America, 23*(1), 31–46.

Harvis, K.A. (1990). Care plan approach to dementia. *Geriatric Nursing, 11*(2), 76–79.

Jacob Perlow Hospice. (1991). *Functional assessment staging (FAST) adapted for Alzheimer's disease.* New York: Author.

Lee, V.K. (1991). Language changes and Alzheimer's disease: A literature review. *Journal of Gerontological Nursing, 17*(1), 16–20.

Lindgren, C.L., Burke, M.L., Hainsworth, M.A., & Eakes, G.G. (1992). Chronic sorrow: A lifespan concept. *Scholarly inquiry for nursing practice: An international journal, 6*(1), 27–42.

Maas, M.L. (1991). Impaired physical mobility. In M. Maas, K.C. Buckwalter, & M. Hardy (Eds.), *Nursing diagnoses and interventions for the elderly* (pp. 263–284). Redwood City, California: Addison-Wesley.

Mace, N.L., & Rabins, P.V. (1981). *The 36 hour day: A family guide to caring for persons with Alzheimer's disease, related dementing illnesses, and memory loss in later life.* Baltimore: Johns Hopkins University Press.

Martin, E.W. (1990). Confusion in the terminally ill: Recognition and management. *American Journal of Hospice and Palliative Care. May/June 1990,* 20–24.

Martin, E.W. (1991, November). *Confusion in the terminally ill: Diagnosis and management.* National Hospice Organization Annual Meeting, Seattle.

Marzinski, L.R. (1991). The tragedy of dementia: Clinically assessing pain in the confused, nonverbal elderly. *Journal of Gerontological Nursing, 17*(6), 25–28.

Mobily, P.R., & Kelley, L.S. (1991). Iatrogenesis in the elderly. *Journal of Gerontological Nursing, 17*(9), 5–10).

Parkes, C.M. (1978). Psychological aspects. In C.M. Saunders (Ed.) The *Management of Terminal Disease* (pp. 44–64). London: Edward Arnold.

Robinson, K.M. (1989). Predictors of depression among wife caregivers. *Nursing Research, 38*(6), 359–363.

Roubein, L.D., & Levin, B. (1993). Gastrointestinal complications. In J.F. Holland, E. Frei, R.C. Bast, D.W. Kufe, D.L. Morton, & R.W. Weischselbaum (Eds.), *Cancer Medicine* (3rd ed.) (pp. 2370–2380). Philadelphia: Lea & Febiger.

Rubin-Terrado, M., & Kinkenheld, D. (1991). Don't choke on this: A swallowing assessment. *Geriatric Nursing, 12*(6), 288–291.

Sayles-Cross, S. (1993). Perceptions of familial caregivers of elder adults. *Image, 25*(2), 88–92.

Stolley, J.M., Buckwalter, K.C., & Shannon, M.D. (1991). Caring for patients with Alzheimer's disease. *Journal of Gerontological Nursing, 17*(6), 34–38.

Walsh, T.D. (1990). Symptom control in patients with advanced cancer. *American Journal of Hospice and Palliative Care, 7*(60), 20–29.

Walsh, T.D., & Brescia, F.J. (1990). Clinitron therapy and pain management in advanced cancer patients. *Journal of Pain and Symptom Management, 5*(1), 46–50.

Willoughby, J., & Keating, N. (1991). Being in control: The process of caring for a relative with Alzheimer's disease. *Qualitative Health Research, 1*(1), 27–50.

Wilson, H.S. (1989). Family caregiving for a relative with Alzheimer's dementia: Coping with negative choices. *Nursing Research, 38*(2), 94–98.

Cardiovascular and Pulmonary Diseases

Cardiovascular Disease

Cardiac problems in advanced cancer are discussed in chapter14.

Patients who are terminally ill from cardiovascular disease are principally those with: (1) advanced congestive heart failure; and (2) acute myocardial infarction, with extensive damage to the myocardium. The patient with congestive heart failure (CHF) may be managed well at home during much of the course of illness, while the patient with acute myocardial infarction (AMI) may live for several days in a cardiac care unit. In either case, care is focused on palliation of cardiac symptoms; extraordinary measures are not used. It is therefore essential that all legal documents concerning the patient's wishes about resuscitation be completed, and that all concerned parties clearly understand the patient's wishes.

Providing palliative care may be philosophically difficult for some staff in critical care units, where the goal is preserving life at all costs

(Fowler, 1990). Even when it is clear that the primary goals of care are to insure comfort and dignity, there is sometimes difficulty in determining what is palliative, what is aggressive, and what lies in-between. There is disagreement about whether, for example, antibiotics, vasoactive, or anticoagulant drugs should be withdrawn or given, whether or not—or how much—sectioning should occur, whether intravenous hydration should be given, and whether sedating doses of opioids for patients in acute respiratory distress are a form of euthanasia (Campbell & Field, 1991; Graham, 1989; Makielski & Broom, 1992; Solomon et al., 1993).

Because of increasing numbers of patients surviving AMI, the incidence and prevalence of CHF is increasing (Quaal, 1992). Although CHF is commonly classed as left or right ventricular failure, patients with end-stage CHF are likely to have both left and right—or biventricular—failure (Braunwald, 1987). Important symptoms of advanced CHF may include dyspnea on exertion *and* at rest, edema, chest pain, difficulty sleeping (including paroxysmal nocturnal dyspnea), nocturia, cognitive deficits, headache, weakness, and fatigue (Quaal, 1992). Pain, discomfort, or other problems stemming from other etiologies are also common and, in the context of heart disease, these may not be readily recognized or treated (Gu & Belgrade, 1993).

Dyspnea is usually associated with left ventricular failure and is related to pulmonary congestion and increased airway resistance (Laurent-Bopp, 1989a). The slight congestion and breathlessness of early CHF can progress to pulmonary edema and feelings of smothering, tachycardia, agitation, and pink, frothy hemoptysis (Quaal, 1992). In addition to therapy intended to maintain or minimize deterioration of the patient's cardiac status (e.g., diuretic, antiarrhythmic, vasodilator), the following measures (Laurent-Bopp, 1989b; Matthews, 1984; Quaal, 1992) can be taken.

- The patient should sit in a high Fowler's position for several hours at a time.
- Oxygen is given through a face mask.
- An opioid, usually morphine, is given. Patients with advanced CHF living at home should have morphine or another opioid on-hand. (In cancer care, crises appear to occur more often at night; in CHF, respiratory crises *do* occur more often at night.) Opioids function to improve the quality of respirations and to relieve anxiety.

Dyspnea is likely to increase when death is imminent, and it may be necessary to give sedating doses of opioids as the patient struggles to breathe and becomes increasingly agitated.

It may seem irrelevant to discuss diet with these patients at a time like this. However, failure to maintain sodium restrictions can have a distinct effect on the speed with which a patient develops pulmonary edema, and thus experiences breathing difficulty. Sodium restrictions are therefore maintained. Fluid restrictions, except for when the patient is hyponatremic, or with respect to sodium content of the fluids, are not as important to follow (Matthews, 1984).

Systemic edema is associated with right ventricular failure, and while it does not necessarily lead to pulmonary edema, systemic edema adds significantly to the cardiac load. In patients with advanced CHF, who perforce are either bedridden or in a sitting position most of the time, edema is found in the sacral, posterior thighs, or other dependent areas. Ascites also develops, and in some cases is extensive enough that it forces the diaphragm up while the patient is recumbent, and thus limits lung capacity (Laurent-Bopp, 1989a). Ascites also increases intraabdominal pressure, causing nausea and anorexia.

Dyspnea and cardiac function may be further exacerbated by respiratory infection, especially in a bedfast patient. Palliation in this case might include antibiotics and possibly increased diuretics, but not necessarily hospitalization and use of powerful drugs with a high incidence of adverse effects. There is controversy about when antibiotics should and should not be given; and about which antibiotics should be given in end-stage disease.

Another factor in dyspnea, fatigue, and even angina is anemia (Matthews, 1984). Severe anemia may also cause tachypnea and intermittent claudication, and may result in further deterioration of the patient's cardiovascular status.

Common etiologies of chest pain in advanced CHF include angina and AMI and, to lesser extent, pulmonary embolism, stress, and other processes. The characteristics and treatment of these vary. Stable angina is a squeezing or heavy, painful sensation lasting more than two and less than 15 minutes, predictable with a certain degree of activity, and relieved with nitroglycerin. Unstable angina occurs even at rest and is unrelieved with nitroglycerin. AMI is similar in quality, but greater in intensity than angina, lasts longer, and is not relieved with nitroglycerin or rest. Pain from pulmonary embolism is sharp, stabbing, and continuous (Haak & Huether, 1992).

Difficulty sleeping is a frequent complaint of older people, and is also common among people who are depressed (Haber, 1992; Sideleau, 1992)—one or both of which are characteristic of patients with advanced heart disease. Patients with CHF are also likely to have paroxysmal nocturnal dyspnea (PND), the frightening experience of suddenly waking up struggling to breathe (Braunwald, 1987). PND further complicates whatever prior difficulties the patient was having with sleep, anxiety, and depression, e.g., the relatively common fear of dying during sleep. Sitting up and taking oxygen provides relief from the dyspnea, if not from the fear. Since PND is related to fluid imbalance, careful attention to measures to maintain balance is important.

Nocturia, a nuisance for those with little disability, becomes a significant problem for patients with advanced disease, and may in some cases manifest as incontinence (Graham, 1989). Indeed, nights in general are often a problem. Inability or difficulty ambulating and confusion from sleeping medications can make urinating a difficult procedure and result in further loss of sleep. Attention to the patient's fluid balance may help relieve nocturia. For example, taking diuretics in the morning and limiting fluids in the evening may significantly decrease nocturia.

Cognitive deficits and headache are most common in older patients (Haak & Huether, 1992). These may be due to a combination of cerebral atherosclerosis and to the complex of anxiety, depression, insomnia, dyspnea, and other processes active in advanced heart disease. Patients with atherosclerosis are also more likely to have Cheyne-Stokes respirations (Braunwald, 1987). Confusion may be due to dementia or delirium. In delirium, confusion may be reversible, and therefore it is important to determine etiologies (Martin, 1990). (Please see the discussion of confusion in chapter 13.)

Weakness and fatigue are intrinsic to advanced heart disease. At some point in the process of advanced disease, exercise, no matter how light, becomes a liability, and is in no way beneficial to the patient (Matthews, 1984). Hyponatremia—characterized by lethargy, anorexia, weakness, and abdominal cramps—

may develop, often as a consequence of excessive treatment with diuretics. "Cardiac cachexia" also may occur as the patient deteriorates (Braunwald, 1987). In the final stages, a "regime regarded as appropriate in terminal cancer" is often the best approach (Matthews, 1984, p. 177).

Pulmonary Disease

The pulmonary diseases most commonly encountered in terminal care situations are the chronic obstructive pulmonary diseases (COPDs)—emphysema and bronchitis. The general principles of care for these usually apply as well to patients with other diagnoses, such as pulmonary fibrosis, coal worker's pneumoconiosis, silicosis, etc. Patients with cystic fibrosis are almost always cared for by staff, and on units dedicated to that disease, and are not discussed in this chapter.

Chronic bronchitis is an airway or bronchial disease characterized by an increase in the size and number of submucous glands of the large bronchi, increase in the number of goblet cells of the mucosa, and thickening of the bronchial submucosa. Inflammatory changes and, later, fibrosis occur. Secretions pool and plug first small, then larger bronchioles. The net result is air moving through less space and more mucus. Chronic cough and expectoration are the cardinal symptoms, and as the disease progresses, dyspnea increases (Dettenmeier, 1992; Kersten, 1989; Petty, 1991). Concurrently, retained mucus and other processes incline the patient to frequent respiratory infections which, in turn, worsen the patients pulmonary status during the infection, and afterwards. Right-sided heart failure is a frequent complication (Kersten, 1989). To this complicated clinical picture, right ventricular failure adds edema, hepatomegaly, and ascites, thus creating further difficulty in breathing. Finally, small airway obstruction contributes to the patient developing emphysema (Kersten, 1989). Chronic bronchitis is marked by a vari-

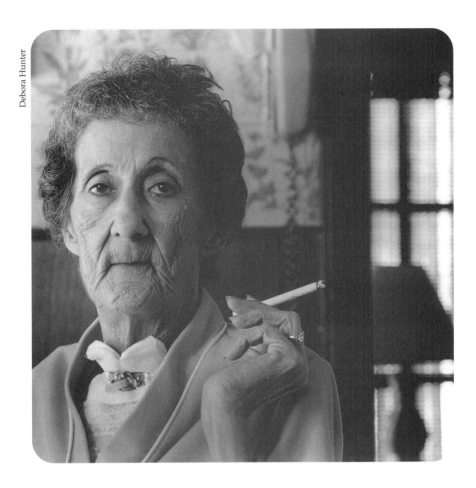

Debora Hunter

able course, with debilitating infections followed by (ever-shorter) periods of recovery.

Emphysema is an alveolar disease, characterized by hyperinflation of the lungs and loss of the alveolar, or gas-exchanging surfaces. The lungs lose elasticity, form bullae (non-functional spaces or vesicles), and air-trapping occurs. Cardinal manifestations are slowly progressive dyspnea with prolonged expiration phase, and cough. Dyspnea/respiratory effort result in first voluntary inactivity as the patient prevents dyspnea and conserves strength, and later involuntary inactivity. Patients with advanced emphysema are sometimes called "fighters" because of their unending struggle to

breathe. Inadequate nutrition is related to the effort required to eat. Malnutrition and inactivity, coupled with dyspnea, result in a characteristically wasted appearance. Respiratory infections increase in frequency and severity. Right ventricular failure may occur as death nears. The course of emphysema is characterized by a steady decline, with periods of acute exacerbation from infections or bronchitis (Dettenmeier, 1992; Kersten, 1989).

Caring for patients with advanced and terminal COPD means caring for bedfast, dyspneic, anxious patients with exhausted and sometimes resentful families. Because the illness is chronic and slowly progressive, by the time the patient is terminal, the family usually (but not always) has experience in providing care and dealing with equipment. Family resentment is sometimes related to family dynamics unrelated to illness, sometimes to physical and psychological exhaustion (COPD is a noisy disease), and sometimes to the fact that some patients continue to smoke as long as they are able to lift the cigarette to their lips and despite the spectacular coughing that results from each inhalation.

The medical management of far-advanced COPD, which usually encompasses both bronchial and alveolar disease, may include bronchoactive drugs (e.g., anticholinergics), mucokinetic agents, methylxanthines (e.g., theophylline, aminophylline), and anti-inflammatories, such as corticosteroids (Petty, 1991). Note that the therapeutic and lethal doses of theophylline are close, and that advanced disease increases the likelihood of adverse reactions (Johanssen, 1994). Antibiotics are used intermittently. Oxygen is necessary and, frequently, so is suctioning (Flenley, 1984). Oxygen must be carefully managed, since ventilatory drive is decreased by increasing oxygen.

Anxiety is almost universal in patients with far-advanced COPD (Johannsen, 1994). Management is complicated by patient's susceptibility to the respiratory depressive effects of opioids, sedatives, and hypnotics (Flenley, 1984). Behavioral interventions are hampered by the physiological etiology of at least some of the anxiety, i.e., oxygen hunger.

The patient's environment should contain a minimum of irritants. Tobacco or other smoke, dust, pollen, high ozone levels, and strong perfumes all have an adverse effect on patients with COPD. Air should not be completely dry as with some forms of indoor heating or air conditioning. Some patients require a humidifier. Days in which the humidity is high are difficult for patients with COPD. In hot climates, air conditioning is essential during summer months.

Adequate fluids are important in keeping

secretions liquefied. Postural drainage, percussion and the like are not possible in patients with end-stage COPD. Suctioning may be necessary, but in some patients creates great difficulties with coughing. Dyspnea is such that patients are unable to remain in any position other than semi-Fowler's. Oxygen is usually administered at 2–3 L/minute 18–24 hours/day via nasal cannula or mask.

Patients with advanced COPD are always at risk for respiratory infections. Patients at home should have their temperature taken at least daily, and lung sounds and sputum should be regularly evaluated for signs of infection.

Patients should rest before meals. Meals should be small and high in protein. Gas-forming, difficult to chew, and very hot or very cold foods should be avoided. Fluid intake must be maintained.

Most patients with COPD die in the hospital. The struggle to breathe as death approaches is more than most families are able to handle. Pneumonia is probably the most frequent cause of death.

References

Braunwald, E. (1987). Heart failure. In E. Braunwald, K.J. Isselbacher, R.G. Petersdorf, J.D. Wilson, J.B. Martin, & A.S. Fauci (Eds.), Harrison's principles of internal medicine (eleventh ed.) (pp. 905–916). New York: McGraw-Hill.

Campbell, M.L., & Field, B.E. (1991). Management of the patient with do not resuscitate status: Compassion and cost containment. Heart and Lung, 20(4), 345–348.

Dettenmeier, P.A. (1992). Pulmonary nursing care. St. Louis: Mosey-Year Book.

Flenley, D. (1984). Palliative care in respiratory diseases. In D. Dole (Ed.), Palliative care: The management of far-advanced illness. Philadelphia: The Charles Press.

Fowler, M.D.M. (1990). Ethical issues in critical care: This mortal coil. Heart and Lung, 19(1), 100–101.

Graham, I. (1989). Edema. In T.D. Walsh (Ed.), Symptom control. Oxford: Blackwell Scientific Publications.

Gu, X., & Belgrade, M.J. (1993). Pain in hospitalized patients with medical illnesses. Journal of Pain and Symptom Management, 8(1), 17–21.

Haak, S.W., & Huether, S.E. (1992). The person with

angina pectoris. In C.E. Guzzetta & B.M. Dossey (Eds.), *Cardiovascular nursing: Holistic practice* (pp. 221–249). St. Louis: Mosby-Year Book.

Haber, J. (1992). Management of depression and suicide. In J. Haber, A.L. McMahon, P. Price-Hoskins, & B.F. Sideleau (Eds.), *Comprehensive psychiatric nursing* (4th ed.) (pp. 549–581). St. Louis: Mosby-Year Book.

Johanssen, J.M. (1994) Chronic obstructive pulmonary disease: Current comprehensive care for emphysema and bronchitis. *Nurse Practitioner, 19*(1), 59–67.

Kersten, L.D. (1989). *Comprehensive respiratory nursing.* Philadelphia: W.B. Sanders.

Laurent-Bopp, D. (1989a). Pathophysiology of heart failure. In S.L. Underhill, S.L. Woods, E.S.S. Froelicher, & C.J. Halpenny (Eds.), *Cardiac nursing* (2nd ed.) (pp. 220–227). Philadelphia: J.B. Lippincott Company.

Laurent-Bopp, D. (1989b). Heart failure. In S.L. Underhill, S.L. Woods, E.S.S. Froelicher, & C.J. Halpenny (Eds.), *Cardiac nursing* (2nd ed.) (pp. 561–570). Philadelphia: J.B. Lippincott Company.

Makielski, M., & Broom, C. (1992). Administering pain medications for a terminal patient. *Dimensions of Critical Care Nursing, 11*(3), 157–161.

Martin, E.W. (1990). Confusion in the terminally ill: Recognition and management. *The American Journal of Hospice and Palliative Care, 7*(3), 20–24.

Matthews, M. (1984). Palliative care in cardiovascular diseases. In D. Doyle (Ed.), *Palliative care* (pp. 171–187). Philadelphia: The Charles Press.

Petty, T.L. (1991). Definitions of airflow disorders and implications for therapy. In G.G. Burton, J.E. Hodgkin, & J.J. Ward (Ed.), *Respiratory care: A guide to clinical practice* (3rd ed.) (pp. 931–936). Philadelphia: J.J. Lippincott Company.

Quaal, S.J. (1992). The person with heart failure and cardiogenic shock. In C.E. Guzzetta & B.M. Dossey (Eds.), *Cardiovascular nursing: Holistic practice* (pp. 302–354). St. Louis: Mosby-Year Book.

Sideleau, B.F. (1992). Management of organic mental disorders. In J. Haber, A.L. McMahon, P. Price-Hoskins, & B.F. Sideleau (Eds.), *Comprehensive psychiatric nursing* (4th ed.) (pp. 599–630). St. Louis: Mosby-Year Book.

Solomon, M.Z., O'Donnell, L., Jennings, B., Guilfoy, V., Wolf, S.M., Nolan, K., Jackson, R., Koch-Weser, D., & Donnelly, S. (1993). Decisions near the end of life: Professional views on life-sustaining treatments. *American Journal of Public Health, 83*(1), 14–23.

Epilogue

The underlying purpose, or mission, of terminal care is to facilitate an internal and external physical, psychosocial, and spiritual environment in which the terminally ill patient and his or her loved ones have the opportunity for reconciliation with God, others, and self. Terminal care thus provides the opportunity to realize, through these reconciliations, what may be termed, in our philosophical and religious traditions, "the purpose of life." As we know—all too well—not everyone achieves these ends. Some never experience any reconciliation. Yet the work goes on, for our charge in this work is to comfort "all the comfortless" (Saunders, 1978, p. 202).

An Exploration of the Purpose or Mission of Terminal Care

To "facilitate" means to make easier, or to help *toward* something. In caring for people who are dying, the nurse makes it easier for the patient to move toward reconciliation; the nurse does not *make* it happen. Expecting all patients and families to do well (however "well" might be defined) is to guarantee failure and, ultimately, disappointment and/or cynicism.

The "internal environment" refers to the patient's physical, psychosocial, and spiritual experiences in the process of dying. Pain and other symptoms should be managed; patients should be made to feel secure in the knowledge that they are neither physically or psychologically alone; opportunities should be provided for patients, their families and loved ones to rediscover, or further explore, the life of the spirit.

The "external environment" refers to the patient's surroundings, especially to other people, such as family and friends—and includes the nurse. At least as important as the presence of these individuals is the way in which they interact, and the psychosocial and spiritual atmosphere they create around them. Moreover, the physical, psychosocial, and spiritual well-being of these individuals too must not be ignored.

"Reconciliation with God" presupposes that all beings were or are of God, and that many have fallen, or feel fallen, away from that vital connection. To come back into harmony with God, or with whatever our concept of that eternal connection is, allows us to discover (or rediscover) a transcendent inner self that exists beyond the pale of the fears, anxiety, and resignation that are the hallmark of so many lives.

Charles Kemp: TERMINAL ILLNESS: A GUIDE TO NURSING CARE. © 1995 J. B. Lippincott.

"Reconciliation with self" refers to acceptance of those aspects of life that we wish were not so. There is no life without regrets. Some regrets revolve around mistakes and missed opportunities; others around things over which we have had no control. In most cases, there is no way to change what was, and so accepting ourselves is the sole alternative.

"Reconciliation with others" means to restore relationships. Terminal illness brings an immediacy that may result in healing relations with others that were lost or broken. At times, however, it is not possible to reach this reconciliation because the object of our efforts is dead, or because they may be incapable of participating in such an experience. In these cases, the goal is to accept that the relationship was, and is, broken, which brings with it another type of reconciliation.

Earlier, in the Preface to this book, I wrote that, in this work, we approach the fulfillment of "an ancient and essential human function: the priestly function of accompanying another through suffering, and to the awesome finality of death."

"In all their affliction he was afflicted, and the angel of his presence saved them; in his love and in his pity he redeemed them; he lifted them up and carried them all the days of old."

ISAIAH 63:9

Finally, caring for people who are dying is an expression of faith.

References

Saunders, C.M. (1978). *The management of terminal disease.* London: Edward Arnold.

Index